Pharmacology Application in Athletic Training

Pharmacology Application in Athletic Training

Brent C. Mangus, EdD, ATC

Program Director
Undergraduate Athletic Training Program
University of Nevada, Las Vegas
Las Vegas, Nevada

Michael G. Miller, EdD, ATC, CSCS

Program Director
Graduate Athletic Training Education Program
Western Michigan University
Kalamazoo, Michigan

With Consultant
Kimberly A. Melgarejo, PharmD
Borgess Medical Center
Kalamazoo, Michigan

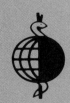

F. A. Davis Company • Philadelphia

F. A. Davis Company
1915 Arch Street
Philadelphia, PA 19103
www.fadavis.com

Printed in the United States of America

Last digit indicates print number: 10 9 8 7

Acquisitions Editor: Christa Fratantoro
Developmental Editor: Jennifer Pine
Production Editor: Jessica Howie Martin
Design and Illustration Manager: Joan Wendt

As new scientific information becomes available through basic and clinical research, recommended treatments and drug therapies undergo changes. The author(s) and publisher have done everything possible to make this book accurate, up to date, and in accord with accepted standards at the time of publication. The author(s), editors, and publisher are not responsible for errors or omissions or for consequences from application of the book, and make no warranty, expressed or implied, in regard to the contents of the book. Any practice described in this book should be applied by the reader in accordance with professional standards of care used in regard to the unique circumstances that may apply in each situation. The reader is advised always to check product information (package inserts) for changes and new information regarding dose and contraindications before administering any drug. Caution is especially urged when using new or infrequently ordered drugs.

Library of Congress Cataloging-in-Publication Data

Mangus, Brent C.
Pharmacology application in athletic training / Brent C. Mangus, Michael G. Miller ;
  with consultant, Kimberly A. Melgarejo.
    p. ; cm.
  Includes bibliographical references.
  ISBN 10: 0-8036-1127-7 (alk. paper)   ISBN 13: 978-0-8036-1127-6
  1. Pharmacology.   2. Athletic trainers.
  [DNLM: 1. Pharmaceutical Preparations—Handbooks.   2. Doping in Sports—Handbooks.
  3. Physical Education and Training—Handbooks. QV 39 M277p 2005]
  I. Miller, Michael G.   II. Title.
RM300.M1843 2005
615′.7—dc22

2004027947

Dedication

This book is dedicated to two different groups of people. First, my family who has given me so much with their unconditional love, patience, and understanding: Brenda, Dusty, Meesha, Bennie, & Nola who are my motivation in life. Second, to the many students who have inspired and encouraged me to be better every day of every year. Many of these students have gone on to professional careers in one of the allied health professions. A special thanks to Allan L., Mick K., Terry G., Mark S., Mark H., Robert N., Troy M., Morgan C., Rick P., Ken F., Tedd G., Ty D., Tim C., Inga V., Shahin G., Joe S., Heidi S., Joe R., Stephanie L., Jack P., Matt S., Yasuo, Kenji, Yutaka, Mika, Misai, Mo, Heidi H., Shawn G., SamIam, Eddie C., Chris B., Brian E., Phil E., Cari C., Gail T., Jeff B., Shawna B., and many other students who will attend the university to study and learn each new school year.

Brent C. Mangus

I would like to thank Brent for providing me the opportunity to work on this project. Your knowledge, experience, and guidance allowed this task to be less troublesome than I anticipated. To my parents, Terry and Joyce, for their endless love and inspiration. To Kim, without your contributions, love and devotion, I would not have been able to complete this project. I would also like to thank the graduate athletic training class of 2005 for their assistance with the ancillary materials. Finally, a special thanks to Bill H., David B., Jack S., Kyle B.

Michael G. Miller

*F*or over 50 years, certified athletic trainers (ATCs) have been employed in traditional settings such as professional sports, universities, colleges, and high schools. As part of the evolution of this field, much like other health professions (e.g., nursing, physical therapy, chiropractic), ATCs are received as allied-health professionals and work alongside colleagues in physical therapy clinics, hospitals, corporate and industrial settings, and other "non-traditional" settings. The ATC is also considered a physician extender and works even more closely with the physician, helping the active population stay healthy. In all of these settings, ATCs are working with people who want to recover from injury or sickness as soon as possible. Because of this close working relationship, many patients are now asking questions about types of medications and how they work to aid in the recovery or healing of their illness or injury. In specific instances, the use of medications can be an integral part of the healing process. An ATC must now understand the many facets of pharmacology: how drugs work in the body, the indications and adverse effects that might affect rehabilitation or participation, the types of drugs that are typically abused, the availability of prescription and over-the-counter drugs (OTCs), the legal aspects of medicines, and emergency situations that involve medications. Although the ATC cannot be expected to know all of the implications of every medication on the market, it is important that ATCs know where to look for applicable drug information.

Having taught courses in pharmacology to athletic training students in approved athletic training curriculums for over 10 years and utilizing a variety of related text books, we wanted to provide a more direct approach for the athletic training student to learn about this topic. With the publication of the National Athletic Trainer's Association (NATA) Educational Competencies, pharmacology has now become required course content area in the education of athletic trainers. We have striven to present the major areas of cognitive skills most likely to be used in professional practice. It was also important to get input and direction from a number of sources when writing this text. We have combined the efforts of university faculty, team physicians at both the university and the high school levels, and a practicing pharmacist to put together a text that provides the information an ATC needs to work knowledgeably in a chosen practice setting.

With pharmacology issues cropping up more frequently in the athletic training setting, especially medication protocols, it's important to understand that the ATC is *not* the person who prescribes medications to athletes, but is, in many instances, the person who answers the first line of questions from the athlete. Although ATCs cannot prescribe medications, they should always keep in mind the legal implications of drug use by people with whom they daily work. The laws concerning medications and the ATC's role vary from state to state. It is important for ATCs to fully investigate all the legal aspects of their profession in the state in which they practice. In most states, the ATC can legally "administer" medication to an athlete under the auspices of a physician, but it remains the responsibility of the ATC to ensure that the athlete is completely informed about the prescribed drug. The ATC is to educate the athlete and communicate with the physician regarding the medical needs of the individual.

This text is designed to discuss the overall pharmacological aspects of common medical conditions that athletic trainers may encounter in their careers. The information presented focuses on aspects relevant to the ATC. Many chapters provide scenarios and specific information that come from real-life situations experienced by ATCs practicing in a variety of settings. Since many certified athletic trainers have an excellent relationship with athletes in their care, we have included chapters on performance enhancements and social drugs to better educate the ATC on the adverse and possible long-term effects of such drugs. To assist educators in preparing their course materials, we have developed an Instructor's Guide and Test Bank to accompany this text. These ancillaries are provided on CD-ROM and are made available to educators who adopt our book.

Pharmacology will continue to change as new drugs are developed and our knowledge about how drugs work increases. We fully recognize that no textbook can totally keep pace with so dynamic a field, but we attempted to provide as up-to-date information as possible. We welcome any suggestions or ideas to improve this work in future additions. Please feel free to contact us with your suggestions through F.A. Davis Publishers or directly.

Brent C. Mangus, EdD, ATC
Michael G. Miller, EdD, ATC, CSCS

Contributors

Mark Hoffman, PhD, ATC
Undergraduate Athletic Training Program Director
Sports Medicine Laboratory Director
Oregon State University
Corvallis, OR

Craig Graham, MD
Team Physician
Oregon State University
Corvallis, OR

Brent S. E. Rich, MD, ATC
Team Physician
Arizona State University (1993–2003)
2002 United States Olympic Team
1998, 2002 United States Paralympic Team

Michael Koester, MD, ATC
Primary Care Sports Medicine Fellow
Vanderbilt University
Nashville, TN

John G. Robinson, M.D.
Cottonwood Hospital
Anesthesia Department
Murray, UT

Reviewer List

Scott Doberstein, MS, LATC, CSCS
Athletic Training
University of Wisconsin—La Crosse
La Crosse, WI

Michael G. Dolan, MA, ATC, CSCS
Sports Medicine
Canisius College
Buffalo, NY

Brett Massie, EdD, ATC
Athletic Training
Miami University of Ohio
School of Education and Allied Professions
Cincinnati, OH

Mary Meier, MS, LAT
Athletic/HHP
Iowa State University
Ames, IA

Mark A. Merrick, PhD, ATC
Athletic Training
The Ohio State University
Columbus, OH

Chris Schmidt, MS, ATC
Athletic Training
Azusa Pacific University
Azusa, CA

Chad Starkey, PhD, ATC
Athletic Training
Northeastern University
Boston, MA

Elizabeth H. Swann, PhD, ATC
Sports Medicine
East Carolina University
Greenville, NC

Sharon West, PhD, ATC
Athletic Training
University of the Pacific
Stockton, CA

Acknowledgements

We would like to thank a number of people who have helped us throughout the writing of this book. First, we need to thank Christa Fratantoro, Acquisitions Editor at F.A. Davis Company, for giving so much time and energy to this project. Christa was willing to listen to the original idea for this book and help us bring it to fruition. In addition, at F.A. Davis, Jennifer Pine worked diligently with us to get the information into a final format and worked with us through the entire publishing process.

We have had numerous people assist us with different parts of the book. Kim Melgarejo, PharmD., who worked with us as our pharmacist consultant throughout the writing. She was very helpful in making sure our drug nomenclature was correct, provided relevant suggestions for the chapters regarding specific drug information, and assisted with the creation of the drug reference guide.

Throughout the book, we had a number of guest authors assisting with writing part of or entire chapters. Those people include Mark Hoffman, ATC/R, PhD; John Robinson, MD; Michael Koester, ATC, MD; Brent Rich, ATC, MD; and Craig Graham, MD. We appreciate the time and effort of all these busy professionals in the writing of this book.

During the development and refinement phases of writing this book, a number of certified athletic trainers were employed as reviewers. Their input and suggestions were very helpful in finalizing each chapter. We would like to thank each of them for the time and effort they put into helping us produce this quality final product.

Brief Contents

Detailed Contents

Part 3

Commonly Abused Drugs in Sports

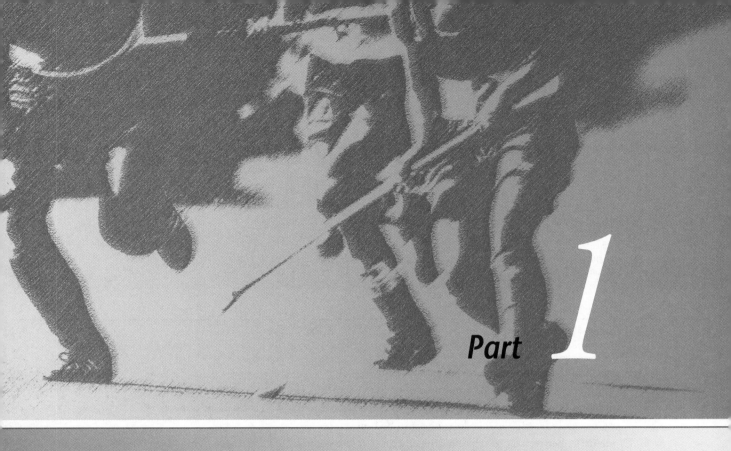

Part 1

Introduction to Pharmacology

1

Historical and Legal Issues

Chapter Objectives

After reading this chapter, the student will be able to:

1 Learn about the origins of pharmacy and medicines.
2 Recognize the Food and Drug Administration (FDA) approval process.
3 Understand the laws governing pharmacy in the professional setting and their ramifications.
4 Recognize and identify the schedules of controlled substances.
5 Differentiate between a prescription drug and an over-the-counter (OTC) drug.
6 Recognize and identify the parts of an OTC label.
7 Differentiate among chemical, brand, and generic names of drugs.
8 Recognize and identify common medical abbreviations.
9 Locate and identify various agencies that produce drug information.
10 Determine the roles and responsibilities of medical professionals as they relate to pharmacy.

Chapter Outline

History of Drugs and Pharmacy
Legal Foundations
United States Food and Drug Administration
Over-the-Counter Products
Naming of a Drug
Generic and Brand-Name Drug Ingredients
Medical Abbreviations
Drug Information
    Pharmacists

Poison Control Centers
    Reference Books
    Websites
Pharmacy in Athletic Training
Scenarios from the Field
What to Tell the Athlete
Discussion Topics
Chapter Review

*D*id you ever wonder how drugs and medicines came into existence? How did rules and regulations governing the formation and distribution of drugs develop? Drugs and medicines were created or developed to heal the sick and injured and protect people who are at risk of sickness or dis-

ease. They have been used by the human race for thousands of years.

As an athletic trainer, you need to understand the origins of medicines and how the laws that govern them protect patients, including your athletes. In addition, it is imperative to learn and understand the differences among classifications of drugs: which medications can be prescribed only by a physician and which can be bought at the local pharmacy or store. Most importantly, you need to know whom to contact for drug information and drug emergencies. This chapter will focus on the origins of drugs and medicines, their current classifications, and basic laws that surround the usage and distribution of drugs in the athletic setting.

*H*istory of Drugs and Pharmacy

The origins of drugs and medicines and the development of pharmacy can be traced back to the ancient civilizations of the Tigris and Euphrates river basin region[6] (Figs. 1–1 and 1–2). Around 2100 BC, physicians and priests began to record references to drug therapy on clay tablets. This collection of works left by ancient healers contained formulas and directions for compounding medicines, which, when translated into modern language, resulted in the identification of 250 vegetable and 120 mineral drugs.[6]

According to these tablets, common foodstuffs, such as alcoholic beverages, fats and oils, parts of animals, honey, waxes, and milks were used as *vehicles* (substances used to carry drugs to their site of action) for medicines. Thus, these tablets from ancient civilizations mark the true beginning of pharmacy.

Over time, the Mesopotamian influence spilled into Egypt. In 1500 BC, the Egyptians developed a collection of

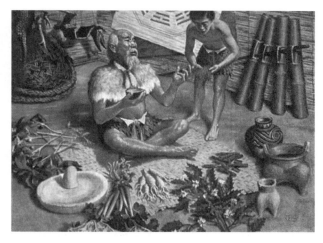

Figure 1–2. Pharmacy in ancient China. Painting by Robert A. Thom. (Courtesy of Pfizer Consumer Group, Pfizer, Inc.)

writings, now commonly referred to as the Ebers Papyrus. The Ebers Papyrus was a 22-yard-long document that described 811 prescriptions and 700 drugs.[6] During this period, the Egyptians also quantitatively defined specific recipes with weights and measures to produce exact formulations of medications. It was at this time that the practice of pharmacy was integrated into daily life.

Between 600 and 330 BC, the Greeks took pharmacy another step forward. True *pharmacopeias* were written. These writings, the forerunners of today's pharmacopeias (treatises documenting the standards for preparation and dispensation of drugs), described how botanicals (extracts derived from plants) were used to make medicines. The *pharmacopeias* specifically listed the drugs' botanical habitats, physical properties, type of actions, medicinal usage, side effects, quantities, and dosages, as well as instructions for harvesting, preparation, and storage of medicinal plants.[7]

Greek physicians eventually became overwhelmed by the responsibilities involved in diagnosing diseases and preparing drug products to treat them. Therefore they found it desirable to rely on the expertise of specialists in the preparation of remedies. It was during this time that the role of the *pharmacist*—a specialist who creates and dispenses medicines for sick people—evolved.

Throughout the Middle Ages and into the Renaissance period, pharmacy continued to grow as a profession. Pharmacy shops appeared and local *guilds* of pharmacists were formed. The guilds were created to maintain a monopoly within the town, protect the quality and integrity of pharmacists' products, control the training and length of service

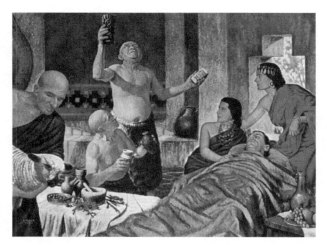

Figure 1–1. Pharmacy in Babylonia, 2600 B.C. Painting by Robert A. Thom. (Courtesy of Pfizer Consumer Group, Pfizer Inc.)

for apprentices, and recognize the status of "master" within the guild.[8]

During the Middle Ages, the practice of pharmacy further improved when it was officially separated from medicine. Emperor Frederick II wrote laws that legally recognized pharmacy as a separate profession. At this time, official schools of pharmacy were created. Students in Montpellier, France studied at the first university program dedicated to the science of pharmacy, with courses taught by prominent physicians. Overall, the Middle Ages gave rise to the most prominent developments in the history of pharmacy.

The settlement of North America brought a new dimension to the pharmacist's profession. The discovery of new plants and the export of knowledge from the indigenous peoples of the Americas fueled a new interest in medicine. As in previous times, most early medical practitioners in North America had no formal training and often dispensed their own types of medicines from their homes. The earliest practicing pharmacy in the North American colonies was thought to be that of William Davis of Boston, opened in the year 1646. However, the first written record of day-to-day pharmacy operations in the colonies was created in 1698 by Bartholomew Browne of Salem, Massachusetts.[11]

During the Revolutionary War, the practice of pharmacy became more standardized. Pharmaceutical activity increased and became a separate but equally important branch of the medical community. The first known mass production of pharmaceutical products began during this period. The Revolutionary War also marked the first attempt to develop a *formulary*—a book that provides standards and specifications for drugs.

As the United States expanded, so did the development of pharmacy. The movement westward produced scores of "pharmacists," both real and fake. Drugstores opened to supply the needs of the migrating population (Fig. 1–3). Charlatans sold "medications" in many forms to cure a variety of ailments. These products often had no therapeutic value. As a result, rules and regulations were adopted in 1804 to govern pharmacy practice and protect the people from unscrupulous practitioners. On the whole, these rules were ineffective. It was not until around 1870 that the American Pharmaceutical Association developed draft regulations for pharmacy practices and sales of pharmaceuticals. Rhode Island was the first state to adopt the rules. One by one, each state followed suit.

The 20th century brought new laws and regulations to the pharmacy profession. The United States Food and Drug Administration (FDA) was established to ensure the safety of drug production, consumption, and distribution. Prescription and over-the-counter (OTC) medication classifications were also developed during this time. Pharmacies

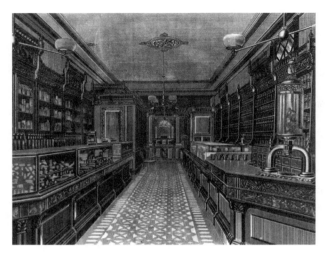

Figure 1–3. Typical pharmacy in 1880. Origin unknown.(Courtesy of the National Library of Medicine.)

opened in almost every community. The pharmacist's scope of practice became highly regulated, and specialized schools similar to those in Europe were opened in the United States.

The current profession of pharmacy still has links to ancient civilizations (Fig. 1–4). New drugs are being still being developed; time-tested compounds are still being manufactured; and laws continue to be enacted to ensure the safety and efficacy of pharmaceutical products. The modern-day pharmacist continues to work in environments similar to the traditional pharmacies of the Renaissance period and, since the 19th century, has also worked in hospitals and industry. As in previous periods, the profession of pharmacy continues to evolve to provide patients with the essential drug therapies and quality drug information they need to treat illnesses and injuries.

Legal Foundations

In the early 20th century, virtually no laws existed to control the sale of medicines, the purity of drug preparations, or the efficacy of medical devices. People could purchase Coca-Cola, a tonic that contained cocaine, an extract of the coca shrub, to help with digestion and respiration. Teething babies were given special soothing syrups (e.g., paregoric) that contained opium. Menstruating women took elixirs of morphine to help with dysmenorrhea.[12] The use of these "medications" was a common practice, and patients sometimes became physically and psychologically dependent on them.

Because of the lack of regulations in this area, the federal government enacted the Pure Food and Drug Act in 1906.

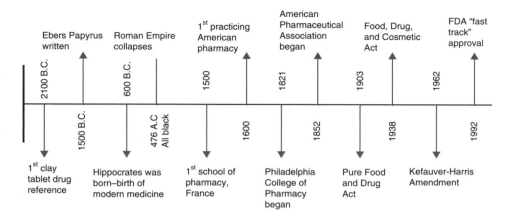

Figure 1–4. Timeline history of the development of pharmacy.

This act prohibited the adulteration and misbranding of foods and drugs that moved in interstate commerce.[1] However, pharmacists were still able to make products containing ingredients of any quality, whether they were efficacious or not. For example, in 1937 sulfanilamide elixir, an oral antibiotic containing deadly diethylene glycol (the main ingredient in automobile antifreeze) was manufactured without safety data for the user. As a consequence, over 100 people died, prompting the federal government to pass the Food, Drug, and Cosmetic Act of 1938. This act stated that all drugs must be safe for human use and be approved before marketing.[1] The act also stated that labels had to contain adequate directions for use and warn users of the habit-forming properties of certain drugs. Drug sellers and manufacturers were forced to comply with the new standards. They had to identify the specific strength and purity of the drug and list on the label any narcotic agents contained in the product. Even so, many drug manufacturers did not differentiate between prescription and nonprescription medicines. Drugs were often mislabeled. As a result, individuals sometimes took prescription drugs without proper medical supervision. In 1952, the passage of the Durham-Humphrey Amendment further enhanced the Food, Drug, and Cosmetic Act of 1938. This amendment codified the distinction between prescription and nonprescription drugs, although, at the time, the legislation was primarily focused on limiting the nonwritten transmission of prescriptions and requests for refills of prescription drugs. The Durham-Humphrey amendment also required that every prescription drug have the following statement on its label: "Caution: Federal law prohibits dispensing without a prescription."

During the 1950s, a popular sleeping pill, thalidomide, was marketed to pregnant women in Europe (the FDA refused to give approval for its use in pregnant women in the United States until it had gathered adequate safety information). After a decade of use in Europe, a positive correlation was established between mothers who ingested thalidomide and the risk of a birth defect called *phocomelia* (the development of seal-like extremities) in children.[1] This birth defect, which affected hundreds of children, resulted in the passage of the Kefauver-Harris Amendment to the Food, Drug, and Cosmetic Act in 1962. The Kefauver-Harris Amendment required manufacturers to test their new drugs for safety and efficacy. The amendment also required that drugs manufactured between 1938 and 1962 be evaluated for safety and efficacy. As a result, many drugs were withdrawn from the market.

In 1970, the Poison Prevention Packaging Act was passed. This act was intended to protect children from accidental poisoning by household substances and drugs. The Poison Prevention Packaging Act requires that drugs dispensed pursuant to a prescription be dispensed in child-resistant containers. The containers must be manufactured so that 80 percent of children under the age of 5 cannot open them, whereas at least 90 percent of adults can.

The Anti-Tampering Act was passed by Congress in 1984 after a number of deaths were caused in the early 1980s by ingestion of OTC medicines that had been contaminated with cyanide. The Anti-Tampering Act requires all OTC products to have tamper-resistant packaging. Packaging can be made tamper resistant by various techniques, including placing a plastic wrapper around the neck of a bottle or gluing an aluminum seal over a container's opening.

Although many laws have been enacted to further public safety, certain drugs warrant even stricter regulation and control. Rigorous regulations have been developed for manufacturing and distribution of specific medications identified by the government as "controlled substances" or "scheduled drugs" because of their potential for addiction and abuse. The Comprehensive Drug Abuse Prevention and Control Act of 1970, otherwise known as the Controlled Substances Act (CSA),[2] governed the use and distribution of these drugs. This law includes regulations for drug abuse rehabilitation programs, a system of registration of manufacturers and distributors of controlled substances, and rules for distribution of these substances.

The CSA also sets forth a five-level scheme or schedules for classifying controlled substances. It is still being used today (Table 1–1). This scheme separates drugs based on their medicinal use and their potential for physical dependence and abuse.

Schedule I drugs are drugs or substances that have a high potential for abuse and are not acceptable for medical use in the United States. Examples of schedule I drugs are heroin and lysergic acid diethylamide (LSD).

Schedule II drugs are drugs or substances that have a high affinity for abuse but are also used medically. Morphine, hydromorphone (Dilaudid), and codeine are examples of schedule II drugs. These drugs may produce severe psychological or physical dependence but are effective in the treatment of pain.

Schedule III drugs are considered to have a lower abuse potential than schedule I and II substances. Some examples of schedule III drugs include acetaminophen with codeine (popularly called Tylenol No. 3) and various hydrocodone combinations such as Lortab and Vicodin.

Schedule IV drugs have an even lower potential for abuse compared to those on schedule III. Common agents in this class are the benzodiazepines, including diazepam (Valium), alprazolam (Xanax), and lorazepam (Ativan).

Schedule V drugs are drugs that have the lowest potential for abuse of all scheduled substances. A common schedule V drug is Robitussin A-C.

Table 1–1

Examples of Scheduled Drugs

Schedule	Drug
Schedule I	Heroin
	Peyote
	Lysergic acid diethylamide (LSD)
Schedule II	Dexedrine
	OxyContin
	Adderall
	MS Contin
	Dilaudid
	Demerol
	Percocet
	Ritalin
Schedule III	Tylenol with Codeine
	Fiorinal with Codeine
	Lortab
	Vicodin
	Esgic with Codeine
Schedule IV	Darvocet
	Restoril
	Valium
	Ativan
	Xanax
	Ambien
Schedule V	Lomotil
	Robitussin A-C

United States Food and Drug Administration

The FDA was created in 1938 to enforce the Food, Drug, and Cosmetic Act of 1938. This agency is responsible for protecting the public's health by ensuring the safety, efficacy, and monitoring of products on the market. This includes making sure that foods are sanitary, safe, and properly labeled; recalling improperly manufactured goods; and inspecting facilities where foods, drugs, or cosmetics are produced. One of the main functions of the FDA is to regulate the drug manufacturing and labeling processes (Fig. 1–5).

It has been estimated that for every 5000 new compounds that enter testing, only one becomes a new product. The drug approval process may take several years. It costs millions of dollars for a pharmaceutical company to manufacture and market a drug. Conversely, in other countries, the approval process may last only 1 year and does not follow the strict regulations of the FDA. Therefore some drugs are available in other countries that are not available in the United States.

Some critics argue that the FDA's stringent and lengthy process limits the public's and the medical community's access to new drugs that address life-threatening and serious illnesses such as AIDS, Alzheimer's disease, and multiple sclerosis. In response to these critiques, in 1992 the FDA established a "fast-track" approval process to decrease the approval time for important therapeutic drugs. This process allows marketing of a drug before the last phase of clinical

| Step 1. Laboratory and Animal Testing (up to 3 years) |
| Step 2. Company Files for Investigational New Drug (IND) with the FDA |
| Step 3. Initiation of Clinical Studies (1 year) Phase 1 – human subjects (volunteer) Goal: to evaluate drug metabolism and side effects |
| Clinical Studies (2 years) Phase 2 – human subjects (patients) Goal: to determine therapeutic effects and dose |
| Clinical Studies (3 years) Phase 3 – human subjects (patients) Goal: to determine safety and efficacy |
| Step 4. FDA Review (2-3 years) |
| FDA Approval of New Drug (Approximately 12 years after initiation) |

Figure 1–5. The FDA approval process for a new drug.

trials, provided that follow-up studies will be performed. The FDA's rationale was that, in certain cases, the unknown risks are balanced by the urgent need for these new drugs.

Another major responsibility of the FDA is to monitor adverse drug reactions. Adverse reactions are unintended effects of drugs. An example of an adverse reaction would be a rash or itch that develops in a patient after he or she takes an antibiotic. The FDA requires that pharmaceutical firms report at regularly scheduled intervals all adverse effects associated with the drugs they sell. The FDA has a reporting system called MedWatch in which health-care professionals can post any occurrences of adverse reactions associated with a drug, its formulation, or its packaging. The MedWatch reporting system documents can be found at *www.fda.gov*.

Over-the-Counter Products

Drugs considered safe for self-administration by consumers without medical guidance are called *over-the-counter* (OTC) drugs. OTC drugs can be found almost anywhere, from drug stores and pharmacies to supermarkets and gas stations. It has been estimated that over 300,000 OTC products are available to the public to treat minor illnesses, injuries, and other problems. The FDA must approve both the ingredients and the information printed on the label of every OTC drug. The drug must also show a low incidence of severe side effects and a low potential for harm when the patient follows all directions for use. Although OTC products are considered relatively safe for general use, they can still produce severe adverse effects if taken incorrectly or if mixed with other OTC or prescription drugs.

A patient who takes an OTC product must read the label carefully. Each OTC label (Fig. 1–6) should contain the following information[1]:

- The name of the product
- The name and address of the manufacturer, packer, or distributor
- A list of ingredients, both active and inactive (inert)
- The quantity of contents
- The name of any habit-forming components contained in the drug
- All warnings and precautions for the user, including whether it is habit forming or is contraindicated for use by pregnant or nursing women
- Adequate directions for use.

Consumers who have questions regarding any of the information found on the label should consult their physician or pharmacist.

Naming of a Drug

One of the most confusing aspects of pharmacology is the naming of each drug. Drugs are typically identified by their chemical, generic, or brand name (Table 1–2).

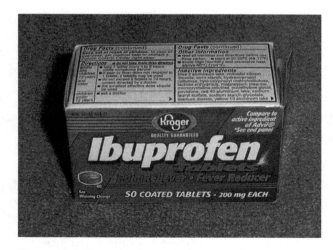

Figure 1–6. Example of generic drug container with printed directions. Courtesy of Kroger Corporation.

Table 1–2

Drugs Commonly Found in the Athletic Setting

Generic Name	Brand Name
acetaminophen	Tylenol
albuterol	Ventolin, Proventil
amoxicillin	Amoxil, Trimox
azithromycin	Zithromax
betamethasone and clotrimazole	Lotrisone
calcium carbonate	Tums
celecoxib	Celebrex
codeine and acetaminophen	Tylenol with Codeine
diazepam	Valium
erythromycin	E-Mycin, Ery-Tab
famotidine	Pepcid
fluticasone	Flovent
furosemide	Lasix
hydrocodone and acetaminophen	Lortab, Vicodin
hydrocortisone (topical)	Cortaid, Lanacort, Cortizone
ibuprofen	Motrin, Advil, Nuprin
ketoprofen	Orudis
naproxen	Naprosyn, Aleve
neomycin, polymyxin B, and hydrocortisone	Cortisporin
omeprazole	Prevacid
oxycodone and acetaminophen	Percocet
pseudoephedrine	Sudafed
rofecoxib	Vioxx
salmeterol	Serevent
triamcinolone	Kenalog

drug is first developed, it is given a *chemical* name. Chemical names are derived from chemical composition and molecular structure. A chemical name is usually long and complex and difficult for everyday use. For example, *N*-acetyl-para-aminophenol is a complex name to pronounce or remember. It is much easier to use its generic name (acetaminophen) or its brand name (Tylenol) instead.

A *generic* name, also known as a *nonproprietary* name, is a shorter name that is assigned to a drug by the United States Adopted Names (USAN) Council. It may have relatively little in common with the drug's chemical or brand name. A generic name is usually given for general recognition and, once assigned, cannot be used for any other drug. The generic name is the preferred name listed in the United States Pharmacopeia (USP).[15] After a drug is given its generic name, the manufacturer assigns the name by which that generic drug will be traded, called a *brand* (trade) or *proprietary* name. This name must be approved by the FDA before the drug is marketed. However, several brand names can exist for drugs of the same generic name. For example, Advil, Motrin, and Nuprin are all brand names for the drug whose generic name is ibuprofen. Because of the various brand names that identify the same product, most healthcare professionals choose to use the generic name when describing a drug. Brand names usually have the symbol (®) after the name and are capitalized (in this text, we will only capitalize the brand name drug), whereas generic names are not capitalized. Any drug on the market, whether prescription or OTC, can be identified by its brand or generic name, or by both.

Generic and Brand-Name Drug Ingredients

Historically, physicians and patients have been reluctant to substitute equivalent generic drugs for brand-name drugs. Manufacturers of brand-name drugs have argued that their drugs are superior in quality and effectiveness to their generic equivalents. However, the products must have the same active ingredient(s) and must be identical in strength and dosage form. Theoretically, generic drugs produce the same desired effects as brand-name drugs.

Brand-name drugs and their ingredients are usually patented for 17 years. After the patent expires, other companies can use the same chemical ingredients to produce a generic equivalent. In order for a generic company to produce a similar-brand-name product, it must submit an abbreviated new drug application (ANDA) to the FDA. This document includes proof of the drug's bioavailability and bioequivalence, as well as information about the manufacturing methods and control of the product the company wishes to manufacture. In other words, the manufacturer must show proof that the generic drug is as clinically effective as the brand-name drug. After it receives FDA approval, the company can release the product to the public.

The FDA recommends that physicians consider prescribing generic drugs when appropriate because they are less expensive to the consumer (most generic drugs cost about one-half to one-fourth the price of brand-name drugs). In fact, all states permit the pharmacist to dispense the generic equivalent of brand-name drugs, if applicable, unless specifically requested by the physician to do otherwise. To determine the equivalency of a generic product to a brand-name product, please refer to an FDA publication entitled "Approved Drug Products with Therapeutic Equivalence Evaluations."[10]

Medical Abbreviations

Most health-care professionals use a written code system consisting of symbols, codes, and abbreviations. This abbreviation system is used to quickly denote commonly used words, phrases, and conditions of medical terminology. Abbreviations are usually standard across professions, and every health-care professional must memorize them for use in medical documentation. In prescribing drugs and medicines, abbreviations are used to denote concepts including frequency, amount, and weight. Table 1–3 provides a common list of drug abbreviations used in the medical and pharmacy professions.

Drug Information

Throughout this text, drugs and their actions will be covered in detail. When questions arise about what course of action or procedure to take regarding a drug, it is imperative that you contact the proper individuals or locate the correct drug information. The references discussed in the next section will help guide you, the athletic trainer, in answering questions about drugs and medicines.

■ Pharmacists

Pharmacists are integral to the medical profession. As health-care professionals, they are trained in the concepts of defining, monitoring, and modifying drug therapy. As a part of a patient's health-care team, pharmacists assess therapeutic needs, prevent adverse drug reactions, develop patient-specific therapy, manage chronic diseases, and monitor follow-up care.[3] The pharmacist understands the actions of drugs: uses, doses, drug and food interactions, contraindications, and many other aspects of each drug agent. Pharmacists are typically educated at the postsecondary level for 6 years, at the end of which they receive a Doctor of Pharmacy (PharmD) degree, and are required to successfully pass a national certification examination. Like many other professionals, pharmacists are also required to pass a state licensure exam. Their scope of practice is therefore geographically defined.

Pharmacists work in a variety of settings, from local drugstores to hospitals, long-term care facilities, managed care, government, and industrial settings. A pharmacist may be part of an interdisciplinary team of physicians, dietitians, social workers, physical therapists, and many other professionals working together in a university or hospital atmosphere. In the athletic training setting, one particular pharmacy is usually used for all prescription and OTC medications. The pharmacist associated with the athletic training setting should be the first choice for soliciting information. If your work setting does not have a designated pharmacist, please contact a pharmacist in your community.

■ Poison Control Centers

Poison control centers (PCSs) are located in all 50 states; are accessible by phone 24 hours a day, 7 days a week; and are free. They provide rapid access to information for assessing and treating poisonings and assist with poisoning prevention. They can answer questions about any potential poison, including medications, chemicals, household products, and biologically produced natural toxins.[5] PCSs handle all calls concerning humans and animals for all different types of poisonings. A PCS can handle emergencies related to insect and snake bites; ingestion of substances such as household products or poisonous plants; identification of different types of drug tablets and capsules; and hazardous material spills. PCSs usually employ specially trained, certified specialists who are nurses, pharmacists, or physicians.

The PCS should be called if you or someone you know has ingested, touched, or been bitten by something you think is poisonous or toxic. Poison control specialists will ask a series of questions and inform the caller on how to solve the problem. For example, they may instruct the caller to seek medical attention, administer ipecac to induce vomiting, or call emergency personnel to the home. When calling a PCS, callers should provide as much detail as possible regarding the description of the product ingested or the source of venom, the amount ingested, and the amount of time that has gone by since ingestion. In most cases, the PCS will ask identifying questions of the caller to assist with follow-up, but the caller can also remain anonymous if desired (Box 1–1). To find the phone number of the nearest PCS, you can

Table 1–3

Common Medical Abbreviations

Abbreviation	Meaning	Abbreviation	Meaning
ā	before	m	meter
a.c.	before meals	mEq	milliequivalent
ad lib.	as desired	Mg	magnesium
AM	morning	mg	milligram
b.i.d.	twice a day	mL	milliliter
c̄	with	mm	millimeter
cap.	a capsule	Na	sodium
CBC	complete blood count	NaCl	sodium chloride
CC	chief complaint	n.p.o.	nothing by mouth
cc	cubic centimeter	OTC	over the counter
cm	centimeter	oz	ounce
dL	deciliter (100 mL)	p̄	after
DM	diabetes mellitus	p.c.	after meals
Dx	diagnosis	PM	afternoon, night
ECG	electrocardiogram	PO	by mouth
ED	emergency department; effective dose; erectile dysfunction	p.r.n.	as needed
		q	every
elix.	elixir	q.d.	every day
FBS	fasting blood sugar	q.h.	every hour
g, gm	gram	q.2h	every 2 hours
GI	gastrointestinal	q.4h	every 4 hours
gtt	drops	q.i.d.	four times a day
Hgb	hemoglobin	q.o.d	every other day
HCT	hematocrit	R/O	rule out
HDL	high-density lipoprotein	Rx	prescription
Hg	mercury	s̄	without
hr	hour	SC	subcutaneous
h.s.	at bedtime	sec	second
Hx	history	SL	under the tongue
IM	intramuscular	stat.	immediately
inj.	inject	Sx	symptoms
IV	intravenous	T	temperature
K	potassium	t.i.d.	three times a day
Kcal	kilocalorie	tbsp	tablespoon
kg	kilogram	tsp	teaspoon
L	liter	VS	vital signs
LDL	low-density lipoprotein		

call the national hotline at 800-222-1222, check your local phone directory, or call directory assistance. You may also locate a PCS by visiting the American Association of Poison Control Centers at *http://www.aapcc.org.*

■ Reference Books

Depending on the scope of their practice, most allied health-care facilities have a variety of written information

Common Questions Asked by Emergency Poison Control Center Personnel

1. Name of person poisoned?
2. Age of person poisoned?
3. What type of poison?
4. How much poison was ingested?
5. Current symptoms?

concerning drugs and medicines. However, it is very important that credible sources be used for gathering drug information. The sources described in the following paragraphs are the texts and guides most commonly used by physicians and pharmacists for information on drugs and other chemicals.

Drug Facts and Comparisons[9] is a very comprehensive and user-friendly reference. It contains comparative drug information and relative costs, and indicates which products are sugar and alcohol free. Basic drug information found in this reference includes drug actions, indications and contraindications, precautions and warnings, administration, and dosage. The text also contains manufacturers' addresses and phone numbers and standard pharmaceutical abbreviations, plus various other reference materials. This reference is updated monthly.

The *Physician's Desk Reference* (PDR)[13] is produced by the pharmaceutical industry and provides detailed descriptions of drugs. This content is identical to the information found in drug package inserts. The PDR also has color photos of over 1000 drug products to assist with identification, and is updated annually. The PDR is easily accessible but sometimes difficult to comprehend because of the complexity of the information it contains.

American Hospital Formulary Service (AHFS) Drug Information[4] is produced by the American Society of Health-System Pharmacists. This reference has detailed monographs on all drugs and general summaries of the drug categories. It provides both FDA-approved and nonlabeled indications. This reference is also updated annually.

United States Pharmacopeia Drug Information (USP DI) is a three-volume set published annually with monthly updates. Volume I, *Drug Information for the Health Care Provider*,[15] provides comprehensive monographs and includes information on veterinary drugs and OTC diagnostic agents. Volume II, *Advice for the Patient*,[16] provides drug information in lay language. Volume III, *Approved*

Drug Products and Legal Requirements,[17] provides equivalence information and legal issues.

Pharmacy in Athletic Training

What are the rules and regulations for athletic trainers regarding dispensing, acquiring, and storing drugs in the athletic setting? To answer these questions, each athletic trainer must first contact his or her state attorney general or state licensing board to determine what, if any, laws regulate medications in the athletic training setting. In addition, the athletic trainer should be aware of federal laws and regulations (promulgated primarily by the United States Drug Enforcement Agency [DEA] and the FDA) that govern controlled substances that may be found in the athletic training room.

There are literally hundreds of federal laws governing the prescription, storage, distribution, and administration of medications. However, athletic trainers should be particularly aware of specific laws that may be applicable in the athletic training setting. For example, any controlled substance in schedules II through V must be securely locked in a structurally sound location to avert theft. All controlled substances found in the athletic training setting must have a complete and accurate written inventory, including the date. If controlled substances are kept in multiple locations, a separate inventory must be on file at each location. Inventory of all controlled substances must be taken at least every 2 years.

If controlled substances are stored in the athletic training setting and dispensed to athletes, it is suggested the athletic trainer contact the state attorney general (for state law guidance) and the DEA (for federal law information) to determine whether special procedures, registrations, or certificates are required. Usually, the team physician solicits this information, because he or she is ultimately responsible for dispensing controlled substances.

To avoid legal liability, the athletic trainer should follow some simple procedures. The athletic trainer should document the following information about each drug administered, whether prescription or OTC, in a logbook (Fig. 1–7):

- Name of the athlete/patient
- Sport
- Age of athlete/patient
- Name of drug
- Dose given
- Quantity prescribed

Athlete Name	Sport	Age	Name of Drug	Dose	Quantity	Indication	Manufacturer	Lot #	Exp. Date	Name of Dispenser	Date
Jimmy John	FB	20	Tylenol	650 mg	2 tablets	Headache	Drugs-R-Us	04566	5/05	Sally Sue	3/10
Tina Tall	WBB	18	Tinactin	1 application	1 tube	Athlete's foot	Drugs-R-Us	09876	5/05	Sammy Saw	3/12

Figure 1–7. Example of pharmacy log used in an athletic training setting.

- Indication (why the drug was given)
- Manufacturer
- Lot number
- Drug expiration date
- Name of person who dispensed the drug
- Date drug was given

In order to properly monitor drug therapy, all drugs should be in single-dose packages with expiration dates stamped on them. If drugs are purchased in bulk, only a 1-day supply should be dispensed. Drugs so dispensed should be placed in a small, secured envelope labeled with the athlete's name and appropriate directions for use.

Many athletes self-administer their medications. They may need assistance with this process. To properly assist the athlete in the drug administration process, the athletic trainer should read all package inserts with the athlete and make sure that the athlete understands the directions for use. OTC and prescription medications should never be made freely available for use or distribution without proper supervision. All medications should be kept in locked offices or storage cabinets and should only be dispensed with physician approval and supervision. Failure to follow these guidelines can predispose athletic trainers to undue legal liability.

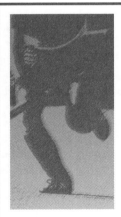

Scenario from the Field

An athlete was seen by the team physician for an infected foot. The physician prescribed an antibiotic. An athletic training student was sent to the local pharmacy to pick up the prescription. The athletic training student then delivered the prescription and told the athlete to read the directions on the bottle and take all the pills. Approximately 24 hours later, the athlete developed an allergic reaction to the medication and sought medical attention in a hospital emergency room. How could have this situation been prevented? Who is financially responsible for the emergency room visit? Who is at fault?

Ideally, athletes should pick up their own prescriptions so that they can talk to the pharmacist. The pharmacist should ask the above questions, make sure that the athlete understands how and when to take the medication, and explain possible side effects. If an athlete cannot pick up his or her own prescription, the prescription should be brought to the athletic training setting and be handed to the athlete in the presence of a physician or other qualified medical professional.

At no time should an athletic training student or staff member deliver or dispense medications to an athlete without proper medical supervision. Athletic trainers should encourage their athletes to pick up their own prescriptions so that they can talk directly to a pharmacist, who will make sure that the athlete understands all aspects of the medication. These policies will ensure that all athletes are given proper medical care and decrease the possible legal or ethical responsibility of the athletic training student, staff, or program.

Scenario from the Field

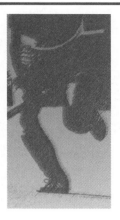

In your job as an athletic trainer, you often dispense Tylenol No. 3 to athletes who have pain and inflammation associated with athletic injuries. Tylenol No. 3 is a prescription medication, and the team physician regularly brings samples of it to the athletic training setting. However, the team physician does not supervise the dispensing of any medication on a regular basis. If an athlete develops dependence or abuses the medication, who is at fault?

State and federal laws mandate that only a physician is allowed to prescribe drugs. Either a physician or a pharmacist may dispense prescription medications. In this case, the athletic trainer should not dispense any prescription medication without written orders and supervision from the team physician. The head athletic trainer, therefore, can be held liable for any allergic reaction, addiction, or other condition associated with the medication that an athlete subsequently suffers.

To help avoid legal liability, it is recommended that the physician develop a document stating that the athletic trainer is an agent of the physician. This document must include the official name and address of the setting, the name of the physician, his or her license number, and a list of individuals who will be allowed to act as agents under the supervision of the physician. At the discretion of the physician, this document may allow athletic trainers some responsibility to store drugs, keep records, call a local pharmacy for restocking purposes, and perform other duties as appropriate. However, it still will not allow athletic trainers to dispense prescription or controlled medications.

Implications for Athletic Trainers

In settings where athletes are under the age of 18, it is recommended that the athletic trainer not administer any drug, even an OTC drug. Instead, in this situation, it is recommended that the athletic trainer discuss all medication issues with the athlete's legal guardian. Referrals can then be made to the appropriate medical personnel or pharmacist for specific drug information.

In the foregoing scenario, an athletic training student was given the task of delivering the medication to the athlete without:

- Determining if the athlete had medical allergies.
- Instructing the athlete on the proper administration of the prescription.
- Determining if the athlete was currently taking other medications.
- Providing information about possible complications from the prescription.

What to Tell the Athlete

As an athletic trainer, you may encounter athletes who regularly obtain OTC products for care of their injuries. Because OTC products can be purchased without a prescription, many athletes do not know the differences among the various products they can consume to treat their injuries. If you were to become aware that an athlete was consistently or stubbornly taking the wrong OTC medication for an anti-inflammatory effect, what would you tell the athlete?

- Let the athlete know which OTC drugs will produce the desired effect and which ones will not.
- Explain the need for taking medication only as directed.
- Explain how to recognize the symptoms of side effects and how to reduce them, such as by ingesting medication with meals.
- Have the athlete consult with his or her physician or pharmacist.

Internet Resource Box

A variety of Websites can be useful in researching medications and their actions. However, not all Websites are reliable. It is your responsibility to select credible sources about drugs and medicines. The following sites are among the most reliable and accurate sources of online information about medicines.

http://www.fda.gov—United States Food and Drug Administration

http://www.cdc.gov—Centers for Disease Control and Prevention

http://www.nih.gov—National Institutes of Health

http://www.dea.gov—United States Drug Enforcement Agency

http://www.hhs.gov—United States Department of Health and Human Services

http://www.safemedication.com—American Society of Health-System Pharmacists

http://www.pharmacyandyou.org—American Pharmacists Association

http://www.aapcc.org—American Association of Poison Control Centers

Discussion Topics

- Is it the employer's responsibility to provide practicing athletic trainers with all state and national drug laws that pertain to the athletic training profession?

- Should controlled substances be kept in the athletic training room?

- Should athletic training students be responsible for distributing medications to athletes?

- What are some of the advantages and disadvantages of having individual dose packages versus bulk containers of medications?

Chapter Review

- The origins of pharmacy date back to ancient civilizations in which botanicals were used to treat illnesses and injuries.

- Pharmacists are educated about all aspects of drugs, injuries, and illnesses.

- The FDA, originally established to govern drug uses and abuses, now regulates the approval processes for thousands of medicines.

- The Poison Prevention Packaging Act and the Anti-Tampering Act require drugs to have child-resistant and tamper-proof containers.

- OTC products are considered safe for the general public; however, not following directions for their use can produce undesired side effects.

- All drugs are given one of three derived names—chemical, brand, and generic. The generic name is the one most commonly used, and is preferred by the United States Pharmacopeia.

- Brand and generic products of the same drug have the same active ingredients and produce the same desired effects, but may differ in the content of inert ingredients.

- When researching information about drugs, there are many valuable sources one can consult, including pharmacists, physicians, and reference texts such as *Drug Facts and Comparisons* and the *Physician's Desk Reference*."

- Poison control centers are available 24 hours a day, 7 days a week in case of emergencies.

- The athletic trainer should be aware of state and federal laws governing the use, distribution, and storing of medicines in the athletic training setting.

- It is the responsibility of the athletic trainer to communicate with athletes and patients about the proper use of medications to alleviate symptoms of athletic injuries.

References

1. Abood, RR, and Brushwood, DB. Federal regulation of medications: Development, production, and marketing. In Pharmacy Practice and the Law, ed. 2. Aspen Publishers, Gaithersburg, Md., 1997, pp. 27–76.
2. Abood, RR, and Brushwood, DB. The closed system of controlled substance distribution. In Pharmacy Practice and the Law, ed. 2. Aspen Publishers, Gaithersburg, Md., 1997, pp. 109–136.
3. American College of Physicians–American Society of Internal Medicine. Pharmacist scope of practice. Ann Intern Med 136: 79–85, 2002.
4. American Society of Health-System Pharmacists: American Hospital Formulary Services (AHFS) Drug Information. American Society of Health-System Pharmacists, Bethesda, Md., 2001.
5. Benson, BE. Poison information centers. In Malone, PM, Mosdell, KW, et al. (eds): Drug Information: A guide for pharmacists. Appleton & Lange, Stamford, Conn., 1996, pp. 357–387.
6. Cowen, DL, and Helfand, WH. Ancient antecedents. In Pharmacy: An Illustrated History. Harry N. Abrams, New York, 1990, pp. 17–26.
7. Cowen, DL, and Helfand, WH. The classical world. In Pharmacy: An Illustrated History. Harry N. Abrams, New York, 1990, pp. 27–38.
8. Cowen, DL, and Helfand, WH. The middle ages. In Pharmacy: An Illustrated History. Harry N. Abrams, New York, 1990, pp. 39–58.
9. Drug Facts and Comparisons. Facts and Comparisons, St. Louis, Mo., 2001.
10. U.S. Department of Health and Human Services, Food and Drug Administration: Electronic Orange Book Approved Drug Products with Therapeutic Equivalence Evaluations. *http://www.fda.gov/cder/ob/default.htm*
11. Kremers, E, and Urdang, G. The North American colonies. In Sonnedecker, G (ed), Urdang's History of Pharmacy, ed. 4. Lippincott, Philadelphia, 1976, pp. 145–162.
12. Liska, K. Federal Laws: The FDA and testing: Penalties for illicit use. In Drugs and the Human Body with Implications for Society, ed. 4. Macmillan, New York, 1994, pp 69–93.
13. Physicians' Desk Reference, ed. 56. Medical Economics, Montvale, N.J., 2002.
14. USP Dictionary of USAN and International Drug Names, 2002. United States Pharmacopeia, Rockville, Md., 1998.
15. United States Pharmacopeia Drug Information (USP DI), ed. 18. Vol 1, Drug Information for the Health Care Professional. United States Pharmacopeial Convention, Rockville, Md., 1998.
16. United States Pharmacopeia Drug Information (USP DI), ed. 18. Vol 2, Advice for the Patient. United States Pharmacopeial Convention, Rockville, Md, 1998.
17. United States Pharmacopeia Drug Information (USP DI), ed 18. Vol 3, Approved Drug Products and Legal Requirements. United States Pharmacopeial Convention, Rockville, Md., 1998.

Chapter Questions

1. The origins of pharmacy began approximately 4000 years ago within this ancient civilization:
   A. Europe
   B. Mesopotamia
   C. Greece
   D. Egypt

2. The earliest pharmacy practice was thought to be established in the United States in the year:
   A. 1646
   B. 1776
   C. 1804
   D. 1870

3. The Pure Food and Drug Act of 1906 was enacted to:
   A. Prohibit misbranding of foods and drugs.
   B. Regulate drug distribution.
   C. Regulate compounding pharmacies.
   D. Ensure drug safety.

4. The Durham-Humphrey Amendment of 1952:
   A. Codified the OTC and prescription drug classifications.
   B. Mandated drug efficacy.
   C. Set forth testing procedures for new drugs.
   D. Required anti-tampering precautions.

5. Drugs that produce the highest affinity for abuse but also can be used medically are called:
   A. Schedule I drugs.
   B. Schedule II drugs.
   C. Schedule III drugs.
   D. Schedule IV drugs.

6. Which of the following disclosures is NOT required but can be found on an OTC label?
   A. Name of the product
   B. Inert and active ingredients
   C. Habituation warnings
   D. Expiration date

7. A generic drug name:
   A. Is shorter than the chemical name.
   B. Is used for general recognition.
   C. Is also called the "nonproprietary" name.
   D. All of the above.

8. Generic equivalent drugs can be substituted for brand-name drugs if:
   A. The drug is similar in dose and strength to the brand-name drug.
   B. The drug has dosage, strength, and active ingredients that are identical to those of the brand-name drug.
   C. The generic drug is similar in color and size to the brand-name drug.
   D. The patient requests the brand-name drug.

9. When calling the poison control center, it is imperative that you provide the following information:
   A. Name, type of poison, and amount ingested
   B. Type of poison, amount ingested, and address
   C. Name, closest living relative, types of poison, and amount ingested
   D. Only what you think is appropriate

10. This reference guide provides a detailed description of a drug similar to the information found within the drug package insert:
   A. Drug Facts and Comparisons
   B. American Hospital Formulary Service Drug Information
   C. U.S. Pharmacopeia Drug Information
   D. Physician's Desk Reference

Pharmacokinetics and Pharmacodynamics

2

Chapter Objectives

After reading this chapter, the student will:

1 Understand and be able to define the term "drug."
2 Know about the process by which drug compounds are attached to receptor sites located on or within the cell.
3 Be able to differentiate between the agonist and antagonist effects of a drug on living tissues.
4 Understand the differences in individual responses to drug therapy.
5 Understand the onset of action and duration of action that drugs exhibit when administered to living tissues.
6 Understand and be able to identify the various forms of in which a drug can be administered.
7 Be able to differentiate among the different types and sites of drug administration.
8 Understand how drugs are absorbed, metabolized, distributed, and excreted.
9 Be able to identify the variety of human physical characteristics that may affect drug responses.

Chapter Outline

*E*ach year over-the-counter (OTC) and prescription drug administration rates increase. As more and more new drugs, both prescription and OTC, are developed for a variety of maladies, the athletic trainer needs to be more knowledgeable about how these drugs affect the human body. It is important to understand the different methods of delivering drugs to the tissues of the body and how these methods affect how the drug is metabolized and utilized by the body.

This chapter will explain how drugs are used to treat,

prevent, and diagnose disease and illness, a field of study known as *pharmacotherapeutics*. Specifically, this chapter will focus on two subcomponents of pharmacotherapeutics: *pharmacokinetics* (how the body assimilates, incorporates, and eliminates a drug) and *pharmacodynamics* (how a drug affects the body). By gaining a basic understanding of the pharmacotherapeutics of both prescription and OTC drugs, you can explain to athletes why it is important to take medications as prescribed by the physician. You will also have a better understanding of how drugs work within the body, why they work, how long a drug remains active, and what the potential drug adverse effects are; and be able to address many of the other general questions athletes typically ask when they are taking a drug.

What Is a Drug?

A drug is a chemical that interacts with and affects living organisms to produce a biological response. In other words, a drug alters physiological functions by replacing, interrupting, or potentiating existing cellular functions. For example, caffeine, a drug found in coffee, tea, soft drinks, and other foods, can produce a stimulant effect on the central nervous system (CNS) by attaching to CNS receptors and essentially overriding the fatigue messages being sent to the brain from various neurotransmitters. The actions of caffeine at the cellular level allow it to assist with headache relief and induce alertness in individuals. (For more specific actions of caffeine, see Chapter 12).

The effects that drugs produce on an organism can be either primary or secondary in nature. A primary drug effect is a desired therapeutic effect. It is the reason why a health-care professional prescribes a drug. For example, the health-care professional may give a patient aspirin to relieve fever.

Secondary effects are all other effects that result from the administration of that drug. Secondary effects may be desirable or undesirable, depending on the individual's medical condition and specific reaction to the drug. For example, with aspirin, desirable secondary effects include analgesia, anti-inflammatory properties, and inhibition of platelet aggregation. Undesirable secondary effects include stomach upset and nausea.

It is important to understand that a drug cannot endow a tissue or cell with properties it does not inherently possess. As mentioned earlier, a drug can potentiate, interrupt, or replace a function of the cell, but cannot perform a completely new function in the cell.

Pharmacodynamics

The previous section discussed the definition of a drug. To gain a better understanding of a drug, one also must consider the physical actions of the drug on the cells and systems of the body. The process of determining the site in which drugs act and the mechanism in which this action occurs is called *pharmacodynamics*. In this section, we will discuss how drugs bind to receptors, how doses are determined, and how to identify the time response and length of time a drug is active within the body.

■ Receptor Sites

Drugs can be either *endogenous*—originating within the body, such as hormones produced by the thyroid, or *exogenous*—originating outside the body and not related to the body's natural hormone production. Most drugs do not produce changes everywhere in the body, but act at specific locations in tissues or organs. For a drug to act specifically, there must be a mechanism or site at the cellular level to which the drug, regardless of its size, shape, weight, or chemical structure, can attach and produce an effect. This mechanism of action between the drug and cellular components is commonly referred to as a *drug-receptor interaction*. A *receptor* is a component of a cell to which a drug binds to produce an effect. In most cases, receptors are located on or within the cell and are identified by their protein structure.[1]

When a drug is introduced into the body, it circulates through the bloodstream and attaches to a corresponding cell receptor. However, not all drug-receptor interactions have *affinity* (the force that makes two agents bind or unite) for all drugs. Each drug has a chemical structure that searches for target-specific cell receptors. When a specific drug molecule finds a corresponding receptor, it binds relatively easily. The binding of drugs to receptors is usually associated with the "lock and key" analogy, in which the receptor is the lock and the drug is the key (Fig. 2–1). When a drug fits into a lock, it will exert its effects within that cell. Occasionally, several drugs, or "keys," can fit the same receptor. The competition for the receptor therefore depends on the affinity (binding power) of the drug for that receptor.[18] A drug with a high affinity will bind readily to the receptors even if the drug concentration is low. A drug with a low affinity usually requires higher drug concentrations before binding to receptors can occur.

A drug that interacts with a receptor to produce a pharmacological response is known as an *agonist*. Agonist drugs

Drug molecules–"key"

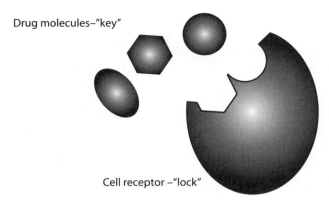

Cell receptor –"lock"

Figure 2–1. "Lock and key" receptor analogy. The cell receptor has a specifically shaped "lock" or binding site that will accept only a same-shape "key" drug molecule.

are said to have both affinity and *efficacy* (the capacity to elicit a response).[1] Conversely, drugs that interact or bind with a receptor but do not produce a pharmacological response or prevent any effect of an agonist are called *antagonists*. Antagonist drugs are sometimes referred to "blockers" because they occupy the receptors and prevent agonist drugs from causing a change in cellular activity. An antagonist drug is said to have affinity but not efficacy.

■ Dose Response

The action of a drug on cellular activity is characterized by several variables, one of which is the dose or amount of the drug given. When a dose is administered, levels of the drug within the body usually increase gradually and smoothly. The lowest dose capable of producing a perceivable response is called the *threshold*. It varies according to the properties of the drug. The maximal effect of the drug is the greatest response produced regardless of the dose administered. When, after the maximal effect is reached, the dose of a drug increases, its efficacy will not increase. Instead, the incidence of associated adverse effects will increase. Hence, drugs have certain limitations regarding the amount that can be given over a period of time.

Dose-response curves are an appropriate method of evaluating and comparing the efficacy and potency of related drugs. *Potency* is the amount of drug necessary to produce a desired pharmacological effect. A more potent drug requires a lower dose and a less potent drug requires a higher dose to produce the same pharmacological effect. For example, it takes a higher dose of drug B (aspirin) to elicit the same pain-relief response as drug A (morphine) (Fig. 2–2). Therefore drug A is said to have a higher potency than drug B and a smaller dose of drug A can be given to bring about pain relief. Another example is the comparison between corticosteroids. Both hydrocortisone and dexamethasone are efficacious, but dexamethasone is approximately 20 times more potent than hydrocortisone. In this specific case, a larger dose of hydrocortisone will be required to create the desired response.

■ Time Response

When a drug is introduced into the system, its effects are not instantaneous. A period of time must elapse before the drug-

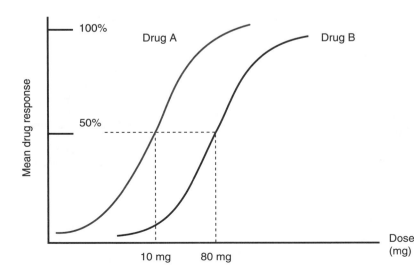

Figure 2–2. Typical dose response curve. At a mean response of 50 percent, it takes a higher dose of drug B to elicit the same response as drug A. Drug A therefore exhibits more potency.

induced effects occur. Some drug effects occur relatively quickly; others manifest their action over days. Moreover, the length of the drug-induced effect is not infinite. Metabolic processes occur in the body that affect the concentration of the drug and alter the therapeutic effect. In determining the time response of a dose, three factors must be considered: latency, maximal effect, and duration of action (Fig. 2–3).

Latency, sometimes referred to as "onset of action," indicates the time required for a drug to produce an observable effect after being administered. *Maximal effect* is the length of time it takes for the drug to reach peak efficacy. *Duration of action* refers to the period of time over which a drug produces a response after a single dose. These metrics are influenced by a variety of attributes including (1) the specific route of administration (e.g., oral or intramuscular), (2) the *solubility* of the drug (the rate at which the drug is absorbed into the bloodstream from the site of administration), (3) how fast the drug is distributed to the site of action, and (4) the time it takes to be inactivated and excreted from the body.

▨ Therapeutic Index

Although drug potency can determine the dose required to achieve a desired effect, it does little to determine drug safety. Ultimately, drugs need to be administered in safe dosage ranges that will elicit the desired response without producing toxic or lethal effects. The range in which desired effects are produced is called the *therapeutic index* (Fig. 2–4). The therapeutic index is useful in determining the safety parameters of doses and is expressed by the ratio between the median effective dose (ED_{50}), the dose required to produce a response, or effect, in 50 percent of the test subjects, and the toxic dose (TD_{50}), the portion of the population in which 50 percent of individuals exhibit adverse effects. To be considered clinically relevant, the therapeutic index should be greater than 1:1, with higher numbers producing safer or less toxic drugs.

▨ Plasma Dose Response

Generally, the level of response to a particular dose of a drug at the site of action is correlated with the plasma or serum level of that drug. The therapeutic window of a drug can be calculated over time by the plasma or serum concentrations of that drug (Fig. 2–5).We will assume that the concentration of a drug in the plasma is the same as the concentration of the drug at the site of action. When a dose is first administered, it can be detected in the plasma but may not have high enough concentrations to produce a pharmacological response. This period is said to be below the *minimal effective concentration* (MEC). As the drug concentration increases above the MEC, so does the intensity of response at the cellular level. The length of time the drug concentration remains above the MEC is termed the *duration of action.* It is the optimal range for the drug to produce its desired response. Drug plasma concentrations that exceed the level of the therapeutic window may produce toxic responses and

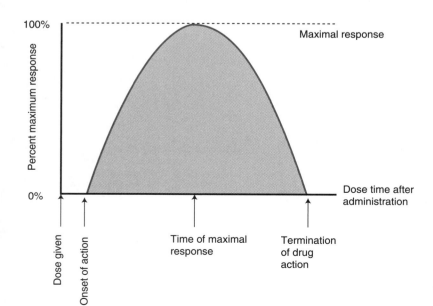

Figure 2–3. Typical time response curve. After initial administration (single dose), the drug concentration will not be immediately measurable. A period of time will elapse before the drug concentration increases, reaches its potential, and then gradually decreases until it is eliminated from the body.

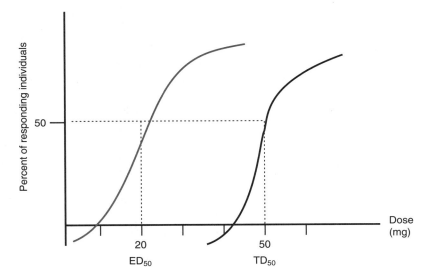

Figure 2–4. Therapeutic index. The ED_{50} of this specific dose is 20 mg and the TD_{50} is 50 mg. The therapeutic index for this particular drug is 2.5.

are not considered safe. The point at which concentration reaches the toxic range is called the *minimum toxic concentration* (MTC).

Some drugs have a very narrow therapeutic window. These drugs require more monitoring because an increase in the dose could be toxic or lethal. A drug with a narrow therapeutic window must be administered at appropriate times and under the proper conditions to maintain an effective level without putting too much of the drug into the body at one time.

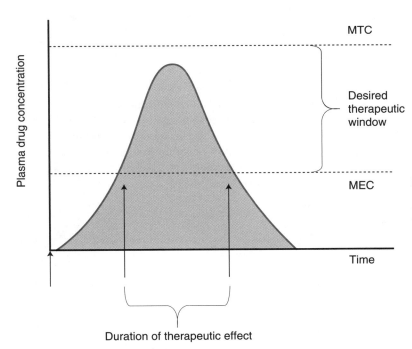

Duration of therapeutic effect

Figure 2–5. Plasma response curve. The period of time during which the plasma drug concentration is above the MEC but below the MTC produces the desired therapeutic range (time in which the drug concentration in plasma must be maintained).

Dose – once administered, a measurable amount will be found in the plasma but cannot produce a pharmacological response

MEC – any drug concentration below this line will not produce a desired drug response

MTC – any drug concentration above this line will produce a toxic response

Half-Life

After a drug is administered, it will remain in the system and produce its effects for a finite period of time. During this period, the drug will be slowly metabolized and eliminated from the body. The rate of metabolism and excretion determines the drug's *biological half-life* ($t_{1/2}$). Half-life is calculated by determining the time required to reduce by one-half the amount of the drug present in the body. In other words, half-life is the amount of time required for 50 percent of the drug remaining in the body to be eliminated.[3,12,15]

The concept of half-life is important for several reasons. First, all drugs have different and distinct half-lives, from minutes to hours or days, depending on chemical properties. Second, it allows comparisons for drug elimination rates. Finally, it determines the frequency with which multiple doses of a drug can be safely administered to produce or sustain the MEC. For example, the half-life of Vicodin (an oral agent used for the treatment of pain) is 3 to 4 hours. Because of the short half-life, the drug is usually taken every 4 to 6 hours instead of once or twice per day to ensure adequate pain relief.

One final point must be made about half-life. Half-life does not change with the drug dose, meaning that it will always take the same amount of time to eliminate one-half of the drug present in the body even if the athlete takes half of the dosage (e.g., one tablet of ibuprofen instead of two) or more than the recommended dosage.

Pharmacokinetics

Thus far in this chapter, we have discussed what constitutes a drug, how it binds to cellular receptors, and the various quantitative methods used to measure the effectiveness of a drug. Different processes or events occur from the time a drug is introduced into the body until it is completely eliminated. This concept is called *pharmacokinetics*. It describes what the body does to or with a drug. Pharmacokinetics is concerned with four processes: absorption, distribution, metabolism, and excretion (Fig. 2–6).

Absorption

As mentioned previously, a drug can exert its effects directly at the site of administration. However, most drugs are not administered at the site of action. For example, many drugs are taken orally. Therefore they must be absorbed into the bloodstream and carried to the site of action. The speed, rate, and extent at which a drug is absorbed and produces its pharmacological action is dependent on the physical and chemical

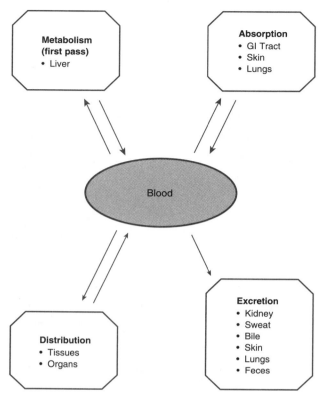

Figure 2–6. The pharmacokinetic process. (Adapted from Lehne, RA. Pharmacokinetics. In Pharmacology for Nursing Care, ed 3, p. 30. Copyright 1998, with permission from Elsevier Science.)

properties of the drug. Such properties include the solubility of the drug, the surface area of the intended site of action, and, most importantly, the specific route of administration.

The major classes of administration are (1) *enteral*, (2) *parenteral*, (3) *respiratory*, and (4) *topical* (Table 2–1).

Enteral

Oral ingestion is the most commonly selected, safest, most convenient, and most economical route of administering medication. When medication is taken by mouth, the onset of drug action usually occurs within 1 hour. The drug is absorbed in several areas along the gastrointestinal (GI) tract. Gastric absorption begins when a drug that has been swallowed enters the stomach. How long a drug remains in the stomach, the pH of a patient's stomach acid, and gastric motility into the small intestine determine the amount of drug absorbed. Slowing down gastric emptying increases drug absorption and speeding up gastric emptying

Table 2–1

Routes of Drug Administration

Route Category	Route	Site	Example
Enteral	Sublingual	Under tongue	Nitroglycerin
	Buccal	Oral mucosa	Miconazole (antifungal)
	Oral	Mouth	Ibuprofen
Parenteral	Subcutaneous	Beneath skin	Insulin
	Intramuscular	Into muscle	Morphine
	Intravenous	Into vein	Phenytoin (anticonvulsant)
	Intrathecal	Into spinal fluid	Bupivacaine (anesthetic)
	Intra-articular	Into joint	Dexamethasone (corticosteroid)
	Intrasynovial	Into joint fluid	Triamcinolone (corticosteroid)
Inhalation	Intrarespiratory	Into lung	Albuterol
Topical	Transdermal	On skin surface	Nicotine patch
Ophthalmic	Intraocular	Into eye	Timolol (antiglaucoma agent)
Otic	Intraotic	Into ear	Cortisporin (antibiotic)
Miscellaneous	Rectal	Into rectum	Acetaminophen
	Vaginal	Into vagina	Clotrimazole (antifungal)

decreases it. Administering drugs on an empty stomach (with water to ensure dissolution) facilitates rapid delivery to the small intestine. Drugs are absorbed more readily in the small intestine because of its alkaline pH and large surface area.

By contrast, the oral mucosa, with a vast capillary blood supply, can dissolve certain drugs rapidly by the *sublingual* or *buccal* route. Drugs taken sublingually (e.g., nitroglycerin for angina) are placed under the tongue, where they dissolve in the saliva. Sublingual administration is often used in individuals who have difficulty in swallowing or who cannot be given drugs rectally.[9] Drugs placed under the tongue are absorbed through the mucosal lining into the venous system and enter the systemic circulation within minutes, without preliminary passage through the liver.

Preliminary passage, or *first-pass metabolism,* can be described as the process by which a drug is ingested orally and then absorbed from the gastrointestinal tract into the portal venous system (Fig. 2–7). The drug must then pass through the liver before reaching the general systemic circulation. As a result of this process, many drugs are metabolized or broken down into inactive agents by the liver, which decreases the amount of active drug that is able to reach the site of action. For example, lidocaine, if given orally, is almost completely metabolized be the liver. This makes oral administration impractical and requires that the drug be introduced into the body by other methods.

Drugs can be administered orally in many forms, including *solutions, capsules,* and *tablets.* Oral solutions—drugs in

liquid form—are easier to swallow than drugs in solid forms. They may have coloring, flavoring, or sweetening agents and are usually dissolved in water. *Syrups* are a type of solution that contains high concentrations of sucrose or other sugars. Because water-soluble drugs are hard to dissolve in syrups, most often the drug is dissolved in water first and the flavoring syrup is added later. *Elixirs* are solutions in which the drug is dissolved in alcohol. The alcohol content usually ranges from 5 to 40 percent.

Capsules consist of one or more drugs plus various inactive substances in powder form, enclosed within a gelatin shell. The gelatin capsule can be either hard or soft and is intended to be swallowed whole. *Tablets* are the most commonly used solid dosage form. They can be swallowed whole or chewed. Tablets can also be coated (*enteric coated*) to delay the release of the drug and avoid gastric irritation. Enteric-coated tablets remain intact in the stomach but dissolve in the small intestine. These tablets are used to protect drugs from acid and pepsin in the stomach and to protect the stomach from discomfort.

Sustained-release capsules or tablets are specially coated and are designed to release a drug over a period of time. Individuals who want to decrease the number of daily doses often use sustained-release products. However, these products are usually more expensive. Allegra D, an antihistamine used for allergies, and Biaxin XL, an antibiotic, are examples of sustained-release products.

Drugs may also be absorbed in the lower gastrointestinal tract via suppository form. A *suppository* is a solid or semi-

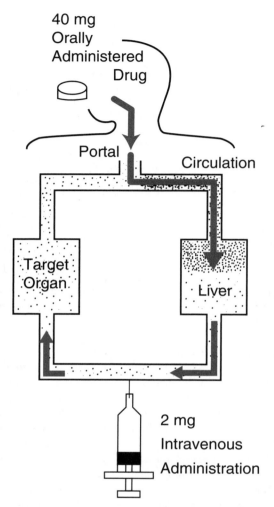

Figure 2–7. First-pass effect. (From M.E. Winter, Bioavailability. In M.E. Winter, M.A. Koda-Kimble, and L.Y. Young [eds], Basic clinical pharmacokinetics, 2d ed. Applied Therapeutics, Vancouver, Wash., 1988, with permission.)

solid compound that is inserted into a body orifice (rectum or vagina). Once inserted, the suppository melts as it reaches body temperature or dissolves into the aqueous secretions of the body cavity. Suppositories can produce local effects and, if used rectally, can also produce systemic effects. Common rectally administered medications include acetaminophen, aspirin, and anti-nausea preparations.

Parenteral

Parenteral administration means to give a drug by any non-oral route, usually by an injection directly into an internal body compartment or cavity. This route of administration usually allows the drug to be delivered directly to the target site. The action of the drug is therefore more predictable. In addition, parenteral administration is not subjected to first-pass metabolism in the liver. Common parenteral routes include subcutaneous, intramuscular, intravenous, intrathecal, and intra-articular.

A drug administered subcutaneously is usually injected beneath the skin into the connective tissue or fat deposits within the dermis. One example of this type of drug is injectable insulin, used by persons with diabetes. Drugs injected by this route can be slowly dispersed and absorbed into the bloodstream. However, only a small amount of a drug can be injected in this manner because of possible local irritation and the small volume the dermis can hold. A primary advantage of subcutaneous administration is that patients with proper training can inject themselves without the assistance of a health-care provider.

A drug injected into the skeletal muscle is absorbed more quickly than a subcutaneous injection because of the close proximity of blood vessels in the muscles. Common intramuscular agents include vaccines and pain medications. Drugs administered intramuscularly can cause local irritation, pain, soreness, and tenderness. Thus, different sites on the muscle are preferred for repeated injections.

Intravenous injections (drugs administered into the veins) produce an almost immediate response because they initially avoid the liver metabolism process. This method of drug introduction enables a drug to be delivered directly to target tissues. A drug administered intravenously can be precisely controlled in regard to quantity and reaches its target site rapidly. Most drugs are administered into the veins with intravenous cannulas (IVs) to produce the desired effects. This method of administration is convenient for prolonged drug therapy. However, any miscalculation of a drug dose can produce undesired consequences and make care difficult after administration.

Intrathecal injections are administered directly into the spinal cord or cerebrospinal fluid and can bypass the blood-brain barrier. Drugs commonly used by this route include narcotic analgesics, local anesthetics, antibiotics, anticancer agents, and antispasmodic drugs.

Intra-articular and intrasynovial injections are administered into the joints and synovial fluid, respectively. The sites normally injected are the elbow, knee, shoulder, wrist, and hip. The medications are usually anesthetics, antimicrobials, or corticosteroids.

Inhalation

Drugs administered by inhalation are in the form of gases or fine mists (aerosols). Because of their large surface area and rich blood supply, the lungs are an effective means of absorbing and transporting medications into the bloodstream rapidly.[8] The small particles of these drugs ensure that gaseous exchange is not impeded within the lungs. This method of drug delivery is useful for applying medications directly to the alveolar and bronchial tissues for treatment of pulmonary conditions. Special inhalation devices are used to propel the agents into the alveolar and bronchial tissues. Common inhalation drugs include albuterol (Proventil), fluticasone (Flovent), and betamethasone (Beclovent), used in the treatment of asthma. Inhalation will be discussed further in Chapter 7, Respiratory Drugs.

Topical

Drugs administered topically are usually applied to the skin or mucous membranes. Lipid-soluble products are absorbed more readily through the skin than water-soluble products. Absorption of medications through the skin is inhibited by the epidermis, so drugs have a difficult time reaching the systemic circulation.[2] Because of poor absorption, many medications are applied topically to treat problems on the skin. Topical drugs are usually manufactured as either ointments, creams, or transdermal patches. All these forms may produce either local or systemic effects.

Transdermal patches are controlled-release devices that may contain any number of drugs for local or systemic absorption. They are attached to the skin by an adhesive layer that ensures proper drug contact with the skin surface. For transdermal patches to be clinically effective, the drug must be able to permeate the skin, be nonirritating and nonsensitizing, and be unaffected by enzymes in the epidermis.[7,11] In addition, mixing the drug in some type of oily base increases solubility and permeability through the dermis.[8] Transdermal agents provide a slow, controlled drug release that is effective in maintaining a relatively constant plasma level of the drug. Common transdermal agents include nicotine and estrogen patches. Drugs may also be administered transdermally via iontophoresis.

Ointments and creams are semisolid preparations for external use only. They include Neosporin and hydrocortisone. They can be easily spread and act as emollients, making the skin more pliable. Ointments and creams serve as protective barriers to prevent substances from coming in contact with the skin, and also as vehicles in which medications can be incorporated.

Powders are mixtures of finely divided drugs or chemicals in dry form that can be applied topically.

■ Distribution

Before a drug can act on a specific receptor, it must pass through the different biological layers, then be transported to the site via the bloodstream. Passage through these layers depends not only on the characteristics of the drug itself—ionization, solubility, and size—but also on the rate of flow of the blood that carries the drug to its site of action. For example, a medication is taken orally to act on specific receptors located on the heart muscle. The drug must initially pass through various GI membranes, enter the bloodstream, pass through the liver, be distributed throughout the entire body via the bloodstream, reenter membranes on the heart, and eventually attach to a specific heart receptor. As you can see, this process takes time. Also, a portion of the active ingredient in the drug is lost by this process.

A brief review of cell physiology is warranted here to provide a better understanding of drug distribution through the biological membranes of the body. The typical cell membrane consists of a bimolecular layer of lipid (fatlike) molecules with protein molecules randomly embedded and protruding from one or both sides of the membrane. The protein molecules serve as carriers or receptors for drugs, and the lipid molecules permit fat-soluble molecules to pass easily into the cell while impeding water-soluble molecules. However, the cell membrane does allow some small-diameter water-soluble molecules (such as electrolytes and alcohol) to pass through specialized pores on the membrane.

The ability of a drug to cross cell membranes through the lipid barrier depends on the physical and chemical properties of the drug molecule. Most drugs exist as either weak organic acids or weak organic bases. When dissolved by body solutions, they form weak electrolytes. However, these electrolytes do not dissociate (form ions) completely in aqueous solution, but exist in solution as a mixture of *ionized* (charged) and *nonionized* (uncharged) forms. Ionized forms (e.g., ketoprofen) are usually water soluble and have difficulty passing through the cell membrane, whereas nonionized forms (e.g., dexamethasone) are lipid soluble and allow easier passage. The relative lipid solubility of the nonionized portion of a drug will determine if the drug will (1) be absorbed into the bloodstream, (2) be distributed throughout the body, (3) be able to cross the cell membranes and act within, and (4) be readily excreted in the urine.

How the drug passes through the cell membrane depends not only on ionization but also on the mode of transportation (Table 2–2). There are three common modes of transportation that most drugs use to cross cell membranes, either individually or using a combination of modes: filtration, diffusion, and active transport. The process of *filtration* allows small water-soluble molecules and ions to easily pass through cell membranes with small pores. Consequently, larger-diameter (lipid-soluble) molecules are unable to pass through the cell membrane by filtration. Instead, lipid-soluble molecules *diffuse* through the cell by dissolving in the lipid portion of the membrane. Diffusion is the most common method of travel across the membrane.

Larger water-soluble molecules also have a more difficult time crossing the cell membrane by filtration. In order for these molecules to gain access to the cell, they need an active transport carrier or an energy-requiring system. Molecules outside the cell that do not have the specific physical and chemical properties to gain access into the cell must bind with a carrier that will transport them within the cell. After it deposits the molecules, the carrier is then free to return to the cell membrane to attach to another molecule. Only molecules with specific chemical properties can be actively transported, and only a certain number of molecules can be transported at one time.

Metabolism

Thus far, we have discussed the mechanisms by which a drug is absorbed and distributed throughout the body to produce a biological or therapeutic effect. However, a drug stays in the body for only a finite period of time before it is eliminated, as explained previously in the discussion of the half-life of a drug. *Biotransformation*, or metabolism, is the process of ridding the body of foreign substances. More specifically, biotransformation is the breakdown of an original drug compound into metabolites, which are then eliminated. The rate of metabolism is different for all individu-

als. Some metabolize the same drug at a slower rate than others. Factors such as disease, starvation, smoking, and age affect the rate of metabolism and the speed with which drugs are eliminated from the body.

The primary organ of metabolism is the liver,[3,16] which has a specialized network of enzymes whose function is to metabolize drugs or foreign compounds. When a drug enters the hepatic enzyme system, it can lose some or all of its original pharmacological activity. In most cases, when a drug is metabolized, the end product is usually more water soluble than the original drug and is easily eliminated from the body.

Excretion

As stated previously, a drug can stay within the body only for a certain period of time before it is eliminated. The main routes for drug elimination are through the urine, bile, and feces. Drug compounds may also be eliminated through the lungs and the salivary, sweat, and mammary glands. The main emphasis in this section is on drug elimination through the urine.

The kidney is the major organ of excretion.[14] The process of excretion through the kidney is by glomerular filtration. Approximately 180 liters of plasma fluid are filtered each day, with 178.5 liters reabsorbed and 1.5 liters eliminated in the urine.[19] As blood flows through the *glomerulus*, drugs are forced through the capillary wall and into the renal tubules. The glomeruli of the kidneys can easily filter unbound (water-soluble) drugs, but cannot filter protein-bound compounds as easily. Lipid-soluble compounds are reabsorbed after filtration and are not eliminated in the urine.

The relative pH of urine also determines whether a compound will be reabsorbed or excreted. Weak acids are eliminated faster in alkaline urine; weak bases are eliminated faster in acidic urine. One final factor controlling the rate of

Table 2–2			
Modes of Drug Transportation Across Cell Membranes			
	Filtration	**Diffusion**	**Active Transport**
Drug size	Small	Small or large	Small or large
Solubility	Water or lipid	Lipid	Water or lipid
Energy requirements	No	No	Yes
Movement against a concentration gradient	No	No	Yes
Drug passage rate determined by:	Size and concentration gradient	Solubility and concentration gradient	Energy, transport carrier saturation, and structural specificity

excretion is patient health. Patients with kidney disease or insufficient kidney function must be cautious when taking medications. Decreased kidney function leads to decreased elimination, causing the drug to accumulate and potentially cause toxicity.

Factors Affecting Drug Response

In a perfect world, all drugs would elicit the same response when administered. However, several factors contribute to the diversity of drug reaction within individuals. These factors are age, weight, gender, and time of administration. Therefore allied health professionals should be aware of individual characteristics and monitor or make adjustments to drug therapy.

Infants and older adults are more sensitive to drugs. Infants have immature hepatic enzyme systems and therefore have trouble metabolizing drug therapy. Because of this, intensified drug responses and increased drug action duration often occur in infants. Although infants are considered by some people to be "small adults," they need only a fraction of the average adult dose.

Older individuals are usually hypersensitive to drug effects. Drugs usually remain in the body for extended periods, which increases drug intensity and toxicity. The cardiovascular and urinary system functions are diminished and the ability of the liver to metabolize compounds is lessened. In addition, older adults usually have a higher proportion of fat, which serves as a storage facility for lipid-soluble drugs. Finally, the protein-binding capabilities decrease with age and the number of unbound drug compounds is increased. Cautious estimates of dosages are always indicated for older adults.

Gender and weight may also contribute to different drug responses. It was once thought that women were more sensitive to drugs than men because of their higher fat content and height and mass differences. Subsequent research has shown that both genders respond equivalently to drugs, provided that dosing is based on weight. Usually, the larger the person, the higher the dose he or she can receive.

The time of drug administration can influence the absorption, distribution, and elimination of drug compounds. Drugs are more rapidly absorbed before a meal than after because the GI tract is free of food substances. If gastric irritation is of primary concern, administration with food will lessen the side effects but also delay the response. Some medications must be administered on an empty or full stomach for proper absorption. Always follow the directions for administration to ensure proper drug activity.

Barriers to Drug Distribution

As drug molecules are distributed throughout the bloodstream, they sometimes encounter barriers that limit their accessibility. Two specific barriers, the *blood-brain barrier* and the *placental barrier*, are used as protective mechanisms. These barriers inhibit or deter certain chemicals in the bloodstream that can be dangerous or toxic to the individual or to a fetus. In order to enter the brain, a drug must first cross specific capillary walls and glial cells, then pass through the extracellular fluid compartment, and finally enter the neuron cell membrane. The capillary walls and glial cells are tightly woven with a special architecture that impedes the movement of drugs into or out of the brain. Drugs that are mostly lipid soluble may be able to enter the CNS by diffusion through the capillaries in the brain or through the cerebrospinal fluid (CSF). Additionally, water-soluble or charged molecules that use the active transport system can at times enter the brain or CSF, but they do so at a much slower rate.

The placenta, with its rich blood supply, serves as the respiratory, digestive, and excretory organ for the developing fetus. Unlike the blood-brain barrier, the placental barrier is nonselective and is permeable to most lipid- and water-soluble drugs. Consequently, drugs that are of therapeutic value for the expectant mother may be harmful or toxic to the fetus. Therefore pregnant women should take drugs only on physician recommendation.

Drug Safety

Whenever a drug is administered, it is important that the athletic trainer follow certain guidelines to prevent serious harm or unnecessary side effects. Nurses commonly use the *Five Rights of Drug Administration* when working with drugs. The five rights are right drug, right patient, right dose, right route, and right time.[13] Along with the five rights, the following reminders should be consciously made each time a drug is administered:

- First, make sure that the drug within the container is the actual drug prescribed or bought. Talk to the pharmacist to ensure that the drug prescribed is the drug dispensed.
- Second, read the directions carefully. Many drugs are delivered into the body by various routes. All administration directions must be followed precisely for the drug to be effective.

Scenario from the Field

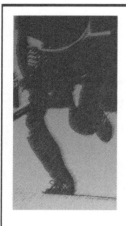

An athlete comes into the athletic training room complaining of shoulder pain. After making an assessment, the athletic trainer provides the athlete with several sample packets of Tylenol. Each packet contains two 325 mg tablets. The athletic trainer forgets to provide the athlete with proper instructions. The next day, the athlete returns and says the pain is subsiding but he is out of Tylenol. After questioning the athlete, the athletic trainer determines that the athlete was taking 2 packets every 6 hours.

The athlete in this case study was using the correct drug to alleviate pain but was taking much more than the recommended dose. He was taking 650 mg 4 times per day for a total of 5200 mg. The maximum recommended daily dose of Tylenol is 4000 mg. If the athlete continued this regimen for longer than a week, he could have sustained liver damage or other toxic conditions

In addition, the athletic trainer provided multiple single doses of an OTC drug rather than one dose.

To correct this problem, it is recommended that both the athlete and the athletic trainer carefully read the directions on the package label, and that the trainer follow the laws and regulations about administering OTC medications in the athletic training setting.

- Third, if a drug dose if missed, read the directions to determine when the next dose should be administered.
- Fourth, store the medication in the setting described on the label. Certain drugs deteriorate if stored in the wrong temperature, in excessive humidity, or in lighted conditions.
- Finally, make sure that all drugs are properly stored in a safe place away from children and either have safety seals or are packaged in child-resistant containers.

Know the patient's medical history. Many drugs have the potential to cause severe effects if taken concurrently. Combining drugs may intensify the actions of one drug.

This is referred to as *potentiation*. For example, a patient is given a prescription for a muscle relaxant such as Robaxin, Skelaxin, or Flexeril that can cause drowsiness and dizziness. If this patient consumes alcohol, these effects are potentiated. This is why certain prescriptions contain warning labels advising the user not to consume alcohol. Conversely, one drug may cancel the effects of another, a process referred to as *antagonism*. This sometimes occurs when prescription drugs are taken in combination with OTC or herbal medications. Therefore it is important to talk to a physician or pharmacist to determine the compatibility of multiple drug administrations.

Discussion Topics

1. What route is the most common method of taking OTC and prescription drugs? What are the factors that an athlete should be aware of when taking drugs via this route?

2. How does half-life affect the therapeutic window of a drug?

3. Can more than one drug be administered to an athlete for an illness or injury?

4. Can a second dose of a drug be administered if the first dose does not produce any noticeable desired effects?

5. How does a drug know where to go in the body to produce its desired effects?

Chapter Review

- Drugs are compounds that are used to produce biological reactions within the body.

- Most drugs need a receptor to travel to within the cell.

- The three most common mechanisms that a drug uses to pass though a cell membrane are diffusion, filtration, and active transport.

- The efficacy of a drug is usually measured by dose-response curves.

- Once a drug is administered, it will act for only a finite period of time.

- The therapeutic index determines a drug's desired effects.

- Half-life is the amount of time it takes to reduce the amount of a drug in the body by one-half.

- The primary routes of drug administration are enteral, parenteral, respiratory, and topical.

- Distribution and metabolism are dependent on cell and large-organ characteristics.

- Most drugs are eliminated from the body via the kidneys.

- Several factors can affect drug response. They include age, gender, weight, and time.

- The blood-brain barrier and placenta act as protective mechanisms in drug distribution.

- Please read and follow drug label directions carefully for storage and administration recommendations.

References

1. Bourne, HR, and Roberts, JM: Drug receptors and pharmacodynamics. In Katzung, BG (ed): Basic and Clinical Pharmacology, ed 5. Appleton & Lange, East Norwalk, Conn., 1992, pp 10–34.

2. Ciccone, CD. Drug receptors. In Pharmacology in Rehabilitation, ed 2. FA Davis, Philadelphia, 1996. pp 15–31.

3. *Ibid.*, pp 32–43.

4. *Ibid.*, pp 44–57.

5. Evans, T, Hepler, JR et al.: Guanine nucleotide regulation of agonist binding to muscarinic cholinergic receptors: relation to efficacy of agonists for stimulation of phosphoinositide breakdown and calcium mobilization. Biochem J 232:751–757, 1985.

6. Fantl, WJ, Johnson, DE, et al.: Signaling by receptor tyrosine kinases. Annu Rev Biochem 62:453–481, 1993.

7. Finnen, MJ, Herdman, ML, et al.: Distribution and subcellular localization of drug metabolizing enzymes in the skin. Br J Dermatol 113:713–721, 1985.

8. Gillis, CN: Pharmacologic aspects of metabolic processes in the pulmonary microcirculation. Ann Rev Toxicol 26:183–200, 1986.

9. Gong, L, and Middleton, RK: Sublingual administration of opoids. Ann Pharmacotherapy 26:1525–1526, 1992.

10. Jaffe, RC: Thyroid hormone receptors. In Conn, PM (ed): The Receptors, vol 1. Academic Press, New York, 1984, pp 141–176.

11. Kao J, Patterson FK, et al.: Skin penetration and metabolism of topically applied chemicals in six mammalian species, including man: An *in-vitro* study with benzo(a) pyrene and testosterone. Toxicol Appl Pharmacol 81:502–516, 1985.

12. Keller, F, and Scholle, J: Criticism of pharmacokinetic clearance concepts. J Clin Pharmacol Ther Toxicol 21:563–568, 1983.

13. Lehne, RA: Drug legislation, development, names, and information. In Pharmacology for Nursing Care, ed. 3. WB Saunders, Philadelphia, 1998 pp 7–11(7).

14. Lehne, RA: Pharmacokinetics. In Pharmacology for Nursing Care, ed. 3.WB Saunders, Philadelphia, 1998, pp 29–48.

15. Levy, RH, and Bauer, LA: Basic pharmacokinetics. Ther Drug Monit 8:47–58, 1986.

16. Pang, KS, Xu, X, et al.: Determinants of metabolic disposition. Annu Rev Pharmacol Toxicol 32:623–669, 1992.

17. Raffa, RB, and Tallarida, RJ: The concept of a changing receptor concentration: implications for the theory of drug action. J Theor Biol 115:623–632, 1985.

18. Ross, EM: Pharmacodynamics: Mechanisms of drug action and the relationship between drug concentration and effect. In Gilman, AG, Rall, TW, et al. (eds): Goodman & Gilman's The Pharmacological Basis of Therapeutics, ed 8. Pergamon Press, New York, 1990, pp 33–48.

19. Sherwood, L: Urinary system. In Human Physiology: From Cells to Systems. West Publishing Company, St. Paul, MN., 1989, pp 462–509.

Chapter Questions

1. The force that binds or unites drug molecules is called:
   A. Agonist
   B. Affinity
   C. Endogenous
   D. Receptor

2. The "lock-and-key" analogy represents:
   A. The process of a drug binding to a receptor.
   B. The affinity of a drug for a receptor.
   C. The biological reaction produced by a drug receptor binding to a drug.
   D. The inability of a drug to bind successfully to its specific receptor.

3. The potency of a drug refers to:
   A. The maximal perceivable response to a specific dose.
   B. The ability of a drug to exert its effects.
   C. The difference between the doses of two drugs.
   D. The amount of a drug needed to produce a pharmacological effect.

4. What is the therapeutic index of a drug with an ED_{50} of 50 and a TD_{50} of 125?
   A. 25
   B. .40
   C. 2.5
   D. 12

5. An individual is directed to take a total of 1.6 grams of ibuprofen in 4 equal increments throughout the day. Each tablet is 200 mg. Which of the following is the correct oral administration of the drug?
   A. 2 tablets every 4 hours
   B. 2 tablets every 6 hours
   C. 6 tablets every 4 hours
   D. 2 tablets every 2 hours

6. The duration of action of a drug is dependent on which of the following?
   A. The dose of the drug
   B. The rate of biotransformation
   C. The length of time above the minimal effective concentration
   D. The health of the individual
   E. All of the above

7. Which of the following internal organs is initially responsible for metabolizing drug compounds?
   A. Kidney
   B. Liver
   C. Small intestine
   D. Stomach

8. Which of the following statements about kidney excretion is correct?
   A. Weak acids are eliminated faster in alkaline urine.
   B. Strong bases are eliminated faster in alkaline urine.
   C. Strong acids are eliminated faster in alkaline urine.
   D. Weak bases are eliminated faster in alkaline urine.

9. Which of the following is NOT an advantage of parenteral over enteral administration of a drug?
   A. Rapid onset of drug action
   B. No direct gastrointestinal contact
   C. Direct administration of the drug to the site
   D. Safest method of drug delivery

10. The ability of a drug to cross a cell membrane depends on:
    A. The active transport system.
    B. Water solubility.
    C. The ionization of the drug receptor.
    D. The diameter of the receptor.

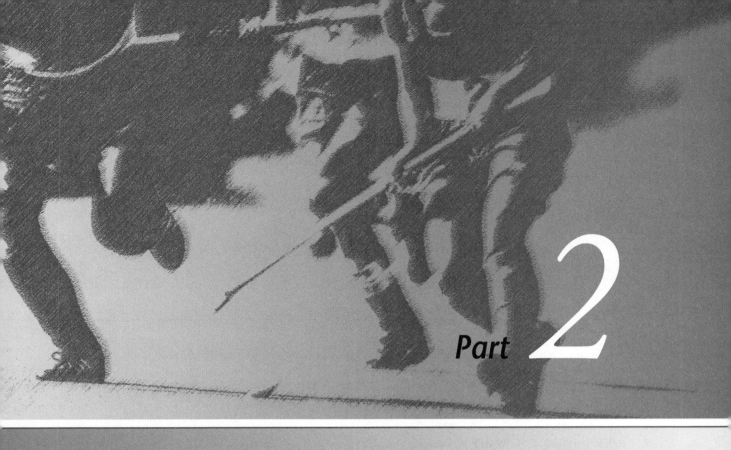

Part 2

Prescription and Over-the-Counter Drugs

3

Anti-inflammatory Medications

Chapter Objectives

After studying this chapter, the student should understand the following basic principles of this drug class:

1 History of anti-inflammatory medications
2 Basic mechanism of action
3 Practical and theoretical advantages of COX-2 inhibitors over other NSAIDs
4 Common adverse effects of NSAIDs
5 Indications for use of NSAIDs and corticosteroids in acute and chronic conditions

Chapter Outline

*A*thletic trainers administer therapeutic modalities such as ultrasound, ice, and electrical stimulation on a daily basis. The goal of treatment is to bring about a rapid and complete resolution of injuries in order to expeditiously return athletes to competition. The treatment for each injury is typically devised and agreed on by the athletic trainer and the team physician, with each drawing on his or her past expe-

rience and knowledge of the current literature to develop the most beneficial rehabilitation plan. In recent years, that treatment plan has increasingly (and often reflexively) included prescription or over-the-counter (OTC) non-steroidal anti-inflammatory medications (NSAIDs).

Electrical modalities, ultrasound, ice, heat, and therapeutic exercise all have accepted and valued roles in the rehabilitation of musculoskeletal injuries. Athletic trainers use these modalities regularly and are usually well aware of their effects, benefits, indications, and contraindications. However, the role of anti-inflammatory medications such as corticosteroids and NSAIDs in the rehabilitation process is not well defined or thoroughly understood.

The use of NSAIDs for the treatment of sports-related injuries, as well as other complaints (particularly osteoarthritis), continues to rise. In 2001, sales of NSAID prescriptions reached $10.9 billion in the United States alone.[47] This figure does not include sales of OTC drugs such as aspirin, ibuprofen, naproxen sodium, and ketoprofen. (Aspirin is technically an NSAID, but is not included in the generic term, which describes the newer agents.) It was recently estimated that more than 1 percent of the US population uses NSAIDs (other than aspirin) daily.[62]

Although NSAIDs are considered relatively safe medications, such widespread use means that a significant number of individuals who take them are unable to tolerate certain side effects. Although gastrointestinal (GI) toxicity has been estimated to occur in only about 2 cases per 10,000 NSAID prescriptions dispensed,[34] this extrapolates to the rather startling figure of 14,000 yearly cases of serious GI complications, based on the over 70 million NSAID prescriptions filled in 1991.[6] Such complications have led to the continued search for "safer" agents such as the cyclooxygenase-2(COX-2) inhibitors that have been introduced in recent years.

Considering that athletic trainers cannot prescribe or dispense prescription or OTC medications, why is this an important topic?[101] If the athletic trainer understands the actions, indications, and side effects of corticosteroid and NSAID use, he or she can continue to play a pivotal role in *all* aspects of an athlete's treatment and rehabilitation plan. A thorough understanding of drug actions, interactions, and effects also enables the athletic trainer to educate athletes about the treatment plan and any symptoms resulting from anti-inflammatory drug therapy.

In the high school and college setting, athletic trainers may be particularly influential regarding the use of OTC NSAIDs by young athletes. A recent study of high school football players revealed that 75 percent of those surveyed had used NSAIDs in the previous 3 months and 15 percent of the respondents were daily NSAID users.[97] The daily users often used the drugs prophylactically before practices and games.

The Inflammatory Response

There are two basic injury categories seen in sports. *Macrotrauma* results from a single, high-force traumatic event. Examples include compound and comminuted fractures, joint dislocations, and tendon ruptures. *Microtrauma* is the result of chronic, repetitive stresses to local tissues (most often tendons). Often classified as overuse injuries, microtraumas typically involve repetitive activities such as throwing, swimming, or distance running. A variety of intrinsic and extrinsic factors contribute to the initial insult and may perpetuate the subsequent inflammatory response (Box 3–1).

Inflammation is the response of vascular tissue to physiological damage and can be divided into three components: acute inflammation, the immune response, and chronic inflammation (Fig. 3–1). The acute inflammatory cascade is set into motion by the initial tissue insult. Grossly, acute inflammation is recognized by the classic and familiar signs of pain (*dolor*), heat (*calor*), erythema (*rubor*), swelling (*tumor*), and loss of function (*functio laesa*).

Inflammation signals the initiation of the healing process and is one facet of the three phases of human tissue response, which include (1) the acute vascular inflammatory phase, (2) the repair-regeneration phase, and (3) the maturation phase.[60] Typically, within 48 hours of the initial trauma, fibroblasts begin the process of wound repair and collagen synthesis. The response prevents the extensive spread of injury-causing agents to nearby tissues, disposes of cellular debris, and sets the stage for the repair process.

BOX 3–1

Factors in Acute and Chronic Sports Injuries

Intrinsic Factors

Anatomic malalignment

Strength imbalance

Poor flexibility

Muscle weakness

Growth (growth cartilage, inflexibility)*

Previous injury

Poor conditioning

Psychological factors (immaturity, stress)*

Extrinsic Factors

Training errors

Poor or improper equipment

Poor or incorrect sport technique

Environment

Playing surface

Psychological factors (pressure from coaches, parents, peers)*

---

*Particular concerns in pediatric and adolescent populations

ACUTE INFLAMMATION

> Pain
> Heat
> Swelling
> Erythema
> Loss of Function

IMMUNE RESPONSE

> Vascular Response
> Repair
> Maturation

CHRONIC INFLAMMATION

> Vascular Damage
> Tissue Hypoxia/Degeneration

Figure 3–1. The inflammatory response.

Cellular injury signals the release of chemical mediators, such as histamine, serotonin, anaphylatoxins, bradykinin, thromboxane, leukotrienes, and prostaglandins, after a short period of vasoconstriction. These chemical mediators increase cellular and capillary permeability and stimulate capillary vasodilation and blood flow. The changes in vascular permeability directly result in edema, caused by the flow of proteins and fluid into the interstitial space. There is also activation of the immune system and humoral response mechanisms. The increased blood flow and vessel permeability allow neutrophils to migrate to the site of injury. Once the leukocytes arrive at the site of inflammation, evidence suggests that they are drawn to "adhesion factors" on the walls of certain vessels and cells. The expression of such adhesion factors increases at times of inflammation and allows the leukocytes to target specific areas.

Activation of neutrophils at the injury site by lysosomal enzymes results in the generation of high concentrations of oxygen free radicals.[89] These free radicals are quite unstable and extremely reactive, attacking the phospholipid structure of cell membranes and resulting in the formation of arachidonic acid metabolites. Once this process is set in place, chemotactic factors are produced, resulting in further migration and activation of leukocytes and potentiating the inflammatory response. It is this continued potentiation that likely plays a role in the development of chronic inflammation.

Chronic inflammation is usually the product of either vascular disruption (in acute injuries) or intermittent tissue hypoxia (Fig. 3–2).[59] Theoretically, such tissue hypoxia might result from the typical cyclic loading of athletic activity and stimulate the release of oxygen free radicals.[57] Leadbetter terms this "sports-induced inflammation" and defines it as "a localized tissue response, initiated by injury or disruption of vascularized tissues exposed to excessive mechanical load or use."[60] Sports-induced inflammation may resolve spontaneously or become a significant limitation to activity. The factors that contribute to its evolution into a chronic injury are poorly understood, but may involve the continued release of local chemotactic factors and a "failed healing response," which leads to the formation of granulation tissue or tissue degeneration.[58]

Two other important substances in the inflammatory process are tumor necrosis factor (TNF) and interleukin-1 (IL-1). Produced predominantly by mononuclear cells and macrophages, they are potent contributors to inflammation

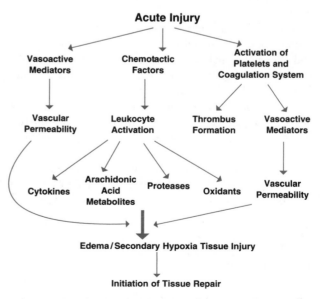

Figure 3–2. The cycle of chronic injury and inflammation.

and are the principal mediators of the immune response to endotoxins produced by bacterial infections. When released because of musculoskeletal injury, they activate and mobilize leukocytes, increase the expression of adhesion molecules, and induce production of the enzymes cyclooxygenase and lipoxygenase, which catalyze the creation of prostaglandins and leukotrienes. Also, TNF and IL-1 likely contribute to the fibrosis and tissue degeneration of chronic inflammation.

There is accumulating evidence that the immune system plays a role in both the acute and chronic inflammatory responses.[59] The immune system is activated when the inflammatory response liberates antigenic substances.[30] These antigenic substances are recognized as foreign tissue by the immune system and eliminated. A complete discussion of the immune response is beyond the scope of this review; however, the immune response certainly results in further amplification and potential propagation of the inflammatory response.

By definition, the inflammatory response is essential to the resolution of the injury. Even so, excessive edema coupled with vascular damage can disrupt the flow of oxygen to the healthy tissue surrounding the injury site. The resultant hypoxia can lead to further tissue damage, appropriately referred to as secondary hypoxic injury.[53] The following discussion will shed light on the specific roles played by various chemical mediators in the inflammatory response and how anti-inflammatory medications may affect that process.

■ Eicosanoids

As noted earlier, the prostaglandins, thromboxane, and the leukotrienes all play a role in the inflammatory response. They are members of the eicosanoid family, derivatives of the 20-carbon fatty acid molecule *arachidonic acid* (Fig. 3–3). Arachidonic acid is a component of cell membranes and must be released from the membrane before it is synthesized into an eicosanoid. Once freed from the membrane, arachidonic acid can be converted through an enzymatic process to either a leukotriene or a common prostaglandin precursor. That precursor may then be converted to thromboxane or to one of a variety of prostaglandins (Box 3–2).

■ Leukotrienes

Leukotrienes are synthesized from arachidonic acid by the action of the enzyme lipoxygenase. The leukotrienes consist of a family of chemicals that function to mediate chemotaxis, increase vascular permeability, and activate leukocytes.[33] Several different lipoxygenase enzymes have been discovered; however, 5-lipoxygenase appears to have the

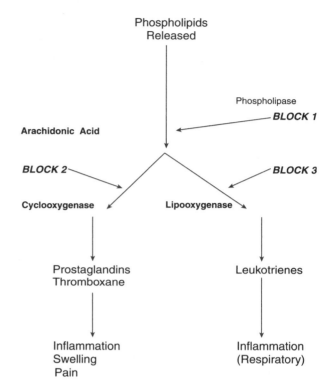

CELL MEMBRANE [DISTURBED/DAMAGED]

Figure 3–3. The eicosanoid cascade. Examples of blocking agents: (*1*).Corticosteroids block the metabolism of phospholipids to arachidonic acid; (*2*). NSAIDs (aspirin and celecoxib) block the metabolism of arachidonic acid into prostaglandins; 3. Lipooxygenase inhibitors (Singular) block the metabolism of arachidonic acid to reduce inflammation.

most clinical relevance as it catalyzes the production of leukotriene B4 (LTB4), leukotriene C4 (LTC4), leukotriene D4 (LTD4), and leukotriene E4 (LTE4). LTB4 is a potent chemoattractant for leukocytes and promotes the migration of neutrophils into the extravascular space.[68] LTC4, LTD4, and LTE4 make up the slow-reacting substances of anaphylaxis (SRS-A), which induce smooth-muscle constriction, particularly in bronchial tissue.

Early attempts at producing pharmacologic agents that block leukotriene production proved too nonspecific or toxic for therapeutic use.[33] The past decade has seen great strides in the development of safe and effective leukotriene inhibitors. Zileuton (Zyflo) acts as a direct 5-lipoxygenase inhibitor; zafirlukast (Accolate) and montelukast (Singulair) are leukotriene-receptor inhibitors. These drugs are indicated for the treatment of asthma and currently have no role as systemic anti-inflammatory medications.

BOX 3–2

Major Actions of the Eicosanoids

Prostaglandins

Mediation of inflammation
Capillary vasodilation
Sensitization of pain receptors
Fever mediation
Protection of gastric mucosa
Inhibition of gastric acid secretion
Uterine muscle contraction
Alteration of renal blood flow
Inhibition of platelet aggregation
Bronchoconstriction

Thromboxane

Promotion of platelet aggregation and release
Potent vasoconstriction

Leukotrienes

Chemoattractants for inflammatory cells
Leukocyte activation
Increased vascular permeability
Potent bronchoconstriction
Synthesis of the slow-reacting substances of anaphylaxis (SRS-A)

▒ Prostaglandins

The enzyme cyclooxygenase is responsible for the biosynthesis of arachidonic acid to prostaglandin H (PGH). From that point, PGH can be converted into numerous different prostaglandins, which are responsible for a variety of actions in almost every tissue of the body, playing various roles in a multitude of physiological processes. Thromboxane is also a product of PGH through the action of the enzyme thromboxane synthase. The relevant actions of these chemicals are examined in the following discussion.

A thorough review of the actions of the prostaglandins can be quite confusing because there are numerous subsets, many of which have antagonistic actions. These natural substances serve as a good reminder of the delicate balance in which the human body functions. As discussed later in this chapter, this delicate balance can be greatly affected by the administration of medications that block the production of these substances. The following discussion is focused on the important physiological properties of prostaglandins in the context of NSAID and corticosteroid use.

Mediation of Inflammatory Process

The term "mediation" is important in describing the inflammatory activities of prostaglandins. By themselves, prostaglandins do not appear to be capable of increasing vascular permeability, but prostaglandin E_2 (PGE_2) and prostaglandin I_2 (PGI_2) may increase edema and leukocyte migration through local capillary vasodilation. In addition, prostaglandins act synergistically with bradykinin and other autacoids to sensitize pain receptors to mechanical and chemical stimulation. Interestingly, PGE also exerts an anti-inflammatory effect by inhibiting the release of hydrolases and lysosomal enzymes from neutrophils.

Fever Mediation

Body temperature set point is regulated by the hypothalamus and can be influenced by a variety of conditions, including fever, inflammation, malignancy, and exercise. Prostaglandins have been implicated in the role of fever mediation. Cytokines increase the synthesis of PGE_2, which, through increases in cyclic adenosine monophosphate, triggers the hypothalamus to elevate body temperature. Supportive evidence for this action is found in animal studies, which have shown that injection of specific prostaglandins into the cerebral ventricles causes an increase in body temperature.[84]

Gastric Protection

Prostaglandins interact in a number of ways to protect the delicate lining of the gastrointestinal system. PGE and PGI inhibit gastric acid secretion and may have an anti-ulcer effect. Prostaglandins also appear to have the property of cytoprotection, defined as the ability to protect the gastric mucosa from exposure to harmful substances. This cytoprotection likely results when PGE stimulates gastric mucus formation. The PGE_1 analog misoprostol (Cytotec) suppresses gastric acid secretion and has been found to be effective in the prophylaxis of gastric ulcers in patients on NSAID regimens.[68] Arthrotec is a formulation of misoprostol (200 μg) combined with the NSAID diclofenac sodium (50 mg and 75 mg).

Reproductive System

In the uterus, prostaglandins act to stimulate the contraction of the smooth muscle layer, known as the myometrium. This smooth muscle contraction serves two important purposes.

During childbirth, prostaglandin-stimulated contractions of the myometrium aid in propelling the baby through the birth canal. They are also released at the end of the menstrual cycle to facilitate the shedding of the uterine lining through the stimulation of muscular contractions. These continuous contractions can result in ischemic pain, referred to as dysmenorrhea. Prostaglandins are also employed in "ripening" the cervix for the induction of delivery at term and as abortifacients that act to expel the fetus from the uterus for elective termination of pregnancy.

Renal Blood Flow

During exercise, the autonomic nervous system releases chemicals into the bloodstream that act as potent vasoconstrictors in many peripheral tissues, including the kidneys. Prostaglandins serve to dilate renal blood vessels, counteracting those chemicals and thus maintaining a constant flow of blood to the kidneys.[72] Through alterations in renal blood flow and direct effects on the renal tubules, prostaglandins also influence salt and water excretion. Prostaglandins likely also affect the release of renin, a substance released from the renal cortex in response to hypotension. The renal effects of the prostaglandins appear to be more significant in patients whose kidneys are functioning abnormally.[51]

Hemostasis

A specific prostaglandin, prostacyclin, is released by the internal lining of the blood vessels. This substance appears to inhibit the aggregation of platelets on blood vessel walls. Thromboxane, produced in platelets, functions as a powerful inducer of platelet aggregation to aid in the clotting mechanism.[33] Therefore, thromboxane and prostacyclin have an antagonistic relationship. This is a good example of how prostaglandins naturally attenuate the actions of other chemicals in a variety of tissues.

Pulmonary Effects

The smooth muscles of the bronchial tree are quite reactive to prostaglandins and leukotrienes. PGF and PGD_2 contract bronchial smooth muscle, whereas PGE causes it to relax. LTC4 and LTD4 are potent bronchoconstrictors and also stimulate mucus secretion and edema in the bronchi. These inflammatory effects are best illustrated by the pathogenesis of bronchial asthma.

*A*nti-Inflammatory Medications

Ever since the bark of willow trees was boiled to cure ague (fever) centuries ago, the power of anti-inflammatory medications has been appreciated. However, that power has long included a variety of adverse effects, with GI toxicity chief among them. From the creation of phenylbutazone in that late 1940s, through the synthesis of indomethacin in the 1960s, to the recent introduction of the selective COX-2 inhibitors, the goal has been to improve efficacy while limiting toxicity.

In the latter half of the 20th century, chemists used aspirin as a prototype to develop the group of drugs now known as NSAIDs. The main goal of this research was to produce agents that do not present aspirin's sometimes severe adverse effects, yet maintain its potent anti-inflammatory properties. Although there are differences in potency, specificity, and specific mechanisms of action, all NSAIDs inhibit the activity of cyclooxygenase in some manner.[30] This inhibition is not an irreversible reaction like that caused by aspirin, but is instead dependent on drug concentration.[74]

Along with blocking cyclooxygenase, NSAIDs are thought to have additional properties, including modulation of T-cell function, inhibition of inflammatory cell chemotaxis, lysosomal membrane stabilization, and free radical scavenging.[5,74] Although some NSAIDs offer theoretical pharmacologic advantages, no single agent appears to be superior to another in diseases such as rheumatoid arthritis or osteoarthritis.[37,94,98] However, efficacy can vary greatly among individuals. Therefore, if an individual does not respond to a specific NSAID within 1 to 2 weeks of initiating therapy, another agent should be started. Nonresponsiveness to one particular NSAID does not preclude response to another agent within the same class.

Due to recent changes in the area of anti-inflammatory drugs, we recommend students also consult an up-to-the-minute drug resource.

▨ Aspirin

Aspirin (acetylsalicylic acid) is a derivative of salicylic acid. Salicylic acid, in turn, is created from salicin, a substance found in the bark of willow trees. Both the medicinal benefits and adverse effects of willow bark have been known for more than 2000 years. Aspirin was first synthesized by a Bayer Company chemist in the late 19th century. It proved to be far less of a gastric irritant than salicylic acid and was introduced to the marketplace in the spring of 1899. Heralded as a wonder drug, it quickly became one of the most widely used pharmaceutical products in the world. Aspirin use has declined in recent years since the introduction of a number of newer anti-inflammatory agents. However, aspirin remains the standard against which these new medications are judged.

Surprisingly, aspirin's mechanism of action has only been known since 1971, when John Vane discovered that the aspirin molecule transfers a functional group onto the cyclooxygenase enzyme.[96] As a result, the enzyme is irreversibly inhibited and is unable to bind arachidonic acid. The enzyme can no longer convert arachidonic acid to prostaglandins and thromboxane. The leukotriene pathway, however, is unaffected.

■ Effects of Aspirin

After the ingestion of aspirin, typically 3000 to 6000 mg per day for anti-inflammatory action, a series of chemical events results from the blockage of cyclooxygenase. The decrease in prostaglandin production leads to a corresponding reduction in inflammation and edema. The inhibition of prostaglandin and thromboxane synthesis may not be the only effect that aspirin has on the tissues. In some systems aspirin may impinge on the formation of 12-HETE, a leukotriene derivative that acts as a chemotactic agent. Aspirin may also reduce inflammation and pain through its influence on the migration of chemical potentiators such as neutrophils and monocytes.[51]

Aspirin use may also produce negative consequences. In the gastrointestinal tract, aspirin can cause gastric upset, bleeding, and even ulcers. Various studies have shown an incidence of these symptoms in anywhere from 2 to 40 percent of patients, depending on the parameters of the investigation.[51] It does not appear that these gastrointestinal side effects are caused by the inhibition of prostaglandin synthesis alone, although this area is not without controversy.[51,74]

The mechanism of gastric irritation appears related to the direct effect of aspirin on the lining of the stomach.[61] Unbuffered aspirin lowers the electrical potential of the gastric membrane, which then affects the flow of hydrogen ions. Davenport's theory contends that this disruption of hydrogen ions triggers a series of events that leads to gastric erosion and bleeding.[51] Studies have shown that enteric-coated aspirin does not cause as many abnormalities in the stomach lining because of its buffering action.[51] Mild gastrointestinal upset can often be avoided if aspirin is taken with a meal because of the "buffering" action of the food.

Aspirin use may also result in complications such as prolonged bleeding time and tinnitus. Prolonged bleeding time results from the inhibition of thromboxane. Because aspirin irreversibly binds to cyclooxygenase, the decreased platelet function lasts from 4 to 6 days (the platelet life span) after aspirin intake.[74] In addition, many people taking high doses of aspirin develop a ringing in their ears. This condition, referred to as tinnitus, is probably caused by an effect on the inner ear rather than the central nervous system (CNS), and may be an indication of aspirin toxicity.

Because of the high incidence of GI and other adverse effects and the availability of safer, efficacious OTC medications such as acetaminophen, ibuprofen, and naproxen, aspirin use continues to diminish. Although it is certainly not as "trendy" as modern alternatives, in those who tolerate it, aspirin remains a potent and effective anti-inflammatory and analgesic agent.

■ Reye's Syndrome

First described in 1963, Reye's syndrome is a rare and potentially devastating acute illness that usually strikes children after a viral infection. For several years, epidemiological data suggested a relationship between Reye's syndrome and aspirin use by children infected with either the influenza or chickenpox virus. Despite the lack of firm scientific evidence, for more than 20 years medical professionals have warned against using aspirin in children with probable viral illnesses. Thus, we have seen a great rise in the use of ibuprofen and acetaminophen as antipyretics.

The incidence of Reye's syndrome has diminished dramatically over the past decades, although it has been suggested that this decline began before the decrease in the use of aspirin.[30] Although no definitive cause-and-effect relationship has been established, it appears prudent to disallow the use of aspirin and other salicylates by anyone under 18 years old who may have a viral infection.

Although the cause of Reye's syndrome is unknown, it is known that the illness impairs mitochondrial function, resulting in liver and neurological damage.[99] In 1974, Lovejoy et al. proposed a five-stage system on which to chart the symptoms of Reye's syndrome (Table 3–1). Reye's syndrome is a potentially fatal condition and the symptoms must be treated as a medical emergency; however, a diagnosis can be made only through various laboratory tests.

■ Aspirin-Sensitive Asthma

An unusual complication of aspirin use, aspirin-sensitive asthma may be associated with the development of vasomotor rhinitis and nasal polyps. On exposure to even small

Table 3–1

The Five Clinical Stages of Reye's Syndrome

Stage	Signs and Symptoms
1	Vomiting, lethargy, indifference
2	Delirium, combativeness, hyperventilation
3	Light coma, hypoventilation, intact pupillary response, decorticate posturing
4	Deep coma, apnea, decerebrate posturing, pupils fixed and dilated
5	Seizures, flaccidity

Adapted from Lovejoy.[63]

quantities of aspirin, affected people may develop nasal congestion and acute, often severe bronchospasm. The prevalence of this disorder is unknown. There is an almost universal cross-reactivity with other NSAIDs, particularly ibuprofen, indomethacin, fenoprofen, naproxen, and mefenamic acid. As yet there are no reports of sensitivity to the selective COX-2 inhibitors. The mechanism for this reaction has not been elucidated, but it may be related to the preferential shunting of arachidonic acid into the lipoxygenase pathway, resulting in the production of bronchoconstricting leukotrienes. Patients can be desensitized over time with daily administration of aspirin. Cross-tolerance to other NSAIDs usually occurs as well.

▌Acetaminophen

Although not an anti-inflammatory agent, acetaminophen (Tylenol) is an important drug and deserves our attention because of its clinical usefulness. Discovered in 1877, it has analgesic and antipyretic properties through its actions on the CNS. Acetaminophen has no anti-inflammatory properties because it cannot inhibit cyclooxygenase in the peripheral tissues.[77] As a result, it also does not present complications such as gastrointestinal disturbance or prolonged bleeding time. Therefore acetaminophen is indicated for mild pain and fever in people for whom aspirin is contraindicated because of Reye's syndrome risk (see previous text) or who cannot tolerate aspirin or NSAIDs. The usual dosage of acetaminophen is 325 to 650 mg at 4-hour intervals.

Acetaminophen can be toxic if abused. The minimum toxic dose in adults is 5 to 15 g.[28] Overdoses or prolonged overuse (5–8 g per day for several days) may result in severe hepatic damage or death.[5] The liver damage appears to be produced by a metabolite of acetaminophen. In therapeutic doses, the toxic metabolite is detoxified by glutathione; however, with extreme intake, if the glutathione drops below 30 percent of normal values, tissue necrosis occurs.[28]

*N*SAIDs

▌COX-2 Inhibitors

A major breakthrough in NSAID development began in the early 1990s with the discovery of two separate cyclooxygenase (COX) isoenzymes. Initially it was believed that COX-1 was a "housekeeping" protein, and that COX-2 was expressed only at sites of inflammation.[12] Although this theory does not completely reflect physiological reality, it is illustrative for the purposes of our discussion. COX-1 is primarily present in the platelets, where it regulates vascular homeostasis, and in the endothelial cells of the GI tract, where it regulates gastric cytoprotection. COX-2 is primarily induced at sites of inflammation by cytokines, endotoxins, growth factors, and other substances.[23] COX-2 is also expressed in some brain and renal tissue. Among the many anti-inflammatory effects of corticosteroids is the inhibition of COX-2 expression (see discussion in the following paragraphs).

The discovery of COX-2 and its expression primarily in inflammatory tissues raised the possibility of creating a selective COX-2 inhibitor that could block the production of proinflammatory prostaglandins without interfering with gastric protection or platelet activity. The COX-1 and COX-2 isoenzymes differ by only a single amino acid.[36] The smaller valine residue in COX-2 allows an inhibitor to bind and prevent the conversion of arachidonic acid to prostaglandin. Many NSAIDs demonstrate preferential inhibition for COX-2 in vitro, including piroxicam, indomethacin, nabumetone, meloxicam, and etodolac. Actual clinical activity cannot be predicted from these laboratory assays, but the latter three agents have been found to have fewer GI side-effects than other NSAIDs.[36,66]

The selective COX-2 inhibitors currently available are celecoxib, rofecoxib, and valdecoxib, and more will certainly follow. Although the new drugs have not proven more effective than the less expensive, less selective agents, they have apparently fulfilled their promise of limiting GI toxicity. One early study found rofecoxib to have a lower ulcer-producing rate than either ibuprofen or placebo.[56] Other large double-blind studies found similar results with both rofecoxib and celecoxib.[13,85,87] The COX-2 inhibitors probably have renal adverse effects similar to those of the nonselective NSAIDs, but data are limited.

Additional uses for these drugs may be indicated pending future research. Celecoxib is currently approved for the reduction of adenomatous colorectal polyps in familial adenomatous polyposis.[12] The expression of COX-2 has been found to be upgraded by tumor promoters as well as inflammatory mediators.[83] Therefore, there may be a role for COX-2 inhibitors in the prevention or suppression of colon cancer, which is often characterized by COX-2 expression.[49] Epidemiologic data also suggest delayed expression or progression of Alzheimer's disease with NSAID use; studies show increased COX-2 expression and inflammation in the brain related to Alzheimer's.[64,73]

Benefiting from positive early studies and aggressive marketing campaigns, celecoxib and rofecoxib have become quite popular. In 2001, 24.5 million prescriptions were filled for celecoxib and 23.7 million for rofecoxib, making them the 10th and 13th best-selling drugs in the United States, and generating $3.1 billion and $2.6 billion, respectively.[78] However, recent reports in both the medical literature and lay press have not been complimentary. In 2002, a scathing editorial in the *British Medical Journal*[48] and an article in the *Washington Post*[78] both echoed questions that had already been raised regarding the veracity of a celecoxib trial known as the CLASS study.[85] The editorial termed the study "overoptimistic short-term data" and called the authors' data "misleading," alleging that the authors omitted disappointing long-term data.

Today there continues to be much debate in the medical community regarding the COX-2 inhibitors. Rofecoxib use was found to increase the risk for myocardial infarction by 300 percent in one large comparison study[13] and has recently been associated with aseptic meningitis.[14] Apart from these apparent concerns, many are troubled by the high cost of these medications as compared to that of generic NSAIDs (Table 3–2). Only further research and longer-term use will sort out many of these confusing implications of COX-2 use. For the time being, their use should be restricted to those who have failed to achieve good results with multiple other NSAID classes, or who are at high risk for GI complications (Box 3–3).

■ Topical NSAIDs

As previously mentioned, the focus of COX-2 inhibitor development has been to improve or maintain NSAID efficacy while limiting potentially harmful or intolerable side effects. Topical application of NSAIDs is an alternative method of administration. It delivers the drug to the desired location while avoiding high systemic concentrations and drug interactions. Drug blood levels are less than 10 percent of those achieved after oral administration, but are present in muscle and subcutaneous tissue.[24] The most commonly encountered adverse effect is a local rash.[41] Data also suggest that there are fewer renal and GI effects.[24,25,41]

Many studies have found objective and subjective improvements in patient symptoms with topical NSAID use.[1,2,31,80,90] The majority of these investigations have compared a single agent with a placebo.[1,31,80,90] Interestingly, a number of researchers have found that, although patients subjectively report improved symptoms, physician evaluations of their responses showed no significant change. These findings imply that there may be some benefit to the use of topical NSAIDs during the rehabilitation process because the injured individual perceives less pain and disability.

In a quantitative systemic review, Moore et al.[67] concluded that topical NSAIDs are effective in alleviating acute soft-tissue injury pain with adverse effects similar to those of placebo. Currently, there are no commercially marketed formulations of topical NSAIDs available for retail sale. However, a number of agents have been studied and may be compounded by a licensed pharmacist. Studies have looked at the use of topical formulations of naproxen, piroxicam, ketoprofen, indomethacin, diclofenac, and ibuprofen.

The initial research appears promising, and more data will certainly follow. The limited adverse effect profile of

Table 3–2

Comparative Costs of a 15-Day Course for a Few Selected Drugs

Drug	Dosage*	Cost ($)†
Celebrex (celecoxib)	200 mg twice per day	76.95
Daypro (oxaprozin)	1200 mg once per day	128.99
Ibuprofen	800 mg four times per day	9.49
Indomethacin	50 mg three times per day	15.99
Naprosyn	500 mg twice per day	53.50
Relafen (nabumetone)	1500 mg once per day	55.99
Vioxx (rofecoxib)	50 mg once per day	60.50

*Dosages given are for maximum anti-inflammatory effect.
†Prices from *http://www.walgreens.com*, accessed April 2004.

Possible Adverse Reactions to NSAIDs

Gastrointestinal

Nausea, vomiting, dyspepsia

Diarrhea, constipation

Gastric mucosal irritation, superficial erosions, peptic ulceration

Increased fecal blood wasting

Major GI hemorrhage

Penetrating ulcers

Small-bowel erosions, "diaphragm" development in small bowel

Hepatic

Hepatotoxicity, hepatitis, fulminant hepatic failure

Renal

Glomerulopathy

Interstitial nephritis

Alterations in renal plasma flow leading to fall in glomerular filtration rates

Interference with diuretic-induced natriuresis

Inhibition of renin release

Edema

Central Nervous System

Headaches

Confusion, hallucinations, depersonalization reactions, depression

Tremor

Aseptic meningitis, tinnitus, vertigo

Hematological

Anemia, bone marrow depression, Coombs-positive anemia, decreased platelet aggregation

Hypersensitivity

Asthma, asthma/urticaria syndrome, urticaria, rashes

Photosensitivity, Stevens-Johnson syndrome

Adapted from Polisson, R: Nonsteroidal anti-inflammatory drugs: Practical and theoretical considerations in their selection. Am J Med. 100 (Suppl2A): 31S–36S, 1996.

Overview of Selected NSAIDs

Dozens of NSAIDs from several different chemical classifications are currently available by prescription in the United States (Table 3–3). Even more are marketed in Europe and Asia. New agents from well-established classifications, reformulations of older drugs, and completely new classes of NSAIDs enter the market on a regular basis. The constant innovation and development of new products seen in NSAID research are a testament to the popularity of the medications and demonstrate that those agents currently available are far from perfect in efficacy and potential adverse effects.

The following section provides a brief overview of a handful of OTC and prescription NSAIDs. These agents have been chosen for discussion based on historical relevance, widespread use, unique clinical aspects, or a combination of all three. There are a number of factors the physician must consider when choosing an NSAID for use by the athlete. An overview of the major factors to consider is listed in Box 3–4. For an exhaustive review of all available NSAIDs the reader is referred to any current pharmacology textbook.

Ibuprofen (Advil, Motrin, Nuprin)

A propionic acid derivative, ibuprofen is the most frequently used NSAID.[6] Introduced to the OTC market in 1985, it is available in 200 to 800 mg tablets by prescription, and 200 mg tablets OTC. Chewable tablets and liquid formulations are also available. It boasts aspirin's potency for analgesic and anti-inflammatory action, but has a lower incidence of side effects. This reduced incidence may be a result of ibuprofen's decreased inhibition of platelet aggregation, which lessens possible gastric bleeding.[84] Ibuprofen is among the most beneficial NSAIDs in easing the pain of primary dysmenorrhea, for which it is effective at doses of 400 mg every 6 hours. It is also frequently used as an antipyretic in adults and children because its longer duration of action makes it a popular alternative to acetaminophen.

Peak plasma levels are achieved within 15 to 30 minutes of ingestion.[30] This rapid onset of action can be quite beneficial for quick relief of pain. However, with a half-life of about 2 hours, ibuprofen must be taken every 6 to 8 hours to maintain effect. An anti-inflammatory regimen requires 2400 to 3200 mg daily, taken in three separate doses. This dosing scheme allows it to be taken at mealtimes, lessening the likelihood of gastric irritation. Sufficient analgesia should be achieved by daily dosages of less than 2400 mg per day. Daily dosage should not exceed 3200 mg. Although ibuprofen is better tolerated than aspirin and indomethacin, approximately 10 to 15 percent of individuals must discon-

these agents is certainly appealing. However, their effects on the initial stages of healing, and their efficacy in certain conditions (bursitis versus tendinitis, acute versus chronic injury) need to be further delineated. The next several years will likely see an explosion in the research and marketing of topical NSAIDs.

Table 3–3

Currently Available NSAIDs, Excluding Aspirin Derivatives

Propionic Acid Derivatives

Fenoprofen calcium (Nalfon)

Flurbiprofen (Ansaid)

Ibuprofen (Motrin, Advil, others)

Ketoprofen (Orudis, Oruvail)

Naproxen (Naprelan, Naprosyn)

Naproxen sodium (Aleve, Anaprox, Anaprox DS)

Oxaprozin (Daypro)

Indoles

Indomethacin (Indocin, Indocin SR)

Sulindac (Clinoril)

Tolmetin sodium (Tolectin, Tolectin DS)

Phenylacetic Acids

Diclofenac sodium (Voltaren, Voltaren XR)

Diclofenac potassium (Cataflam)

Diclofenac sodium/misoprostol (Arthrotec)

Naphthylalkanones

Nabumetone (Relafen)

Oxicams

Piroxicam (Feldene)

Meloxicam (Mobic)

Pyrrolo-pyrrole

Ketorolac tromethamine (Toradol)

Pyranocarboxylic Acid

Etodolac (Lodine, Lodine XL)

Selective COX-2 Inhibitors

Celecoxib (Celebrex)

Rofecoxib (Vioxx)

Valdecoxib (Bextra)

Fenamates

Mefenamic acid (Ponstel)

Meclofenamate sodium (Meclomen)

BOX 3–4

Factors to Consider in Choosing an NSAID

Age of Patient

■ Patients over 60 years of age at increased risk for GI toxicity.

■ Few studies have been conducted on NSAID safety in children. Ibuprofen and naproxen are most often used in this population. There has been some use of indomethacin and sulindac in juvenile rheumatoid arthritis.

Duration of Treatment

■ If long-term use is planned, safety and cost must be balanced and dosing schedule must be considered.

■ Duration of treatment longer than 3 months increases risk of GI toxicity, therefore, medications with superior safety profiles must be considered.

Time of Onset

■ Drugs with shorter half-lives, such as ibuprofen, reach peak plasma levels much sooner than long-acting agents. Therefore, if quick pain-relief is desired, short-acting agents should be used.

Compliance

■ Limited adverse-effect profile, efficacy, and once- or twice-daily dosing all contribute to patient compliance with a medication regimen.

Other Medications

■ All other medications that a patient is taking must be considered (See Table 3–4)

General Health of the Patient

■ The risk of adverse reactions increases greatly with concomitant disease states, particular GI or renal disease.

Cost of Treatment

■ Many factors must be considered in cost because GI bleeding quickly raises the cost of treatment for any patient.

tinue use because of GI symptoms.[30] It should be noted that a large meta-analysis found ibuprofen to have the lowest risk of adverse effects among all nonselective NSAIDs.[27] Additional adverse effects, which are quite rare, include headaches, rash, blurry vision, and thrombocytopenia.

Naproxen (Naprosyn, Aleve)

Also a propionic acid derivative, naproxen is chemically similar to ibuprofen.[30] In one comparison study with ibuprofen, naproxen was found to be marginally superior in decreasing joint inflammation.[71] The sodium salt of naproxen is available as the OTC preparation Aleve, and as Anaprox by prescription. Naproxen sodium is more

Table 3–4

NSAID Drug-Drug Interactions

Drug	Common Use	Interaction
ACE inhibitors	Treatment of hypertension	Decreased renal perfusion
Aminoglycosides	Antibiotics	Decreased renal function
Antacids	Treatment of dyspepsia	Reduced NSAID absorption
Anticoagulants	Prophylaxis/treatment of clotting disorders	Effect prolonged, increased risk of GI bleeding
Barbiturates	Sedation, anxiety disorders	Accelerated NSAID metabolism
Beta-blockers	Treatment of hypertension	Diminished treatment effect
Hypoglycemic agents	Treatment of Type 2 diabetes	Increased hypoglycemic activity
Lithium	Treatment of bipolar disorder	Decreased renal excretion
Phenytoin and valproic acid	Anti-epileptic drugs (AEDs)	Diminished AED metabolism
Potassium-sparing diuretics	Treatment of hypertension	Increased risk of hyperkalemia

readily concentrated in the synovium than naproxen, and therefore may be more efficacious for joint pain and inflammation.[3]

Because of naproxen's long half-life (approximately 12 hours), the daily recommended dosage of 750 to 1000 mg can be taken on a twice-daily schedule. This tends to reduce gastric upset caused by the lesser number of exposures and improves compliance. Peak plasma levels are achieved within 2 to 4 hours.[30] An extended-release formulation (Naprelan) is now available for once daily dosing and is also effective for migraine headache prophylaxis in some individuals.

Naproxen is 20 percent more potent than aspirin with an adverse-effect profile similar to ibuprofen's.[84] Although naproxen is better tolerated from a GI standpoint than indomethacin, the incidence of upper GI bleeding in OTC use is double that of OTC ibuprofen.[30] A dose effect may be the cause of this aberration. Naproxen is eliminated from the body mainly by way of the kidneys. Therefore, like all NSAIDS, it should be used with caution in persons with renal complications.

Indomethacin (Indocin)

Introduced in 1963, indomethacin (an indole derivative) was one of the first NSAIDs developed and continues to be among the most powerful inhibitors of cyclooxygenase.[54] It may also owe its potency to the additional activities of phospholipase A inhibition, reduced migration of PMNs, and decreased proliferation of T and B cells.[30] Although particularly effective in maladies such as rheumatoid arthritis, ankylosing spondylitis, and gout, indomethacin is typically not recommended for use as a simple analgesic or antipyretic because of potentially severe adverse effects.[5] Up to half of people using indomethacin may experience some adverse effects, and almost one-third will discontinue use. Common adverse effects include gastrointestinal symptoms (ulceration, nausea, abdominal pain) and headaches (15 to 25% of patients).[5]

Peak concentrations can be achieved in 1 to 2 hours (in fasting subjects, onset is delayed by food intake) with a half-life of approximately 2.5 hours.[30] Daily dosage ranges from 75 to 100 mg taken in 3 or 4 doses. Prolonged-release formulations are available (75 mg 1 to 2 times per day); however, gastrointestinal and other adverse effects appear to be similar to those seen with the regular formulation.[5]

Indomethacin's use has declined as newer agents with a lower side effect profile have emerged. However, with almost 40 years of evidence-based efficacy in the clinical setting, it remains a popular choice in certain situations. Nonorthopedic uses of indomethacin include suppression of uterine contractions to prevent delivery during preterm labor and intravenous administration in neonates to induce closure of a patent ductus arteriosus.

Phenylbutazone

The significance of phenylbutazone, formerly marketed under the trade name Butazolidin, is now historical rather than clinical. Introduced in 1949, it was widely used for decades, but decreased in popularity with the development of less toxic NSAIDs. Long-term use of phenylbutazone increased the incidence of various blood dyscrasias, including aplastic anemia, and severe hepatic reactions.[74]

Nabumetone (Relafen)

The only nonacid NSAID currently available, nabumetone is converted to an active acetic acid derivative in the liver. The prodrug resembles naproxen in structure. It can be given once a day because the half-life is more than 24 hours. Dosage varies from 1000 mg to 2000 mg per day. The incidence of GI ulceration does appear to be lower with nabumetone than with the other nonselective NSAIDs.[69] As a nonacid prodrug, it produces no local irritation of the gastric mucosa. It also does not undergo enterohepatic recirculation, which may improve its GI profile. Adverse effects may include diarrhea, rash, and heartburn.

Rofecoxib (Vioxx)

A furanose derivative, rofecoxib was introduced in 1999 and is one of only three potent and highly selective COX-2 inhibitors available. It does not inhibit COX-1 and has no effect on platelet function. It is FDA approved for the treatment of osteoarthritis, dysmenorrhea, and acute pain at dosages ranging from 12.5 mg to 50 mg. It is administered once daily because of its nearly 17-hour half-life. Long-term toxic effects, including GI and renal effects, are not yet known because of the drug's relatively recent introduction. Please see the section on COX-2 inhibitors for further discussion on rofecoxib and similar agents.

Ketorolac (Toradol)

Although it is not typically employed for its anti-inflammatory properties, ketorolac, an acetic acid derivative, deserves special mention. It is the only NSAID available for intramuscular or intravenous injection as well as oral administration. Although it also has anti-inflammatory and antipyretic properties, it is most commonly marketed and used as an analgesic, particularly in postoperative patients. As an analgesic, ketorolac offers great promise because it avoids the most common shortcomings of opioids, (i.e., tolerance, withdrawal effects, and respiratory depression). Interestingly, Tokish et al[92] recently reported that 28 of 30 National Football League team medical staffs commonly use ketorolac intramuscular injections on game days for pain relief.

Studies have shown ketorolac to be equal to, or more effective than, opioids in the treatment of postoperative pain.[6,8] Dosages range from 15 to 60 mg and peak plasma concentrations are reached within 30 to 50 minutes. Ketorolac may also be used as a therapeutic adjunct to opioids, allowing for a decrease in opioid requirement. When ketorolac is administered intramuscularly, damage to the gastrointestinal mucosa may still occur. However, doses of 10 to 30 mg given 5 times per day produced less mucosal injury than 650 mg of aspirin given on the same dosage schedule.[5]

Ketorolac use has been linked to acute renal failure in a small number of published reports,[92] but few large studies have been conducted on ketorolac's renal effects. Feldman et al. found a similar incidence (1.1%) of acute renal failure in patients treated with either ketorolac or opioids. However, ketorolac treatment longer than 5 days in duration did show an increased risk of renal failure.[29] Thus, in clinical practice, duration of ketorolac treatment is typically held to less than 5 days. An additional study found ketorolac users to have a higher rate of upper GI bleeding than users of other NSAIDs.[32]

■ NSAID Indications

NSAIDs are commonly used in the treatment of many afflictions, including but not limited to rheumatoid arthritis, spondyloarthropathies, juvenile rheumatoid arthritis, osteoarthritis, gout, and a variety of acute and chronic musculoskeletal injuries (sprains, strains, tendonitis, bursitis). Although our discussion has centered on sports-related use, the majority of research regarding the efficacy of NSAIDs has been conducted on patients with rheumatoid arthritis or osteoarthritis. As mentioned previously, no single NSAID has been found to be superior in the treatment of either condition.[37,94,98]

Given that no one agent has been found superior in a large number of clinical trials involving rheumatoid arthritis or osteoarthritis, we can be assured that no data exist guiding specific NSAID therapy in acute or chronic musculoskeletal conditions. In fact, as we will discuss further, little evidence supports the use of *any* NSAID for *any* injury. Because no one agent is superior to another, the criteria listed in Box 3–4 must be considered when deciding on appropriate NSAID therapy. Cost must also be considered because there is a tenfold difference in price between some agents (see Table 3–2).

Despite decades of widespread use of NSAIDs, some research over the past decade has cast uncertainty on the empiric use of NSAIDs in sports medicine practice. Several studies have concluded that NSAIDs may have the effect of slowing the healing process. In a study conducted by culturing rabbit articular cartilage chondrocytes in the presence of certain NSAIDs, diclofenac and indomethacin (and piroxicam to a lesser degree) inhibited the secretion of proteoglycans.[20] Proteoglycans are extracellular molecules involved in the formation of cartilage, tendons, and ligaments, and are vital to the process of tissue repair. Other studies have shown that indomethacin and aspirin can interfere with the synthesis or transport of connective tissues components.[9,22,39] One recent animal study suggests that the new COX-2 inhibitors may actually delay fracture healing.[86]

A review of studies conducted in the clinical setting is largely inconclusive when looking for direction in NSAID use. Reynolds found worse outcomes at 7 days after injury in patients treated with NSAIDs.[79] DuPont et al. found some positive subjective trends, but no significant efficacy in the treatment of ankle sprains.[26] These results are similar to those of many other studies, including LaBelle et al., which found no evidence to support the use of NSAIDs or corticosteroids in the treatment of lateral epicondylitis.[55] A paucity of randomized studies exist regarding NSAID treatment of chronic conditions such as tendonitis and bursitis. However, few studies point to significant delays in healing or return to competition in NSAID-treated groups.

The decision to use NSAIDs should not be a reflexive one. Although their lack of proven scientific efficacy may discourage some clinicians, NSAIDs are still widely prescribed in sports medicine practice. On an individual basis, they may have positive effects in "cooling down" chronic inflammation, diminishing pain and inflammation associated with chronic injury, or potentially aiding in the rehabilitation of acute injuries through the same means. In reviewing the mechanism of chronic, or "sports-induced," inflammation, one can postulate that NSAIDs (or corticosteroids) may diminish the inflammatory process enough to allow for the resolution of the normal tissue healing process.

Implications for Activity

The athletic trainer should not use NSAIDs impulsively for all athletic injuries. The efficacy of NSAIDs remains a topic of research, and the athletic trainer should remember that there are valid arguments on both sides of the research question. However, NSAIDs are still widely prescribed in sports medicine practice. It may be that the use of NSAIDs provides a period of time during which the body can rest and recuperate while maintaining some movement, which allows the injured tissues to be remodeled in the appropriate fashion. The athletic trainer must be concerned if an athlete continues to use NSAIDs after the healing process should have been complete.

It is unlikely that definitive data will ever emerge on the exact effect of NSAIDs in musculoskeletal injuries. Variations in type and degree of tissue trauma, individual responses, and study outcomes are all difficult to quan-

tify. More importantly, long-term outcome data may be quite misleading because nearly all musculoskeletal injuries eventually resolve without treatment. In fact, one argument against the use of NSAIDs is the self-limiting nature of such injuries. However, for competitive athletes, a difference of 1 or 2 days in return from an injury may be crucial.

Controversy also exists regarding when an NSAID regimen should begin after an acute injury. Some clinicians initiate drug therapy immediately, along with rest, ice, compression, and elevation (RICE), in an attempt to arrest the inflammatory process. Others believe that NSAID therapy should begin no sooner than 48 hours after injury and implementation of RICE.[91] Experts advising against NSAID treatment are concerned that the inhibition of thromboxane production will promote additional bleeding and that early NSAID use may diminish the inflammatory response and delay healing. Evidence on either side of the argument is largely anecdotal and based on clinical experience.

Certainly the inflammatory process is important to the resolution of any injury because it represents the first phase of tissue healing. Thus, NSAIDs must be used judiciously and only in situations in which the presumed benefits outweigh potential risks. This author's current practice is to recommend against the use of NSAIDs in the first 48 hours after acute injury. After that, they are prescribed for use only on an as-needed basis for minor pain and discomfort. Depending on the degree of pain, acetaminophen or prescription-strength analgesics may be helpful. Ibuprofen is typically recommended because it is relatively inexpensive, efficacious, and safe and has a rapid onset of action. In chronic inflammatory conditions, naproxen sodium is recommended twice daily for 10 to 14 days to alleviate pain and break the inflammatory cycle.

■ Adverse Effects

A number of complications and adverse effects of NSAID therapy have been alluded to throughout this chapter, particularly in the section on the new COX-2 inhibitors. Numerous NSAID adverse effects have been reported (see Box 3–3). However, the majority of complications arise in the GI tract and the renal parenchyma. NSAID use may occasionally result in elevation of liver enzymes, but hepatotoxicity is rare. Please refer to the discussion of aspirin-sensitive asthma for pulmonary complications.

It has been estimated that 50 percent of patients on NSAID therapy experience some form of reaction, and 1 to 2 percent of these reactions may be serious.[59] The first week

---

BOX 3–5

*Patient Risk Factors that May Increase the
Likelihood of GI Toxicity with NSAID Use*

Age greater than 60 years

Higher NSAID dose, or use of more than one NSAID
  at a time

Concomitant use of a corticosteroid

NSAID use longer than 3 months

History of peptic ulcer disease

Cigarette use

Alcohol use

---

of therapy with any new NSAID is quite important because most patients who do not tolerate a new agent will develop intolerance during this time frame. Age is also an important factor because only 10 percent of complications occur in patients under 40 years old.[11]

GI toxicity is the most frequently encountered NSAID complication. Up to 20 percent of patients have some GI symptoms and 1 to 2 percent may develop peptic ulcer disease. Shockingly, Hollander reported that 33 to 50 percent of all patients who die of ulcer-related complications have recently ingested NSAIDs.[43] NSAID-related ulceration may be asymptomatic, particularly in older patients, which may increase their risk of serious complications once bleeding develops. Risk factors for GI complications are listed in Box 3–5. The pathogenesis of GI irritation and prophylaxis for NSAID gastropathy are discussed elsewhere in this chapter. Prophylactic use of H2 blockers such as Zantac, Pepcid, Axid, and Tagamet has not been shown to reduce NSAID-related GI ulceration.[59]

Patients with preexisting renal disease are at particular risk for renal toxicity related to NSAID use. Prostaglandins are more critical to the maintenance of renal blood flow in diseased kidneys. Therefore inhibition of prostaglandin production may have deleterious effects on renal blood flow and function. These effects may result in hypertension, edema, exacerbation of congestive heart failure, and reduced renal function. There are many case reports of acute and chronic renal failure, interstitial nephritis, papillary necrosis, proteinuria, and other renal effects.[19] Avoidance of renal toxicity is best carried out by careful patient selection, by limiting dosages, and by carefully following blood pressure and renal function in at-risk individuals.

Implications for Activity

When an athlete is given an NSAID such as aspirin, the athletic trainer should remind the athlete of the possibility of gastrointestinal toxicity as a complication. Typically, athletes will try to play through the adverse effects that are sometimes produced by NSAID use. Signs and symptoms of GI toxicity can include severe stomachache (especially when the stomach is empty), diarrhea, nausea, vomiting, unexpected weight loss, and darkened stools. If the athlete is having problems with any of these signs and symptoms, he or she needs to speak to a physician. The physician may encourage the athlete to have food in the stomach before taking NSAIDs or may even change the type of medication being prescribed.

■ Drug Interactions

A number of drug interactions may occur in patients taking other medications in addition to NSAIDs (see Table 3–2). Fortunately, in a young, athletic population, multiple disease states are rare, and such interactions are typically not of concern. However, the practicing athletic trainer should be aware of such possibilities. Most NSAIDs are extensively bound to plasma proteins and compete for binding sites with other protein-bound medications, resulting in higher drug levels and increased risk of toxicity. Such drugs include the anticoagulant warfarin, oral hypoglycemic agents, digoxin, and antihypertensives.[15,17,95]

Specifically in the kidneys, NSAIDs may reduce the clearance of methotrexate and inhibit lithium excretion. As discussed previously, GI and renal toxicity are particular concerns in NSAID use. Concomitant use of anticoagulants, aspirin, high-dose corticosteroids, or alcohol increases the risk of serious GI pathology.[40] Particular caution must be given to patients on antihypertensive therapy because NSAIDs may diminish their effectiveness. ACE inhibitors, which diminish renal perfusion, may also interact poorly with NSAIDs.

Web Resource

Potential risks of herbal anti-inflammatory medications is the subject of a bulletin by the American Academy of Orthopedic Surgeons.
http://www.aaos.org/

What to Tell the Athlete

Some athletes will not understand which types of OTC drugs produce anti-inflammatory effects and will thus be using products that do not work but still produce adverse effects. It is important for the athletic trainer to be able to discuss with the athlete the types of OTC drugs the athlete may select to gain an anti-inflammatory effect.

The athletic trainer should make the following points when educating the athlete about these drugs:

■ Taking anti-inflammatories with meals can reduce adverse GI effects.

■ There appear to be differences in the potential for adverse effects between OTC and prescription anti-inflammatory medications. These adverse effects need to be communicated to the athlete.

■ To produce maximum effectiveness, anti-inflammatory medications must be taken as prescribed.

■ The overall effects of OTC and prescription anti-inflammatory medications on the inflammatory process are very similar.

■ For the athlete on a budget, a more expensive prescription drug may not be worth the extra cost in controlling a short-term inflammatory reaction.

*G*lucocorticosteroids

■ History

In 1849, Addison first described the importance of the adrenal glands, detailing fatal outcomes in patients with adrenal destruction. Over the next century, Brown-Sequard, Cushing, and others further elucidated the importance of the adrenal glands, their products, and their interactions with the pituitary gland and hypothalamus. With the synthesis of cortisone (compound E) in the late 1940s, the stage was set for the use of corticosteroids as therapeutic agents. Hench and colleagues showed dramatic effects in the treatment of rheumatoid arthritis in 1949.[38]

The practice of injecting anti-inflammatory medications directly into inflamed joints began in 1951 when hydrocortisone acetate crystal suspension became available for trials.[57] In the early 1950s Hollander[44–46] reported in multiple publications his experience of nearly 8000 intra-articular injections. Over the past 50 years the use of many synthetic analogs of adrenal corticosteroids has become essential. However, the role for corticosteroids in the treatment of sports-related musculoskeletal injuries remains unclear.

■ Physiology of Adrenal Corticosteroids

The adrenal glands lie above the kidneys in the retroperitoneum and are essential to the normal function of the human body. The production of adrenal corticosteroids is influenced by the pituitary gland and the hypothalamus. Many of these hormones are released cyclically throughout the day, and times of emotional or physical stress may trigger increased production and release. Each gland consists of two areas: the medulla and the cortex. Epinephrine (adrenaline) and norepinephrine are the main products of the medulla. The cortex is further subdivided into three zones, each producing distinct steroidal hormones. Mineralocorticoids are produced in the *zona glomerulosa.* Their primary function is to maintain the proper balance of electrolytes (chiefly sodium) in the body. The *zona reticularis* is the site of androgen production. Androgens are the precursors of male and female sex hormones and the analogs of anabolic steroids.

Glucocorticoids are products of the *zona fasciculata* and have a multiplicity of actions, because receptor proteins for these hormones are found throughout the body. Although glucocorticoids influence glucose concentration, protein metabolism, epinephrine release, gastric acid secretion, and kidney function, among other actions, our discussion

---

BOX 3–6

Actions of Corticosteroids.

Inflammatory Cycle

Inhibition of phospholipase

Decrease in cytokine expression

Induction of T-lymphocyte death

Mast cell and neutrophil stabilization

Inhibition of COX-2 induction

Inhibition of chemotactic agents

Inhibition of white blood cell migration

Tissue Repair

Inhibition of protein synthesis

Inhibition of fibroblast proliferation

Inhibition of collagen synthesis

centers on their anti-inflammatory actions. The exact mechanisms are not completely understood, but the anti-inflammatory effects of glucocorticoids are thought to result from a variety of intracellular actions (Box 3–6).

Phospholipase is directly inhibited, limiting the availability of inflammatory substrates for both the cyclooxygenase and lipoxygenase enzyme pathways. Evidence also supports the hypothesis that glucocorticosteroids regulate the expression of the COX-2 isoenzyme, thus limiting the production of prostaglandins at two distinct steps in the pathway. Many studies have shown that glucocorticosteroids greatly inhibit the migration of white blood cells to areas of injury, thus greatly limiting the migration of other pro-inflammatory substances to the area. The expression of cytokines such as IL-1 and TNF is also greatly limited. Finally, the enhanced stabilization of cell membranes diminishes capillary permeability and prevents the release of lysosomal enzymes. This effect includes the stabilization of neutrophil membranes, inhibiting their release of inflammatory mediators.

In an animal study by Beiner et al., the potent anti-inflammatory actions of glucocorticosteroids and their subsequent effects on healing were confirmed. They found that, when used to treat muscle contusions, glucocorticosteroids induced an early, transient recovery of the force-generating capacity of the affected muscle. However, long-term findings revealed irreversible damage to the healing muscle, including atrophy and diminished force-generating capacity. It is speculated that such damage results from the initial inhibition of a typical inflammatory response to injury. The attenuated inflammatory response was confirmed by a relative paucity of inflammatory cells seen in the tissue. This study underscores the importance of the inflammatory response in tissue healing.[10]

■ Current Use of Corticosteroids in Sports Medicine

Despite a half-century of use, the efficacy of corticosteroids in the treatment of acute and chronic musculoskeletal injuries is not truly known. In their 1998 review article, Stanley and Weaver state that "inconsistency in the studies on glucocorticosteroid use does not lend adequate support or direction to the sports medicine clinician in their use."[89] A more accurate observation could not have been made. A review of the available literature on corticosteroid use certainly leaves one a bit confused regarding their overall role in the treatment of sports injuries.

Why is there not a better body of literature to give us better insight into the use of these powerful medicines? There are actually several reasons for the lack of good, consistent data. There is no reproducible animal model for "overuse" musculoskeletal injuries. In most animal studies that have been conducted, the animals were relatively healthy. Even if good animal models existed, the application of these results to humans would not always be appropriate. Also, in human subjects, an exact diagnosis is not always possible. The degree to which bursitis, tendonitis, and tenosynovitis each contribute to pain in a certain area may be difficult to quantify without radiographic imaging or tissue diagnosis, thus making it difficult to determine which condition is actually being treated.

Much of the early successful experience with corticosteroids was in the treatment of rheumatoid arthritis. This success led to their use in a variety of other inflammatory conditions, as well as musculoskeletal injuries and osteoarthritis. These medications can be delivered to the desired tissue in a variety of ways. The oral administration of corticosteroids has been used to treat numerous systemic illnesses, such as asthma and juvenile rheumatoid arthritis. Although this route is effective at attenuating the inflammatory process, it also raises the risk of complications, which may include GI bleeding, fluid retention, adrenal insufficiency, and behavioral changes.[82]

If a more direct route to the needed site of action exists, this is preferable because it avoids the more potent adverse effects. Thus, the development of inhaled anti-inflammatory medications in the treatment of asthma has been a major advance. Orally administered corticosteroids currently have no clinically proven role in the treatment of acute or chronic musculoskeletal injuries. Phonophoresis and iontophoresis are two novel approaches to the administration of anti-inflammatory medication. These involve the use of therapeutic ultrasound or electrical current, respectively, in an attempt to "drive" the medication into the underlying inflamed tissues. Although these modalities are often used by athletic trainers and physical therapists, there is a paucity of scientific evidence to validate them, and studies have failed to show greater delivery of medication to the target tissue than that found with topical application alone.[91] Therefore the preferred method of delivery for corticosteroids is injection at the site of inflammation. Although this method limits systemic adverse effects, it is not without risk, as will be discussed in the following paragraphs.

The conflict between the lack of proven scientific efficacy of corticosteroids and their use in clinical practice can be no better illustrated than in the results of studies by LaBelle et al. and Hill et al. Since 1966, 185 articles have been published on the management of lateral epicondylitis ("tennis elbow"). LaBelle et al. carried out a meta-analysis of all of these articles and found that only 18 were randomized and controlled studies. None of these 18 studies met criteria for acceptance as a "valid clinical trial." Therefore the authors concluded that the evidence was insufficient to support the use of corticosteroid injection or NSAIDs for lateral epicondylitis treatment.[55] Three years before the publication of La Belle's findings, Hill (1989) and colleagues surveyed orthopedic surgeons regarding their use of corticosteroid injections. They found that 93 percent of those surveyed would inject a painful elbow epicondyle.[42] Their findings underscore the fact that the use of corticosteroids in sports medicine practice is likely to depend more on personal experience, anecdotal reports, and local practice preferences than on scientific data.

An extensive review of the available literature is beyond the scope of this discussion; however, there are a handful of significant studies that may be used to guide the judicious use of these powerful medications. The primary indication for their use is a chronic inflammatory condition, such as that seen with bursitis and tendonitis (Box 3–7). The goal of the therapy, just as with NSAIDs, is to break the cycle of inflammation and allow proper healing. There is no indication for the use of corticosteroids in the treatment of acute injuries because some degree of inflammatory response is mandatory for tissue healing. Additionally, not all inflammatory tendonopathies are appropriately treated with corticosteroids. For example, injections in and around the Achilles and patellar tendons should be avoided.[59]

In reviewing the literature regarding the use of corticosteroids, one may conclude that evidence, albeit anecdotal in many cases, does support the use of these medications in certain conditions. Many studies support the efficacy of corticosteroid injections in the treatment of stenosing tenovaginitis, trigger finger, and de Quervain's tenosynovitis.[4,35,37] Chronic olecranal bursitis was found to have a more rapid resolution with corticosteroid injection, but side effects included skin atrophy, infection, and chronic pain and were thought to outweigh the benefits of injection in a typically self-limiting condition.[100] An additional study found significantly less swelling at 1 week in injected patients.[88] Interestingly, these results have not been duplicated in treating prepatellar bursitis, in which injection therapy has resulted in frequent surgical removal and infection.[70] Corticosteroids are not indicated for the treatment of acute traumatic bursitis[70] and one may speculate that this is the explanation for the lack of efficacy for steroid injection in prepatellar bursitis.

Plantar fasciitis is also commonly treated with corticosteroid injection. Crawford et al. reported in 1999 that a group treated with corticosteroids showed improvement at one month, but no difference at 3 or 6 months after injection.[21] Although steroid injection has been recommended for a variety of running maladies, including greater trochanteric bursitis, iliotibial band friction syndrome, and retrocalcaneal bursitis, as well as plantar fasciitis,[16] upper extremity conditions are more commonly treated. Elbow epicondylitis, shoulder bursitis, and various tendon maladies of the hands are among the more frequent injuries treated by corticosteroid injection.[59]

Among the reasons for the lack of good scientific evidence demonstrating the efficacy of steroid injections is the variety of regimens regarding the specifics of treatment. Apart from the actual injection site (and that may vary depending on the technique and the skill of the physician), multiple confounding variables may exist. Foremost among these is the proper diagnosis. The number of previous injections, the agent and dosage injected, and the postinjection rehabilitation are also variables.

Most authorities recommend a minimum of 2 weeks between injections and a maximum of 3 injections per site.[59,89] As has been the familiar refrain throughout this section, there are no controlled studies to validate these practices. Pettrone urged that injections be used sparingly because of the risk of collagen breakdown in athletes. Typically, a "relative rest" period of 10 to 14 days after the injection of a corticosteroid is prescribed.[75] This recommendation, in and of itself, raises questions. First, in the treatment of any overuse injury, any period of rest is beneficial to the condition and thus clouds the efficacy of the steroid itself. Second, few athletes are willing, or able, to take 2 weeks off from training or sports participation. The selection bias for steroid treatment singles out those who are more seriously injured, or who have exhausted all other nonsurgical options.

The agent and dosage are subject to the greatest variation among those who perform corticosteroid injections. The most important characteristics of a corticosteroid are its

---

BOX 3–7

Most Common Indications for Injectable Corticosteroids

Prepatellar bursitis
Pes anserine bursitis
Greater trochanteric bursitis
Rheumatoid arthritis
Severe osteoarthritis
Shoulder bursitis
Elbow epicondylitis
de Quervain's tenosynovitis
Plantar fasciitis
Trigger finger

solubility and its duration of action.[59] A soluble, short-acting agent, such as betamethasone sodium phosphate (Celestone) is preferred for paratenonous injections. Intra-articular and bursal injections are appropriate for a less soluble, longer-acting drug such as triamcinolone diacetate. Little guidance is given in the literature regarding drug doses. An additional consideration is the avoidance of corticosteroid preparations that contain additives.[59,89] One additive, phenol, can be caustic to soft tissues and another, sodium bisulfate, has been implicated in anaphylactic reactions in sensitive patients.[59]

Another common type of additive to corticosteroid injections is an anesthetic agent such as lidocaine. This combination of agents is both diagnostic and therapeutic. If effective, the so called "pain ablation test" assures the physician both that the diagnosis was correct and that the medication was delivered to the proper tissue. The patient is also reassured by immediate relief and encouraged that the appropriate therapy has been initiated.

Despite the lack of convincing scientific data, corticosteroids remain popular in the treatment of many chronic inflammatory conditions encountered by the sports medicine clinician. These agents are obviously effective in some conditions because anecdotal evidence keeps their use alive. Although they are probably not as widely used as they have been in the past, they do have a role in the treatment of a few specific conditions. The future should see more controlled, double-blind studies further assessing the role of corticosteroids. At this time, they must be used cautiously and only after more conservative treatment regimens (e.g., ice, activity modification, NSAIDs) have failed. The athlete should be fully aware of the risks and benefits of the treatment and of other treatment options.

Web Resource

This service, which supports the safe, effective, and efficient use of medicines by providing information and advice, contains several articles regarding the use of anti-inflammatory medications.
www.ukmicentral.nhs.uk/aboutukm/index.htm

■ Adverse Effects

Historically, the most feared complication of corticosteroid injection has been tendon rupture. Although there are no controlled studies regarding tendon rupture after corticosteroid injection, numerous anecdotal and case reports exist.[50,52] Such reports have led many experts to suggest avoiding direct tendon injection, as well as avoiding injection around the Achilles, patellar, or biceps tendons.[59]

Although tendon rupture is the most devastating adverse consequence of corticosteroid injection, it was found to be the third most common complication encountered by practicing orthopedists. Bruno and Clark surveyed 52 orthopedic surgeons and found fat necrosis and skin depigmentation to be the most commonly encountered complications.[18] Another survey found similar results, along with infection, peripheral nerve damage, and systemic reactions (vasovagal syncope and transient hypoglycemia).[18] A wide range of potential local and systemic consequences of local corticosteroid injection are listed in Box 3–8.

There are multiple anecdotal reports regarding joint destruction after multiple intra-articular corticosteroid injections. Intra-articular injections are often used in both rheumatoid arthritis and osteoarthritis. Although they are often used for symptomatic pain relief in osteoarthritis, a systematic review failed to find any long-term benefit from steroid injections. Some short-term (1 to 2 weeks in duration) benefit was demonstrated.[93] Some animal models suggest that corticosteroids may have a detrimental effect on cartilage, but there is no pathological evidence in humans to support a diagnosis of steroid-induced arthropathy.

BOX 3–8

Potential Complications of Corticosteroid Injections

Local

Subcutaneous atrophy
Hypopigmentation
Tendon/ligament rupture
Accelerated joint destruction/osteolysis
Flare reactions
Infection/sterile abscess
Peripheral nerve injury
Muscle damage
Vascular injury

Systemic

Transient hyperglycemia
Vasovagal syncope
Psychological problems
Systemic allergic reactions/anaphylaxis
Adrenal suppression
Avascular necrosis

Adapted from Stanley and Weaver[89]

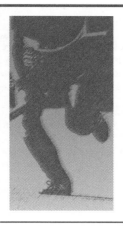

Scenario from the Field

A 16-year-old high school football player was told by his coach to take an anti-inflammatory for the swelling he was experiencing in his knee after an injury in a game on Friday night. The player was told by his mother to take two Tylenol tablets every 4 hours over the weekend. He comes to the athletic training facility on Monday afternoon before practice and explains that he still feels the swelling and thinks it is not getting better even though he is taking plenty of anti-inflammatories. The athlete then confides to the athletic trainer that he has taken more Tylenol than his mother suggested because he thought more would reduce the inflammation faster over the weekend and he would be able to practice on Monday. Now you have to explain to the athlete that Tylenol is not an anti-inflammatory and taking too much can cause health problems.

Discussion Topics

- If a high school athlete's physician wants the athlete to use an OTC anti-inflammatory for a week, what should the athletic trainer consider when discussing what type of anti-inflammatory the player should purchase at the pharmacy?

- What precautions should be pointed out when explaining to athletes the problems with using anti-inflammatory medications before a practice or competition when head injury is possible?

- How would you explain to an athlete why taking an anti-inflammatory with analgesic properties before a practice or competition could be detrimental if the athlete were injured during the practice or competition.

- What are the adverse effects that the athletic trainer should be looking for in an athlete taking anti-inflammatory medications?

- What types of OTC medications might an athlete take to reduce inflammation that are not actually anti-inflammatory? With what types of OTC medications containing aspirin might the athlete be unaware of the aspirin content?

- A 19-year-old college basketball player has patellar tendonitis that has been unresponsive to a week of therapy. He wants a "cortisone shot" like the ones he used to get for the same problem when he was in high school. What are the contraindications for this injection?

Chapter Review

- The inflammatory response prevents the extensive spread of injury-causing agents to nearby tissues, disposes of cellular debris, and sets the stage for the repair process.

- There is evidence that the immune system has a role in both the acute and chronic inflammatory processes.

- Prostaglandins are responsible for a variety of actions in almost every tissue of the body, playing various roles in many physiological processes.

- Reye's syndrome is attributed to a combination of aspirin and viral infection in children and young adults.

- Acetaminophen produces only antipyretic and analgesic effects in the body.

- The goal of the COX-2 inhibitors is to improve efficacy and limit toxicity of drugs used in the inflammatory process.

- NSAIDs do not produce the side effects of opioid drugs but will assist with mild pain.

- NSAIDs have negative interactions with other drugs, both prescription and OTC.

- Corticosteroids can be used as anti-inflammatory agents, but are available only on a physician's prescription.

- Complications of corticosteroid injections can result in tendon rupture and generalized joint destruction.

References

1. Airaksinen, O, et al.: Ketoprofen 2.5% gel versus placebo gel in the treatment of acute soft tissue injuries. Int J Clin Pharmacol Ther Toxicol 31:561, 1993.
2. Akermark, C, and Forsskahl, B: Topical indomethacin in overuse injuries in athletes: A randomized double-blind study comparing Elmetacin with oral indomethacin and placebo. Int J Sports Med 11:393, 1990.
3. Amadio, P, et al.: Nonsteroidal anti-inflammatory drugs: Tailoring therapy to achieve results and avoid toxicity. Postgrad Med 93:73, 1993.
4. Anderson, BC, et al.: Treatment of de Quervain's tenosynovitis with corticosteroids: A prospective study of the response to local injection. Arthritis Rheum 4:793, 1991.
5. Antiarthritic Drugs: Drug Evaluations Annual. American Medical Association, Chicago, 1993, p 889.
6. Anti-arthritic medication usage: United States, 1991. Stat Bull Metrop Insur Co 73(3):25, 1992.
7. Armstrong, RA: Initial results in exercise-induced muscular injury. Med Sci Sports Exerc 22:429, 1990.
8. Barber, FA, and Gladu, DE: Comparison of oral ketorolac and hydrocodone for pain relief after anterior cruciate ligament reconstruction. Arthroscopy 14:605, 1998.
9. Bassleer, C, et al.: Effects of sodium naproxen on differentiated human chondrocytes cultivated in clusters. Clin Rheumatol 11:60, 1992.
10. Beiner, JM, et al.: The effect of anabolic steroids and corticosteroids on the healing of muscle contusion injury. Am J Sports Med 27:2, 1999.
11. Black, HM, et al.: Use of phenylbutazone in sports medicine: Understanding the risks. Am J Sports Med 8:270, 1980.
12. Bombardier, C: An evidence-based evaluation of the gastrointestinal safety of coxibs. Am J Cardiol 89 (suppl):3D, 2002.
13. Bombardier, C, et al.: Comparison of upper gastrointestinal toxicity of rofecoxib and naproxen in patients with rheumatoid arthritis. N Engl J Med 343:1520, 2000.
14. Bonnel, RA, et al.: Aseptic meningitis associated with rofecoxib. Arch Intern Med 162:713, 2002.
15. Brater, DG: Clinical pharmacology of NSAIDs. J Clin Pharmacol 28:518, 1988.
16. Brody, D: Techniques in the evaluation and treatment of the injured runner. Orthop Clin North Am 13:541, 1982.
17. Brouwers, JRBJ, and de Smet, PAGM. Pharmacokinetic-pharmacodynamic drug interactions with nonsteroidal anti-inflammatory drugs. Clin Pharmacokinet 27:462, 1994.
18. Bruno, LP, and Clark, RP: The use of local corticosteroid injections in orthopaedic surgery. Presented at the 56th Annual Meeting of the American Academy of Orthopaedic Surgeons, Las Vegas, Feb 9–13, 1989.
19. Clive, DM, and Stoff, JS: Renal syndromes associated with nonsteroidal anti-inflammatory drugs. N Eng J Med 310:563, 1984.
20. Collier, S, and Ghosh, P: Comparison of the effects of NSAIDs on proteoglycan synthesis by articular cartilage explant and chondrocyte monolayer cultures. Biochem Pharmacol 41:1375, 1991.
21. Crawford, F, et al.: Steroid injection for heel pain: Evidence of short-term effectiveness: A randomized controlled trial. Rheumatology (Oxford) 38:974, 1999.
22. David, MJ, et al.: Effect of NSAIDs on glycosyltransferase activity from human osteoarthritic cartilage. Br J Rheumatol 31 (Suppl 1):13, 1992.
23. Davies, NM, and Skjodt, NM: Choosing the right nonsteroidal anti-inflammatory drug for the right patient. Clin Pharmacokinet 38:377, 2000.
24. Dominkus, M, et al.: Comparison of tissue and plasma levels of ibuprofen after oral and topical administration. Arzneimittelforschung 46:1138, 1996.
25. Doogan, DP: Topical nonsteroidal anti-inflammatory drugs. Lancet 2:1270, 1989.
26. DuPont, M, et al.: The efficacy of anti-inflammatory medication in the treatment of the acutely sprained ankle. Am J Sports Med 15:41, 1987.
27. Eccles, FN, and Mason, J: North of England evidence based guideline development project: Summary guideline for nonsteroidal anti-inflammatory drugs versus basic analgesia in the pain of treating degenerative arthritis. British Medical Journal 317:526, 1998.
28. Ellenhorn, MJ, and Barceloux, DG: Medical Toxicology: Diagnosis and Treatment of Human Poisoning. Elsevier, New York, 1988, p 156.
29. Feldman, HI, et al.: Parenteral ketorolac: the risk for acute renal failure. Ann Intern Med 126:193,1997.
30. Furst, DE, and Munster, T: Non-steroidal anti-inflammatory drugs, disease-modifying antirheumatic drugs, nonopioid analgesics and drugs used in gout. In Katzung, BG, ed.: Basic and Clinical Pharmacology. Lange/McGraw-Hill, New York, 2001, p 596.
31. Galer, BS, et al.: Topical diclofenac patch relieves minor sports injury pain: Results of a multicenter controlled clinical trial. J Pain Symptom Manage 19:287, 2000.
32. Garcia-Rodriguez, LA, et al.: Risk of hospitalization for upper gastrointestinal tract bleeding associated with ketorolac, other nonsteroidal anti-inflammatory drugs, calcium antagonists, and other antihypertensive drugs. Arch Intern Med 158:33, 1998.
33. Glew, RH: Lipid metabolism II: Pathways of metabolism of special lipids. In Devlin, TM, ed.: Textbook of Biochemistry with Clinical Correlations. Wiley-Liss, New York, 1992, p 423.
34. Goodman, TA, and Simon, LS. Minimizing the complications of NSAID therapy. J Musculoskel Med 11:33, 1994.
35. Gunther, SF, et al.: The efficacy of cortisone injection for trigger fingers and thumbs. Presented at the 56th Annual Meeting of the American Academy of Orthopaedic Surgeons, Las Vegas, Feb. 9, 1989.
36. Hawkey, CJ: COX-2 inhibitors. Lancet 353:307, 1999.
37. Heller, CA, et al.: Nonsteroidal anti-inflammatory drugs and aspirin: Analyzing the scores. Pharmacotherapy 5:30, 1985.

38. Hench, PS, et al.: The effect of a hormone of the adrenal cortex (17-hydroxy-11dehydrocorticosterone; compound E) and of pituitary adrenocorticotropic hormone on rheumatoid arthritis. Proc Staff Meet Mayo Clin 24:181, 1949.

39. Henrotin, Y, et al.: In vitro effects of etodolac and acetylsalicylic acid on human chondrocyte metabolism. Agents Actions 36:317, 1992.

40. Henry, D, et al.: Variability in the risk of major gastrointestinal complications from nonaspirin nonsteroidal anti-inflammatory drugs. Gastroenterology 105:1078, 1993.

41. Heynemann, CA: Topical nonsteroidal anti-inflammatory drugs for acute soft tissue injuries. Ann Pharmacother 29:780, 1995.

42. Hill JJ, Jr., et al.: Survey on the use of corticosteroid injections by orthopaedists. Contemp Ortho 18:39, 1989.

43. Hollander, D: Gastrointestinal complications of nonsteroidal anti-inflammatory drugs: Prophylactic and therapeutic strategies. Am J Med 96:274, 1994.

44. Hollander, JL: Intra-articular hydrocortisone in arthritis and allied conditions: A summary of two years' clinical experience. J Bone Joint Surg 35A:983, 1953.

45. Hollander, JL, et al.: Hydrocortisone and cortisone injected into arthritic joints: Comparative effects of the use of hydrocortisone as a local antiarthritic agent. JAMA 147:1629, 1951.

46. Hollander, JL, et al.: Local anti-rheumatic effectiveness of higher esters and analogues of hydrocortisone. Ann Rheum Dis 13:297, 1954.

47. IMS Health. Leading therapy classes by global pharmaceutical sales, 2001. Available at http://www.imshealth.com/public/structure/dispcontent/1,2779,1343-1343-144167,00.html. Accessed October 29, 2002.

48. Juni, P, et al.: Are selective COX 2 inhibitors superior to traditional nonsteroidal anti-inflammatory drugs? (Editorial). British Medical Journal 324:1287, 2002.

49. Kawamori, T, and Rao, CV: Chemopreventative activity of celecoxib, a specific cyclooxygenase-2 inhibitor, against colon carcinogenesis. Cancer Res 58:409, 1998.

50. Kelly, DW, et al.: Patellar and quadriceps tendon ruptures: Jumper's knee. Am J Sports Med 8:375, 1984.

51. Kimberly, RP, and Plotz, PH: Salicylates including aspirin and sulfasalazine. In Kelley WN, et al (eds): Textbook of Rheumatology. WB Saunders, Philadelphia, 1989, p 739.

52. Kleinman, M, and Gross, AE: Achilles tendon rupture following steroid injection: Report of three cases. J Bone Joint Surg 65A:1345, 1983.

53. Knight, KL: Cold as a modifier of sports-induced inflammation. In Leadbetter, WB, et al (eds): Sports-Induced Inflammation. American Academy of Orthopaedic Surgeons, Park Ridge, Ill., 1990, p 463.

54. Knych, ET: Anti-inflammatory agents. In Thomas JA (ed) Drugs, Athletes, and Physical Performance. Plenum, New York, 1988, p 105.

55. LaBelle, H, et al.: Lack of scientific evidence for the treatment of lateral epicondylitis of the elbow—A meta-analysis. J Bone Joint Surg 74B:646, 1992.

56. Laine, L, et al.: A randomized trial comparing the effect of rofecoxib, a cyclooxygenase 2-specific inhibitor, with that of ibuprofen on the gastroduodenal mucosa of patients with osteoarthritis. Gastroenterology 117:776, 1999.

57. Leadbetter, WB: Cell-matrix response in tendon injury. Clin Sports Med 11:533, 1992.

58. Leadbetter, WB: Soft tissue athletic injury. In Fu FH and Stone DA, eds. Sports Injuries—Mechanisms, Prevention, and Treatment. William and Wilkins, Baltimore, 1994, p 733.

59. Leadbetter, WB: Anti-inflammatory therapy in sports injury. Clin Sports Med 14:353,1995.

60. Leadbetter, WB. An introduction to sports-induced soft tissue inflammation. In Leadbetter, WB, et al (eds): Sports Induced Inflammation. American Academy of Orthopaedic Surgeons, Park Ridge, Ill, 1990, p 3.

61. Lehne, RA, et al.: Pharmacology for Nursing Care. WB Saunders, Philadelphia, 1990, p 701.

62. Lichtenstein, DR, et al.: Nonsteroidal anti-inflammatory drugs and the gastrointestinal tract. Arthritis Rheum 38:5, 1995.

63. Lovejoy, FJ, et al.: Clinical staging in Reye's syndrome. Am J Dis Child 128:36, 1974

64. McGeer, PL, et al.: Arthritis and anti-inflammatory agents as possible protective factors for Alzheimer's disease: a review of 17 epidemiologic studies. Neurology 47:425, 1996.

65. McGuire, DA, et al.: Comparison of ketorolac and opioid analgesics in postoperative ACL reconstruction outpatient pain control. Arthroscopy 9:653, 1993.

66. Meade, EA, et al.: Differential inhibition of prostaglandin endoperoxide synthase (cyclooxygenase) isoenzymes by aspirin and nonsteroidal anti-inflammatory drugs. J Biol Chem 268:6610, 1993.

67. Moore, RA, et al.: Quantitative systemic review of topically applied non-steroidal anti-inflammatory drugs. British Medical Journal 316:333, 1998.

68. Morrow, JL, and Jackson-Roberts, L, II: Lipid-derived autacoids. In Hardman, JG, and Limbird, LE (eds): Goodman and Gilman's The Pharmacological Basis of Therapeutics. McGraw-Hill, New York, 2001, p 669.

69. Morrow, JL, and Jackson-Roberts, II, L: Analgesic-antipyretic and anti-inflammatory agents and drugs employed in the treatment of gout. In Hardman, JG, and Limbird, LE (eds): Goodman and Gilman's The Pharmacological Basis of Therapeutics. McGraw-Hill, New York, 2001, p 687.

70. Mysnyk, MC, et al.: Prepatellar bursitis in wrestlers. Am J Sports Med 14:46,1986.

71. Nuki, G: Nonsteroidal analgesic and anti-inflammatory agents. British Medical Journal 287:39, 1983.

72. Oates, JA, et al.: Clinical implications of prostaglandin and thromboxane A2 formation. N Eng J Med 319:761, 1988.

73. Pasinette, GM, and Aisen, PS: Cyclooxygenase-2 expression is increased in frontal cortex of Alzheimer's disease brain. Neuroscience 87:319, 1998.

74. Paulus, HE, and Furst, DE: Aspirin and other nonsteroidal anti-inflammatory drugs. In McCarty, DJ (ed): Arthritis and Allied Conditions: A Textbook of Rheumatology. Lea & Febiger, Philadelphia, 1989, p 507.

75. Pettrone, FA: Shoulder problems in swimmers. In Zarins B, et al. (eds): Injuries to the Throwing Arm. WB Saunders, Philadelphia,1985, p 318.

76. Porro, GB, et al.: Sulglycotide in the prevention of nonsteroidal anti-inflammatory drug-induced gastroduodenal mucosal injury: A double-blind, double-dummy, randomized endoscopic study versus placebo in rheumatic patients. Scand J Gastroenterol 28:875,1993.

77. Rang, HP, and Dale, MM: Pharmacology. Churchill Livingstone, New York, 1987, p 204.

78. Redfearn, S: Journal: Drug sales based on "seriously biased" data. *Washington Post*, June 4, 2002, sect. HE01.
79. Reynolds, JF, et al.: Non-steroidal anti-inflammatory drugs fail to enhance healing of acute hamstring injuries treated with physiotherapy. S Afr Med J 85:517, 1995.
80. Russell, AL: Piroxicam 0.5% topical gel in the treatment of soft tissue injuries: A double-blind study comparing efficacy and safety. Clin Invest Med 14:35, 1991.
81. Ryan, GB, and Majno, G: Inflammation. Upjohn, Kalamazoo, MI, 1977, p 42.
82. Schimmer, BP, and Parker, KL: Adrenocorticotropic hormone; adrenocortical steroids and their synthetic analogs; inhibitors of the synthesis and actions of adrenocortical hormones. In Hardman, JG, and Limbird, LE (eds): Goodman and Gilman's The Pharmacological Basis of Therapeutics. McGraw-Hill, New York, 2001, p 1649.
83. Sheng, H, et al.: Transforming growth factor-beta 1 enhances Ha-ras-induced expression of cyclooxygenase-2 in intestinal epithelial cells via stabilization of mRNA. J Biol Chem 275:6628, 2000.
84. Shires, TK: Anti-inflammatory drugs. In Conn, PM, and Gebhart, GF (eds): Essentials of Pharmacology. FA Davis, Philadelphia, 1989, p 303.
85. Silverstein, FE, et al.: Gastrointestinal toxicity with celecoxib versus nonsteroidal anti-inflammatory drugs for osteoarthritis and rheumatoid arthritis: the CLASS study: a randomized controlled trial. Celecoxib Long-term Arthritis Safety Study. JAMA 284:1247, 2000.
86. Simon, AM, et al.: Cyclo-oxygenase 2 function is essential for bone fracture healing. J Bone Mineral Res 17:963, 2002.
87. Simon, LS, et al.: Anti-inflammatory and upper gastrointestinal effects of celecoxib in rheumatoid arthritis. JAMA 282: 1921, 1999.
88. Smith, DL, et al.: Treatment of nonseptic olecranon bursitis: A controlled, blinded prospective trial. Arch Intern Med 149:2527, 1989.
89. Stanley, KL, and Weaver, JE: Pharmacologic management of pain and inflammation in athletes. Clin Sports Med 17:375, 1998.
90. Thorling, J, et al.: A double-blind comparison of naproxen gel and placebo in the treatment of soft tissue injuries. Curr Med Res Opin 12:242, 1990.
91. Thornton, JS: Pain relief for acute soft-tissue injuries. Available at *http://www.physsportsmed.com/issues/1997/10oct/thornton.htm.* Accessed September 29, 2002.
92. Tokish, JM, et al.: Ketorolac use in the National Football League. Phys Sportsmed 30 (Sept.):19, 2002.
93. Towheed, TE, and Hochberg, MC: A systematic review of randomized controlled trials of pharmacological therapy in osteoarthritis of the knee with an emphasis on trial methodology. Sem Arthritis Rheum 26:755,1997.
94. Towheed T, et al.: Analgesia and non-aspirin, non-steroidal anti-inflammatory drugs for osteoarthritis of the hip. The Cochrane Library, Oxford, England: Update Software; 2001.
95. Verbeeck, RK: Pharmacokinetic drug interactions with nonsteroidal anti-inflammatory drugs. Clin Pharmacokinetic 19: 44, 1990.
96. Vignon, E, et al.: In vitro effect of nonsteroidal anti-inflammatory drugs on proteoglycanase and collagenase activity in human osteoarthritic cartilage. Arthritis Rheum 10:1332, 1991.
97. Warner, DC, et al.: Prevalence, attitudes, and behaviors related to the use of nonsteroidal anti-inflammatory drugs (NSAIDs) in student athletes. J Adolesc Health 30:150, 2002.
98. Watson, MC, et al.: Non-aspirin, non-steroidal anti-inflammatory drugs for treating osteoarthritis of the knee. The Cochrane Library, Oxford, England: Update Software; 2001.
99. Weil, ML: Infections of the nervous system. In Menkes, JH (ed): Textbook of Child Neurology. Lea & Febiger, Philadelphia, 1990, p 327.
100. Weinstein, PS, et al.: Long-term follow-up of corticosteroid injection for traumatic olecranon bursitis. Ann Rheum Dis 43:44, 1984.
101. Whitehill, WR, et al.: Guidelines for dispensing medications. J Athletic Training 27:20, 1992.

Chapter Questions

1. What is the role of eicosanoids in inflammation?

2. Arachidonic acid in the body is converted to which substance(s)?

3. What actions are prostaglandins responsible for in the various tissues of the body?

4. Which syndrome is attributed to a combination of aspirin and viral infection in children and young adults?

5. Acetaminophen produces what effects in the body?

6. What is the goal of the COX-2 inhibitors used in the inflammatory process?

7. Aspirin was derived from what product?

8. What is the most frequently reported complication of NSAIDs therapy?

9. The COX -2 inhibitors are targeted at which of the following?
   A. Central nervous system/neurotransmitters
   B. Blood-brain barrier
   C. Inflammation from arthritis
   D. Muscle spasms

10. With the recent advent of the use of over-the-counter NSAIDs for anti-inflammatory reasons, it is apparent that:
    A. They are superior to aspirin in their action within the body.
    B. There is no evidence that they are any better than aspirin in gaining a therapeutic effect on the system.
    C. There is a high incidence of abuse with these drugs.
    D. Acetaminophen is as good an anti-inflammatory without the side effects.

4

Skeletal Muscle-Relaxant Drugs

It is not uncommon for an athlete to experience muscle strains, trauma, or mild chronic irritation as a result of athletic participation. Sometimes traumatic injury or irritation to muscle tissue has an associated unwanted muscle spasm that can inhibit the progress or participation of an athlete. Trauma-caused muscle spasm typically results in an increase in afferent pain impulses from the traumatized area, which in turn causes an increase in efferent messages from the CNS to the muscle and a resultant chronic tension. Often the athletic trainer uses thermal modalities or other manual techniques to overcome the associated muscle tension. Because the physician, under certain conditions, may treat these symptoms by prescribing a skeletal muscle relaxant, the athletic trainer needs to have a basic understanding of these types of drugs.

Skeletal muscle relaxants can be helpful in managing the symptoms of moderate muscle spasms caused by muscle contusions, strains, and other traumatic muscle injuries. However, it is important to note that there is an ongoing debate in the medical community regarding the effectiveness, or, more correctly, the appropriateness of the use of skeletal muscle relaxants. Some physicians contend that muscle relaxants can be beneficial for short-term muscle spasm, but tend to be overused for patients with chronic pain.[6] Many physicians also point out that, in spite of overwhelming evidence that skeletal muscle spasm is nonexistent; they are continually deluged with seductive incentives to prescribe expensive muscle relaxants.[5] The writer of a letter to the editor of the Journal of the Canadian Medical Association stated, "There is no proof that pain symptoms or decreased range of motion result directly from abnormality or spasm of muscles."[10] These diverse ideas indicate a division in the medical field regarding the use of muscle relaxants in a general sense. Because some team physicians prescribe muscle relaxants to certain athletes, it is important that the athletic trainer be aware of the positive and negative aspects of these drugs. The intent of this chapter is to provide a brief overview of these drugs for the athletic trainer's general awareness of this drug class.

Muscle Spasm and Spasticity

The athletic trainer should understand the difference between muscle spasm and muscle spasticity. The athletic trainer will be exposed more often to muscle spasm because this condition is more commonly a result of irritation or trauma to healthy muscle tissue. *Muscle spasm* resulting from athletic injury trauma results in a loss of range of motion and increased pain in the general area of the tissue damage. *Spasticity* is a generalized rigidity of the musculature. A brief explanation of spasticity will be helpful to the athletic trainer's overall understanding of the two muscular problems.

Muscle spasticity is caused by a central nervous system (CNS) dysfunction more commonly known as an *upper motor neuron lesion*. Spasticity is a muscle stretch reflex that is exaggerated in the individual's limb or limbs. Rapid lengthening of the affected muscle results in a contraction of the stretched muscle. Spasticity is technically not a disease process but a result of motor interruption, typically in the upper motor complex of the CNS.[14] Spasticity is more commonly associated with cerebral palsy, paraplegia, or quadriplegia, and is considered a more permanent disorder. The physician's approach to treating spasticity will be much different than the approach to treating muscle spasms.

During a muscle spasm, involuntary tension is developed in the muscle, and the athlete is unable to completely relax the muscle. As mentioned, this muscle spasm will be affected by the pain impulses from the muscle to the CNS. With an increase in the amount of pain impulses traveling from the muscle, there is a concomitant increase in tension in the muscle. This is commonly referred to as the *pain-spasm-pain cycle* of the injury process. Chronic muscle spasm can result in muscle atrophy in the specific muscle or muscle group.

If the athlete experiences muscle spasm and associated pain that do not allow him or her to get enough rest as is necessary for healing, the physician may prescribe a muscle relaxant. Typically, this will be a centrally acting drug, meaning that the drug works on the CNS somewhere in or along the afferent or efferent pathways of the muscle.

Malignant Hyperthermia

A disorder that is known to be associated with muscle spasms is "malignant hyperthermia" (MH), which has been diagnosed in some athletes and also in individuals who have recently been under anesthesia.[2] In the general population, this disorder is linked to a genetic predisposition that causes the carrier to be more sensitive to the gases used in anesthesia. This increased sensitivity to anesthesia gases causes the person suffering from MH to experience tachycardia, tachypnea, generalized muscular contractures (rigidity), cyanosis, skin mottling, possibly fever, and sometimes hyperthermia. In rare instances, death is possible. Athletes suffering from this disorder are the focus of this explanation.

Malignant hyperthermia is a disorder usually associated with athletes who exercise in hot and humid environments. It results in an excessive breakdown of muscle tissue. When an athlete experiences a reduction in water intake, this can have a negative impact on cellular function or cellular damage. When muscle cells are damaged by a lack of water intake, an imbalance arises in the calcium homeostasis of the cell. This calcium imbalance can lead to muscle necrosis and possibly rhabdomyolysis. The administration of dantrolene in the early stages of MH, in combination with cooling and hyperventilation, can reverse the destructive process.[8] However, often a diagnosis of MH is not made before the athlete begins to experience the effects of this muscle cell breakdown.[1,4]

Athletes who exercise for long periods of time in hot and humid environments need to drink plenty of water and rest periodically. If an athlete exercising in a stressful environment begins to suffer from hyperthermia, CNS difficulties (dizziness, confusion, lapses of consciousness), or other common heat–stress-related symptoms, he or she should stop exercising and have his or her recovery monitored carefully.

The transition from exertional heat stroke to MH is not common, but can occur in individuals with the genetic trait. You will want to monitor the athlete for increased symptoms of tachycardia, tachypnea, cyanosis, skin mottling, and fever when monitoring heat-related stresses. Exertional heat stroke has been associated with MH, and therefore the athletic trainer should be cognizant of this disorder because it could occur during almost any of the sports seasons. When you suspect that an athlete has experienced a significant heat stress situation, it is important to continue to monitor the weight, CNS, and kidney functions of the athlete. Timely and appropriate treatment of this problem will help the athlete and reduce the problems that the athletic trainer and team physician must deal with later.

Muscle-Relaxant Drugs

■ Spasms

The exact mechanism of action of skeletal muscle relaxants is not well known at this time. The use of centrally acting muscle-relaxant drugs is not a frequent first-line treatment in the athletic population. It should also be noted that the specific purpose of muscle relaxants to decrease muscle spasm continues to be questioned as a therapeutic intervention.[3] The use of these drugs may result in a mild general sedative effect, producing an overall relaxation of the entire body.[7,13] This sedative effect results in a reduction of CNS impulses, which reduces the overall activity of the individual muscle. In short, it is not clear that centrally acting muscle-relaxant drugs directly affect the muscles. It is suggested that these drugs create a sedative effect, which allows the athlete to relax, rest, and allow the muscle to repair itself, thus reducing the amount of muscle spasm the athlete experiences.

The centrally acting muscle relaxants are usually combined with an analgesic like aspirin or acetaminophen to assist with associated pain. Physicians use different types of analgesics based on onset of action, duration, and possible adverse effects for the individual.

As can be seen by reviewing Table 4–1, the drugs prescribed for skeletal muscle spasms display a variety of phar-

macodynamic parameters, including onset and duration of action. These factors should be taken into consideration because these drug agents may affect the ability of the athlete to practice or compete. Skeletal muscle relaxants do have a depressing effect on the CNS and therefore can produce sluggishness or even cause the athlete to sleep. Most of the drugs prescribed have an onset of action between 30 and 60 minutes. Knowledge of this will help you explain to the athlete when he or she should take the medication to minimize any associated lethargy. The duration of action varies among these drugs, and this is another important point for the athlete to be cognizant of when trying to participate in rehabilitation programs or attend practices. Drugs with a shorter duration of action will allow participation in rehabilitation and practices. Obviously, drugs with a longer duration of action (12–24 hours) will prevent the athlete from participation in many team activities.

■ Spasticity

Some muscle-relaxant drugs are considered direct acting. These drugs are most commonly used for treatment of spasticity because their efforts are directed to the individual cells. The use of these drugs is common in individuals who have experienced some type of CNS lesion from an accident at birth (cerebral lesion) or some type of spinal cord accident that results in spasticity. If the athletic trainer is working with disabled athletes, he or she may want to learn more about the use of direct-acting skeletal muscle relaxants in this population.

Table 4–1

Drugs Commonly Used to Treat Skeletal Muscle Spasms

Generic Name (Trade Name)	Usual Adult Oral Dosage (mg)	Onset of Action (min)	Duration of Action (hr)
Carisoprodol (Soma)	350 TID and bedtime	30	4–6
Chlorzoxazone (Paraflex, Parafon Forte, others)	250–750 TID or QID	Within 60	3–4
Cyclobenzaprine (Flexeril)	10 TID	Within 60	12–24
Diazepam (Valium)	2–10 TID or QID	15–45	Variable
Metaxalone (Skelaxin)	800 TID or QID	60	4–6
Methocarbamol (Robaxin)	1000 QID	Within 30	24
Orphenadrine citrate (Antiflex, Norflex, others)	100 BID	Within 60	4–6

Source: Adapted from Ciccone, CD: Pharmacology in Rehabilitation. FA Davis, Philadelphia, 2002, p 172, with permission.

Adverse Effects

The muscle relaxants have adverse effects that the athletic trainer should be aware of when talking with the athlete taking these drugs. The main adverse effect is drowsiness.[13] The instructions on the prescription container will indicate that the athlete should not drive a motor vehicle or perform other activities requiring a high level of motor functioning or reaction capabilities. The athlete may also experience lack of muscle coordination, dizziness, headache, or nausea when taking these medications. These drugs are known to become addictive, and the athlete can develop a tolerance to them. Additionally, the muscle-relaxant drugs can have an additive effect with alcohol that creates an increased sedative effect, sometimes resulting in death.[7,11] When skeletal muscle relaxants are taken in combination with antihistamines, other CNS depressants, or monoamine oxidase inhibitors, there is an additive effect creating increased CNS depression (Box 4–1).

Muscle relaxants can be abused by some athletes, can be obtained illegally, and have a potential for dependence.[13] The athletic trainer should encourage the athlete to discontinue the use of these drugs as soon as he or she is able to function without them. Additionally, skeletal muscle relaxants are among the most commonly reported drugs of abuse by health-care professionals.[9] In addition to monitoring your athletes' use of these drugs, you may want to watch for signs of abuse among your fellow athletic trainers and the other health-care professionals you work with on a daily basis. Take the appropriate steps to assist those in need if they are abusing skeletal muscle relaxants or any other drugs.

Implications for Activity

The athletic trainer needs to remind the athlete who uses skeletal muscle relaxants that these drugs have a mild general sedative effect and produce overall relaxation. This general relaxation effect may make the athlete unable to practice or compete because of being tired or even sleepy from the medication. The combination of skeletal muscle relaxants with alcohol or other CNS depressants can be dangerous or even lethal to the athlete. The use of skeletal muscle relaxants by physicians working with athletes is not a common procedure and should be monitored closely.

BOX 4–1

Adverse Effects of Skeletal Muscle Relaxants

Drowsiness (warning against operating machinery or performing activities that require mental alertness)

Dizziness

Blurred vision

Confusion

Hallucinations

Agitation

Headaches

Gastrointestinal problems

    Anorexia

    Vomiting

    Epigastric distress

Allergic reactions

    Skin rash

    Pruritus

    Edema

    Anaphylaxis

List compiled from Waldman, HJ: Centrally acting skeletal muscle relaxants and associated drugs. J Pain Symptom Manage 9:434, 1994.

What to Tell the Athlete

The athlete should understand that the use of muscle-relaxant drugs is not a first line of resolution for muscle tension resulting from trauma or irritation. Skeletal muscle relaxants really treat only the symptoms and not the underlying cause of the problem.[7] Here are some tips for the athletic trainer when educating the athlete about these drugs:

- Before the physician prescribes a skeletal muscle relaxant, thermal modalities and manual techniques should be tried.
- Encourage the athlete to continue scheduled therapy even after the physician has prescribed a skeletal muscle relaxant.
- The overall sedative effect of the drug will reduce the energy level of the athlete.
- Therapy sessions should be scheduled during times when the drug is getting to the end of its duration of action.

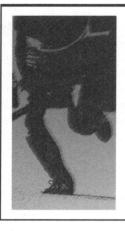

Scenario from the Field

At a university in Utah, athletes reporting minor injuries were admitted to the physician's examination room in the athletic training facility, where they stole pages from the physician's prescription pad. They then wrote their own prescriptions for skeletal muscle relaxants. Because the athletes were well known in their own town, they went to a pharmacy in a nearby, smaller town to have the prescriptions filled. Fortunately, the pharmacist suspected that something was amiss. She made a phone call to the physician of record to inquire about the prescriptions. The athletes were apprehended and charged by the police. This incident illustrates that it is important to maintain security in the physician's examination room.

Discussion Topics

- Why would an athlete abuse a skeletal muscle relaxant during practice, in competition, or during the season?

- Explain the difference between skeletal muscle spasm and spasticity.

- Why would a physician prescribe skeletal muscle relaxants for an athlete?

- Why would a physician not prescribe skeletal muscle relaxants for an athlete?

Chapter Review

- Muscle spasm is typically caused by trauma or irritation to the muscle.

- Muscle spasticity is a result of a CNS lesion.

- Muscle relaxant drugs can act either centrally or directly on the system.

- Centrally acting muscle relaxants are commonly prescribed for muscle spasm in the athlete.

- Prescription muscle relaxants are often combined with an analgesic to reduce the pain associated with muscle spasm.

- Muscle relaxants cause a general sedative effect on the athlete. Some authors believe that the sedative effect allows the athlete to gain proper rest, allowing the muscles the time needed to heal.

- Common adverse effects of muscle relaxants are drowsiness, dizziness, headache, and nausea.

- Muscle relaxants have an additive effect when combined with alcohol; therefore the athletic trainer should discourage any use of alcohol by athletes who are taking these drugs.

- The athletic trainer should work with the physician and the athlete to provide adjunct therapies so that the athlete can overcome muscle spasms.

- The athletic trainer should encourage the athlete to discontinue the use of prescription muscle relaxant drugs as soon as possible.

References

1. Arrington, ED, and Miller, MD: Skeletal muscle injuries. Orthop Clin North Am 26:411, 1995.
2. Bourdon, L, and Canini, F. On the nature of the link between malignant hyperthermia and exertional heatstroke. Med Hypotheses 45:268, 1995.
3. Ciccone, CD: Pharmacology in Rehabilitation. FA Davis, Philadelphia, 2002, p 169.
4. Denborough, M: Malignant hyperthermia. Lancet 352:1131, 1998.
5. Epstein, NL: Benztropine for acute muscle spasm in the emergency department. CMAJ 164(2):203, 2001.

6. Feinberg, SD: Prescribing analgesics: How to improve function and avoid toxicity when treating chronic pain. Geriatrics 55(11):44, 2000.

7. Gutierrez, K: Pharmacotherapeutics: Clinical decision-making in nursing. WB Saunders, Philadelphia, 1999, p 386.

8. Kozack, JK, and MacIntyre, DL: Malignant hyperthermia. Phys Ther 81:945, 2001.

9. Meeker, JE, et al.: Detection of drug abuse by health professionals. Occup Health Saf 71(8):46, 2002.

10. Rush, P, and Epstein, NL: Acute muscle spasm. CMAJ 165: 13, 2001.

11. Smith, CM, and Reynard, AM: Essentials of Pharmacology. WB Saunders, Philadelphia, 1995, p 205.

12. Venes, D (ed.): Taber's Cyclopedic Medical Dictionary, ed. 19. FA Davis, Philadelphia, 2001.

13. Waldman, HJ: Centrally acting skeletal muscle relaxants and associated drugs. J Pain Symptom Manage 9:434, 1994.

14. Young, RR: Spasticity: a review. Neurology 44:S12, 1994.

Chapter Questions

1. What is the difference between muscle spasm and spasticity?
   A. Spasm is usually a result of muscle trauma.
   B. Spasm is usually a result of a CNS lesion.
   C. Spasticity is usually a result of intense activity
   D. Spasticity is usually a result of prolonged muscle contraction.

2. The use of prescription muscle relaxant drugs in combination with which of the following will reduce muscle spasm?
   A. Thermal modalities
   B. Regular practice and activity
   C. Correct sitting posture
   D. Psychological counseling

3. Prescription muscle relaxants have what effect when combined with alcohol?
   A. Additive
   B. Excitatory
   C. No effect
   D. Stabilizing

4. The main adverse effect of muscle relaxants mentioned in this chapter is:
   A. General sedation.
   B. General excitation.
   C. Loss of memory.
   D. Lack of motivation.

5. When is the best time to schedule an athlete who takes muscle relaxants to come in for adjunct therapy?
   A. During the end portion of the drug's duration of action
   B. During the middle portion of the drug's duration of action
   C. During the most relaxed time for the athlete
   D. During the athlete's regular practice session

Drugs for Diabetes Mellitus

5

Chapter Objectives

After reading this chapter, the student will be able to:

1 Differentiate between the two major classifications of diabetes mellitus.
2 Understand the etiology of type 1 and type 2 diabetes mellitus.
3 Recognize the signs and symptoms, adverse effects, and complications of diabetes mellitus.
4 Understand basic glucose metabolism and how insulin affects diabetes mellitus control.
5 Recognize and identify appropriate blood glucose levels for an individual with diabetes.
6 Recognize the benefits of diet and exercise for an individual with diabetes.
7 Identify and recognize the different devices for insulin administration and injection.
8 Differentiate between the types, onset, duration, and peak action of insulin.
9 Differentiate between the types and responses of oral antidiabetic agents for treatment of diabetes mellitus.
10 Recognize the adverse affects of insulin and oral antidiabetic agent therapy.

Chapter Outline

*A*ccording to the American Diabetes Association, approximately 18.2 million people in the United States have diabetes.[1] However, only a third of the individuals with diabetes actually know that they have the disease. It is estimated that 5 to 10 percent who are diagnosed with diabetes have type 1 diabetes and the remaining 90 to 95 percent have type 2 diabetes[1] (Table 5–1). A third type, gestational diabetes, emerges during pregnancy and is usually reversible after delivery.

Diabetes is the sixth leading cause of death in the United States, with 213,000 individuals dying of complications of the disease in the year 2000 alone.[1] Complications include blindness, kidney disease, heart disease, stroke, impotence, and nontraumatic lower limb amputations (Box 5–1). Individuals from specific ethnic backgrounds, such as Latinos, African-Americans, Native Americans, Asian-Americans, and Pacific islanders, are at a higher risk of developing diabetes. Obesity is also a risk factor.

The cost of managing diabetes is increasing each year. In 2002, direct and indirect health-care expenditures of persons with diabetes totaled $132 billion.[1] In order to defray the costs of managing and treating diabetes and its complications, allied health-care professionals and athletic trainers must understand how to effectively treat individuals with the disease. Moreover, proper care and management will allow a person with diabetes to live a more functional lifestyle and decrease or diminish the extent of complications and reliance on insulin or oral antidiabetic agents.

If you have experience working with individuals with diabetes or know someone who has diabetes, you may be aware of the seriousness and restrictions this disease may impose. However, people with diabetes can live functional and active lives. In this chapter, we will explain the etiology of diabetes and common management techniques including blood glucose response and insulin and oral antidiabetic drug therapy. We will also discuss some of the common complications of diabetes and adverse affects of insulin and oral antidiabetic drug therapies.

*D*efinition of Diabetes

The term diabetes mellitus stems from the Latin words *diabetes,* meaning "siphon," and *mellitus,* meaning "sweet." Diabetes mellitus is a condition in which the body cannot effectively regulate blood glucose, commonly called "blood sugar." The disease is characterized by hyperglycemia (high blood glucose) (Box 5–2). Physiologically, there are several mechanisms from which the disease develops, ranging from beta (β)-cell destruction in the pancreas to cellular insulin resistance. The specific type of diabetes depends on the mechanism of etiology. Type 1 diabetes results from the body's failure to produce insulin because of an *autoimmune* pathology. Type 2 diabetes arises from cell insulin resistance or failure of the pancreas to produce enough insulin. Additional information on the etiology of diabetes will be discussed in specific sections of this chapter.

Table 5–1		
Characteristics of Types 1 and 2 Diabetes		
Characteristics	**Type 1**	**Type 2**
Incidence (relative to all persons with diabetes except the gestational type)	10%	90%
Age of onset	Adolescence	Usually >35 years
Onset	Abrupt	Gradual over years
Family history	Usually negative	Usually positive
Etiology	Autoimmune	Unknown—strong genetic association, obesity, sedentary lifestyle
Symptoms	Polyurea, polyphagia, polydipsia, weight loss, ketosis, blurred vision, slow-healing sores, tingling in feet	Can be asymptomatic for years; have similar symptoms to those of type 1 diabetes, including tiredness and dry, itchy skin
Body weight	Usually underweight or normal	Overweight or obese
Insulin levels	Reduced or deficient	Normal or slightly decreased
Management	Insulin, diet, exercise	Diet, exercise, oral antidiabetic agents

cells for energy metabolism and storage, stimulates the uptake of amino acids, and facilitates amino acid conversion into proteins. Insulin also converts triglycerides into free fatty acids to be used as energy by the tissues. When the body's insulin supplies are insufficient, excess glucose accumulates in the blood and is then excreted in the urine. Because the cells cannot uptake glucose, the body is "starved" even though there is plenty of glucose available for energy. To produce the energy required for the body, muscles metabolize glycogen (stored glucose) and the liver metabolizes free fatty acids to form glucose.

Insulin, once it is released from the pancreas, binds with specific insulin receptors located on the cell membrane. Once they are bound, the receptors signal protein messengers (GLUT-4) found inside the cells of skeletal and cardiac muscles, liver, and adipose tissue. These protein messengers migrate to the cytoplasm of the cell membrane, bind with glucose, and allow passage through the cell by passive transport (Fig. 5–1).

Although most cells need insulin to actively transport glucose across cell membranes, some tissues are not dependent on insulin to receive circulating glucose. Because the brain requires a constant supply of glucose for its energy needs, it is freely permeable to glucose at all times. During exercise, skeletal muscles can readily uptake glucose into the cells without the presence of insulin. The liver is also non-insulin dependent, but insulin does enhance the metabolism of glucose.

*G*lucose Metabolism

During digestion, the body converts much of the food we eat into glucose to be used for energy. If glucose is not utilized at the time of digestion, it is stored in the form of glycogen in the liver and muscles. Insulin, produced by β cells of the pancreas, facilitates glucose transport into most

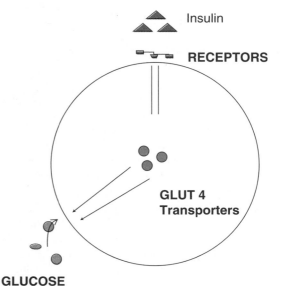

Figure 5–1. Glucose transporters. Receptors on the cell membrane allow insulin to pass into the cell. Insulin then stimulates GLUT transporters to travel to the cell membrane and allow glucose to enter the cell.

Type 1 Diabetes Mellitus

Type 1 diabetes, formally known as insulin-dependent diabetes mellitus (IDDM) and previously called juvenile-onset diabetes, has the lower prevalence of the two types of diabetes. Usually children, teenagers, and young adults are diagnosed with this type of diabetes. It results from an autoimmune destruction of the pancreatic β cells.[6] The β cells of the pancreas, under normal circumstances, produce enough insulin to metabolize fat, carbohydrates, and proteins in the foods that we eat. Destruction of the β cells limits the effectiveness of food metabolism, leading to hyperglycemia, ketoacidosis, and the need for exogenous insulin to sustain life.

The destruction of the β cells is variable, meaning that some individuals have a rapid rate of destruction and others have a slower rate of destruction.[49] Usually the process of cell destruction takes place over weeks, months, or even years. A virus, toxin, or some environmental condition is thought to stimulate the destruction of the β cells; however, the exact process is unclear.

Type 2 Diabetes Mellitus

The etiology of type 2 diabetes, formally known as non–insulin-dependent diabetes and previously called adult-onset diabetes, remains unclear but is thought to stem from insulin deficiency or resistance.[13,35–36,44] Type 2 diabetes can occur at any age, including adolescence, but usually affects older individuals. Individuals diagnosed with type 2 diabetes can have elevated, reduced, or normal insulin levels, but all present with hyperglycemia. Insulin resistance, dysregulated hepatic glucose production, impaired glucose tolerance, and decreasing β-cell function are other factors that contribute to hyperglycemia.

Insulin resistance is thought to be caused by abnormal insulin antibodies, decreased insulin receptor numbers or affinity, postreceptor defects such as deficient GLUT transporters, or abnormal postreceptor signal transduction. With insulin resistance, insulin-sensitive tissues do not readily absorb glucose and serum levels of glucose begin to rise. The increased glucose levels stimulate the β cells of the pancreas to release more insulin. However, the increase in insulin secretion rarely alleviates the high glucose levels. Over time, the β cells become exhausted and fail to secrete insulin at appropriate levels. Autoimmune destruction of the beta cells usually does not occur in type 2 diabetes.

Type 2 diabetes often goes undiagnosed for years (Box 5–3). Hyperglycemia increases gradually, and individuals rarely notice symptoms before they realize they have the dis-ease.[16,20,48] Most individuals with type 2 diabetes are obese, which has been shown to correlate with some form of insulin resistance.[9,29] Insulin resistance may improve with a combination of weight reduction, diet, exercise, and drug therapy to reduce hyperglycemia, but individuals rarely return to normal levels.[15,24,39–40,45] The risk of developing type 2 diabetes increases with age, lack of exercise, and obesity,[19,48] and occurs more frequently in individuals with hypertension or dyslipidemia, members of certain racial and ethnic groups, and women who were previously diagnosed with gestational diabetes.[16,19,48] A strong genetic disposition plays a contributing role in developing type 2 diabetes, although the specific genetic link is not clearly known.[7,33]

Management of Diabetes

The primary goals for managing diabetes are glucose control through education, glucose monitoring, diet, exercise, oral drug therapy, and/or insulin therapy. With proper management, diabetes can be controlled and the complications associated with it can be minimized. Individuals who properly manage their disease can live long, productive, and active lives.

BOX 5–3

Testing Criteria for Asymptomatic Undiagnosed Individuals for Diabetes

1. Testing should be conducted for all individuals over the age of 45. If blood glucose levels are normal, should be repeated every three years thereafter.
2. Testing should be conducted at a younger age or more frequently if the patient:
   A. Is obese (over 20 percent of ideal body weight or have a BMI ≥ 25 kg/m²)
   B. Has relatives with diabetes
   C. Is a member of a high-risk ethnic population
   D. Has delivered a baby weighing more than 9 pounds OR has been diagnosed with gestational diabetes mellitus
   E. Is hypertensive (≥140/90)
   F. Has HDL cholesterol levels <35 mg/dL and/or triglyceride levels >250 mg/dL
   G. Had abnormal glucose values when previously tested

Glucose Monitoring

Individuals with type 1 and type 2 diabetes are strongly encouraged to monitor their blood glucose levels. Normal fasting plasma glucose (FPG) levels are less than 100 mg/dL (Table 5–2). To determine if an individual has diabetes, a fasting plasma glucose test is advised. Values above 126 mg/dL may be indicative of diabetes mellitus and values between 100 mg/dL and 126 mg/dL are considered pre-diabetes (Box 5–2).

Patients with diabetes should monitor their glucose levels daily. Blood glucose levels are measured using self-monitored blood glucose (SMBG) equipment (Fig. 5–2), which can be used any time during the day as needed. Although most diabetes patients use SMBG equipment, clinicians and physicians usually assess glucose concentrations over time using glycosylated hemoglobin levels (HbA1c). HbA1c is an indicator of average glycemic control for a period of 2 to 3 months, and normal values for individuals without diabetes range from 4 to 6 percent. HbA1c is the preferred test because it is least affected by daily fluctuations in blood glucose.[10]

Diet and Exercise

Individuals with type 2 diabetes should be encouraged to monitor their diet and exercise (Table 5–3). Regular exercise, along with diet management, can improve blood glucose control and insulin sensitivity, and possibly lower medication requirements.[12,14,21,37–38,41–42] Exercise can also promote weight loss and reduce body fat,[3] resulting in decreases in cholesterol and blood pressure.[5,18,21,23,27] Exercise and diet may reduce the amount of oral antidiabetic medication or insulin needed for glucose control.[3] In addition, exercise may prevent or delay the onset of type 2 diabetes.[3]

Type 1 diabetes patients should also be encouraged to exercise (Table 5–3) and to monitor their diet to control glucose responses. During rest, approximately 10 percent of muscle metabolic requirements come from glucose. During exercise, almost all metabolic requirements come from glucose, rapidly depleting muscle glycogen stores and increasing peripheral glucose utilization. As the demand for glu-

Table 5–2

Normal Glycemic Values

Average preprandial glucose	<100 mg/dL
HbA1c	<6%

Source: Copyright © 2002 American Diabetes Association. From Diabetes Care, Vol. 25, Supplement 1, 2002; S33-S49. Reprinted with permission from The American Diabetes Association.

Table 5–3

Exercise Recommendations and Guidelines for Individuals with Diabetes

Type of Diabetes	Type of Exercise
*Type 2 (>300 mg/dL without ketones)**	Aerobic: walking, jogging, cycling, cross-country skiing, etc.
Intensity	60–90% maximal heart rate; 50–85% VO$_{2max}$
Duration	20–60 minutes
Warm-up/cool-down	5–10 minutes of light activity
Frequency	3–5 times per week
*Type 1 (>250 mg/dL and ketones present in urine)**	Aerobic: walking, jogging, cycling, cross-country skiing, etc.
	Resistance Training: circuit training programs, light weights and 10–15 repetitions
Intensity	60–90% maximal heart rate; 50–85% VO$_{2max}$
Duration	20–60 minutes
Warm-up/cool-down	5–10 minutes of light activity
Frequency	3–5 times per week

*All individuals with diabetes should avoid initiation of exercise during times of poor glycemic control.
Source: American College of Sports Medicine: Resource Manual for Guidelines and Exercise Testing and Prescription, ed 4. Lippincott Williams & Wilkins, Philadelphia, 2001. Used with permission.

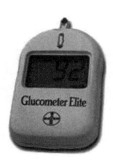
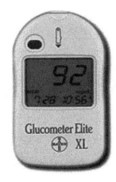

Figure 5–2. Example of a glucose monitoring device. Copyright Bayer Corporation. Used with permission, 2002.

cose increases, hepatic glycogenolysis and gluconeogenesis increases. If exercise commences when insulin levels are insufficient, hepatic glucose production will increase and peripheral utilization will decrease, causing hyperglycemia. After exercise, muscle cells need relatively little insulin to facilitate glucose uptake. This glucose uptake into the muscle cells can last for up to 10 to 12 hours after exercise. If adjustments are not made in diet and insulin therapy, individuals can become hypoglycemic.[32]

People with diabetes who have glucose levels equal to or exceeding 250 to 300 mg/dL should delay exercising because high glucose levels indicate insulin deficiency. In contrast, excess insulin will enhance peripheral glucose utilization by muscles and suppress hepatic glucose output, resulting in hypoglycemia. Individuals who have glucose levels that are close to normal before exercise have a higher chance of developing hypoglycemia and should be instructed to either ingest 10 to 20 g of carbohydrates before exercise or decrease their dose of insulin.

Managing insulin levels during exercise can be difficult for athletes with both types of diabetes. These athletes have to experiment with their insulin and carbohydrate intake to participate safely in exercise. Type 1 and 2 diabetes patients must know the hormonal and metabolic responses of their body to exercising and need to avoid dangerous conditions such as hypoglycemia. To avoid hypoglycemia, type 1 diabetes patients must alter insulin therapy (time, location, dose). Type 2 diabetes patients must alter oral antidiabetic agents (time and dose) or ensure appropriate nutritional intake before or during exercise. In addition, both types 1 and 2 diabetes patients should monitor blood glucose and adjust for exercise intensity and dietary requirements. In many cases, these processes are managed not only by individuals but also by their health-care professionals, including their athletic trainer. Therefore it is the responsibility of the athletic

trainer to become familiar with diet, exercise, insulin, and oral antidiabetic therapies.

▦ Insulin Administration

Insulin is required to treat gestational diabetes, as well as type 1 and sometimes type 2 diabetes, when diet, exercise, and oral antidiabetic agents cannot control symptoms. Regardless of the type of diabetes, insulin dosage must be individualized and balanced with diet and exercise. Insulin was originally manufactured from the pancreases of pigs and cows but now is being replaced by human insulin synthesized using recombinant DNA techniques. With this new technology, a more purified insulin can be prepared biosynthetically that is structurally identical to human insulin and causes fewer allergic reactions (Fig. 5–3).

The absorption rate of insulin (and ultimately the patient's glucose control) can vary with the site of administration.[28] Most patients with diabetes use the upper arms, thighs, abdomen, and buttocks for insulin administration. It is now recommended that insulin be injected in the same anatomical region each day to control for insulin reactions[4] and to ensure similar and consistent absorption (Fig. 5–4). Individuals who exercise should inject insulin into the abdomen to avoid accentuated absorption into exercising muscles.

When storing insulin, one should closely follow the manufacturer's guidelines. Insulin should generally be kept at room temperature; however, when not in use, it should be refrigerated (not frozen). If an individual is traveling for a long period of time in warm weather, insulin can be stored in an insulated container with a cooling agent. Extreme temperatures ($<36°$ or $>86°F$) and agita-

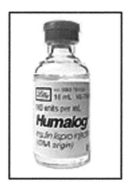

Figure 5–3. Example of an insulin vial. Copyright Eli Lilly and Company. Used with permission, 2002. Humalog® is a registered trademark of Eli Lilly and Company.

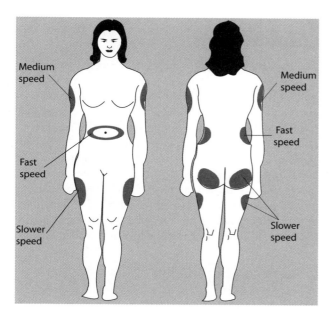

Figure 5–4. Graphic representation of common sites used to inject insulin under normal conditions. Used with permission from the National Institute of Diabetes and Digestive and Kidney Diseases.

tion can produce clumping or precipitation (the separation of solids from a solution or suspension) of insulin and affect potency.

Visual inspection of insulin before administration is necessary. Clumping, frosting, precipitation, or color change may signify a loss of potency. If unsure about the potency of a vial, individuals should always substitute a new vial of the same type. Expiration dates stamped on each vial should remind the user to dispose of any expired insulin.

The type of syringe used to inject insulin is also important. Most manufacturers produce small syringes (27–30 gauge with a length of 5/16 or 1/2 inch) that can hold 1.0, 0.5, 0.25, or 0.3-mL. Syringe capacities of 0.25 mL and 0.3 mL are recommended for pediatric and insulin-sensitive patients who require less than 25 units of insulin before meals or snacks.

Most athletes with type 1 diabetes self-administer their own insulin as needed. However, there may be circumstances under which the athletic trainer may be required to inject insulin. To begin, first clean the injection site with alcohol, moving in a circular fashion outward. Grasp the skin around the injection site to elevate the subcutaneous tissue (about 1″ fat fold) (Fig. 5–5.) With the other hand, position the needle bevel up. Insert the needle at a 45° or 90° angle and release the skin. (Fig. 5–6) Inject the insulin and remove the needle gently at the same

angle used for insertion. Cover the injection site with an alcohol sponge and check the site for any bleeding or bruising.

■ Insulin Injection Devices

Currently, there are several ways to deliver insulin: (1) drawing a dose from a vial with an insulin syringe and needle; (2) an insulin pump; or (3) prefilled insulin pens.

Insulin pumps are a more precise way to mimic normal insulin secretion. An insulin pump, which is a battery-operated device with an internal computer, delivers a predetermined amount of insulin, stored in a reservoir, to a subcutaneously inserted catheter or needle. Insulin pumps are designed to be portable and to deliver a basal amount of insulin throughout the day to replicate insulin secretion from the pancreas, as well as to deliver meal-related boluses (concentrated quantities administered rapidly). Individuals may regulate the amount of insulin pumped depending on their circumstances (e.g., time of meals and exercise). Intermittently, depending on individual habits and insulin responses, the pump's reservoir must be refilled.

Insulin pumps can also be implanted, delivering insulin continuously. Insulin is stored in a reservoir surgically located subcutaneously in the abdomen or the chest wall. However, there can be several complications, ranging from infection to catheter blockage. Currently, the widespread use of implantable pumps is limited.

Prefilled insulin pens are convenient for individuals who

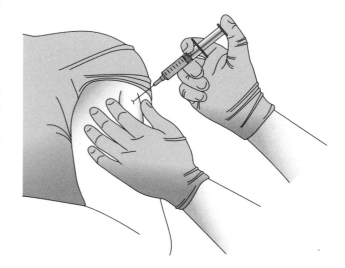

Figure 5–5. Preparing the skin for insulin injection.

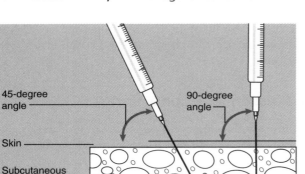

Figure 5–6. Proper placement of the insulin needle for injection.

want to carry insulin discreetly. An insulin pen actually looks like a writing pen and has a cartridge that contains fixed amounts of insulin. Each end of an insulin pen has a specialized function. Located on one end of the insulin pen is a needle similar to the needle found on a syringe. There is a plunger on the other end. To use, the patient selects the desired amount of insulin (measured by a dial on the pen) and then uses the plunger to administer it through the skin. Insulin pens can be disposable or have replaceable cartridges (Fig. 5–7).

Implications for Athletic Trainers

Individuals who have an insulin pump may engage in school/university-sponsored sports. It is recommended that participation in contact sports be limited to decrease the chances of damage to the insulin pump. However, specific decisions to engage in contact sports must be made by the athlete and the physician and may require special protective devices for the insulin pumps.

Insulin Types

Insulin is available in different forms, categorized according to duration and onset of action (Table 5–4). Currently, there are four types of insulin: rapid acting, short acting, intermediate acting, and long acting. Patients with diabetes may combine different types of insulin for glucose management. However, when different types of insulin are mixed, physiochemical changes may occur and therapeutic responses may differ from those obtained by injecting insulin separately. Please consult the physician or pharmacist to ensure proper procedures and precautions for injecting mixed insulin. Injection techniques, site of injection, and patient response may also affect the onset, degree, and duration of insulin activity.

■ Rapid-acting Insulin

Insulin Lispro (Humalog)

The first available rapid-acting insulin that received United States Food and Drug Administration (FDA) approval (1996) was lispro (Humalog). Lispro is administered 0 to 15 minutes before meals because this type of insulin mimics the normal physiologic insulin secretion response after meals.[26] Because lispro has a short duration of action, users may be more susceptible to hyperglycemia and ketosis if insulin administration is inadvertently interrupted.

Insulin Aspart (Novolog)

Insulin aspart (Novolog) is another type of rapid-acting insulin. It is similar to lispro, but its genetic composition differs. Like lispro, insulin aspart controls postprandial (after meals) glucose. It was approved by the FDA in June 2000. Insulin aspart should be administered 0 to 15 minutes before meals.

■ Short-acting Insulin

Regular

Regular (R) insulin has a slightly longer onset of action than rapid-acting insulin. The duration of action is approxi-

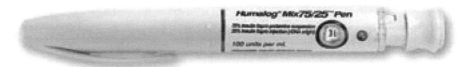

Figure 5–7. Example of an insulin pen. Copyright Eli Lilly and Company. Used with permission, 2002. Humalog® is a registered trademark of Eli Lilly and Company.

Table 5–4

Insulin Types and Actions*

Type	Example	Onset	Peak	Duration of Action
Rapid-acting insulin	Insulin lispro (Humalog)	1/4 hr	1/2–1 hr	2–4 hrs
	Insulin aspart (NovoLog)	5 min–1/4 hr	1–3 hrs	3–5 hrs
Short-acting insulin	Regular insulin (Humulin R)	1/2–1 hr	2–5 hrs	5–10 hrs
Intermediate-acting insulin	Isophane insulin (NPH)	1–2 hrs	6–14 hrs	18–>24 hrs
	Insulin zinc (Lente)	1–3 hrs	6–14 hrs	18–>24 hrs
Long-acting insulin	Insulin zinc, extended (Ultralente)	4–6 hrs	16–24 hrs	24–>28 hrs
	Insulin glargine (Lantus)	1 hr	2–20 hrs	24 hrs

*The times listed in the table for onset, peak, and duration of action can vary according to the individual.

mately 5 to 10 hours. Of major concern for people using regular insulin is the proper timing of premeal administration because of the relatively longer onset of action.[25]

Intermediate-acting Insulin

Isophane Insulin (NPH) and Insulin Zinc (Lente)

NPH and Lente are two similar, related intermediate-acting insulins. The insulin action is dependent on individual responses and glucose level. Fluctuations in absorption of intermediate-acting insulin may alter glucose responses.

Long-acting Insulin

Insulin Zinc Extended (Ultralente)

Ultralente is a long-acting insulin. Because of its delayed-action effects, Ultralente is not recommended for acute glucose control related to meals. Long-acting insulin is usually mixed with short-acting insulin to produce a basal level of insulin between meals. However, administrations are often required twice daily for continuous control of blood sugar throughout the entire day.

Insulin Glargine (Lantus)

Insulin glargine is indicated for children and adults who have type 1 diabetes and those who have type 2 diabetes and need basal insulin to control hyperglycemia. Glargine has no pronounced peak, but instead maintains a basal rate over

a 24-hour period. Insulin glargine is administered usually once daily, at bedtime.

Combination Insulin Products

A variety of combination insulin products are also available. In such products, two different types of insulin, usually short and long acting, are dispensed already mixed in the same vial or insulin pen. This method requires fewer injections per day but still provides the control needed. Some examples include Humulin 50/50, Humulin 70/30, and Humalog 75/25.

Insulin Therapy

An insulin regimen is developed after determining the total daily dose and types of insulin required. Because of the variability, there are a multitude of insulin regimens that a physician may prescribe. A common insulin regimen consists of a mixture of intermediate- and short-acting insulin injected twice daily, before breakfast and before dinner (Fig. 5–8). The morning injection of short-acting insulin is intended to control for glucose responses after the morning meal and the intermediate acting insulin controls glucose responses of the noon meal and provides a basal rate throughout the day. The second injection of insulin controls for the evening meal plus later snacks and also provides a basal rate until morning. This method is preferred for individuals who are newly diagnosed and are still secreting pancreatic insulin. Other individuals who need tighter glucose control may administer 3 to 4 injections over the course of the day, usually at meal times.

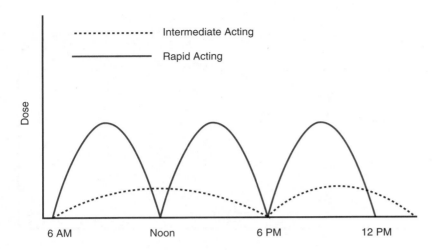

Figure 5–8. Onset and duration of action using a split mixed method of intermediate and rapid-acting insulin.

Athletes with diabetes who require insulin must closely monitor glucose utilization and insulin intake. In most cases, athletes with diabetes can decrease the amount of insulin administered before exercise because of the glucose uptake by the exercising muscles. In addition, athletes with diabetes may be required to snack frequently before or during competition to control glucose levels adequately.

Implications for Athletic Trainers

Athletic trainers must monitor individuals with type 1 diabetes after exercise because exercised muscles can increase the uptake of glucose without the presence of insulin. Unaccustomed or unexpected exercise intensities, in combination with insulin administration, may alter glucose uptake and predispose the athlete to hypoglycemic reactions several hours after exercise. This can occur while the athlete is traveling after a game or practice. Therefore the athletic trainer should have glucagon kits or other glucose sources available in case of this emergency.

Insulin Therapy Adverse Effects

▪ Hypoglycemia

The most common adverse effect of insulin therapy is hypoglycemia, sometimes referred to as insulin shock. Hypoglycemia is a serious and potentially life-threatening condition, most commonly caused by an excess amount of insulin. Other causes of hypoglycemia associated with insulin ther-

apy include a decrease in glycogen stores, skipping meals, or exercise. A person suffering from hypoglycemia may feel weak, drowsy, confused, hungry, or dizzy. Other signs and symptoms include pallor, headache, irritability, trembling, sweating, and tachycardia. In severe cases, the person can lose consciousness and lapse into a coma.

To avoid hypoglycemia, individuals should follow a strict meal regimen, monitor glucose levels regularly, eat snacks if necessary, and learn glucose responses to food and exercise. In addition, all insulin-dependent individuals should carry at least 15 to 20 g of carbohydrates to consume in the event of a hypoglycemic reaction. Some examples are chewable glucose tablets and glucose gel. Medical personnel, athletic trainers, roommates, family members, friends, or other involved persons should also be instructed to use a glucagon emergency kit for situations in which the individual cannot be given carbohydrates orally. Finally, all insulin-dependent individuals should wear a medical alert identification tag.

▪ Diabetic Ketoacidosis

Diabetic ketoacidosis (DKA) is frequently seen in people with type 1 diabetes, with rare occurrences in non–insulin-dependent individuals. DKA results from a shift in metabolism from glucose to nonglucose sources (fatty acids from adipose tissue) for use as energy as a result of insulin deficiency. Glucose levels rise as a result of decreased glucose uptake by the cells. Therefore fatty acids are metabolized and used by the cells as an alternate energy source.

The byproducts of fat metabolism are ketones. As ketones accumulate in the blood, the blood becomes more acidic than the body tissues. The increase in acidity results in the condition called ketoacidosis. Signs and symptoms of DKA include hyperglycemia, thirst, excess urination, fatigue, blurred vision, fruity breath, nausea, muscular stiffness, and difficulty breathing. Other signs are a flushed face, dry skin and mouth, a rapid and weak pulse, and low blood pressure. If the person is not given fluids and insulin immediately, ketoacidosis can lead to coma and potentially death. Individuals who display the symptoms described should check for ketones in the urine, drink fluids, continue with insulin therapy, and contact a physician immediately.

■ Lipohypertrophy

Lumpy or bumpy appearances on the surfaces of injection sites are thought to be from the lipogenic (fat-producing) effects of insulin. Lipohypertrophy usually results after months to years of repeated injections in the same region. In some cases, the injection site even becomes anesthetized from the constant use of the needle. Proper rotation of the injection region may limit development of lipohypertrophy. If it develops, surgical excision may be necessary.

■ Lipoatrophy

Lipoatrophy is the breakdown of adipose tissue at the injection site. This causes skin depression and may delay the effects of insulin absorption. Causes of lipoatrophy include an immune response or using less pure insulin, such as animal-derived insulin.

■ Local Skin Reactions

The prevalence of skin reactions, including pain, swelling, erythema, and itching, has decreased since the development of more purified insulin (insulin made by recombinant DNA technology). Zinc and protamine (additives to increase the duration of action) are thought to be the cause of skin reactions. Skin reactions usually occur in four forms: (1) an immediate flare reaction, (2) as an immediate reaction followed by 4 to 8 hours of erythema, (3) a delayed reaction up to 12 or 24 hours, and (4) a severe inflammatory local reaction.[34] Most individuals become desensitized after the first vial of insulin. For resistant cases, oral antihistamines or a glucocorticoid steroid mixed within the syringe can be tried.[30]

*O*ral Antidiabetic Agents

Initial treatment for individuals newly diagnosed with type 2 diabetes is a diet and exercise program to help them gain control of their high glucose levels and lose weight. If, after a period of time, these modifications are unsuccessful, oral antidiabetic agents may be prescribed.

Until 1995, oral antidiabetic agents were limited strictly to a specific drug class known as sulfonylureas. Now several newer oral medications have been developed to control glucose levels at different sites of the body (Fig. 5–9). The combination of oral antidiabetic medications with a regimen of diet and exercise allows people with diabetes to better manage hyperglycemia. Only if these systems fail is insulin prescribed to control hyperglycemia. The next section will describe the type and pharmacology of oral drugs available for diabetes. For an overview of these oral agents, please refer to Table 5–5.

■ Alpha-Glucosidase Inhibitors

Alpha (α)-glucosidase inhibitors currently include two specific drugs, acarbose (Precose) and miglitol (Glyset). These drugs target the enzymes of the mucosa of the small intestine by inhibiting the breakdown of complex polysaccharides and sucrose into monosaccharides, which are more easily absorbed into the bloodstream. This action results in a slower rate of digestion and lowers the postprandial blood glucose concentrations by up to 25 to 50 mg/dL. Although

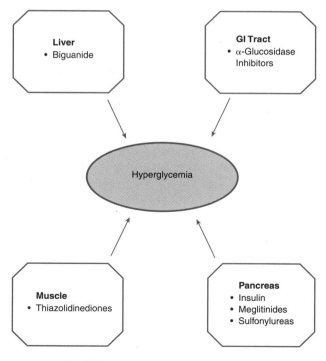

Figure 5–9. Oral antidiabetic agent sites of action. Adapted from Applied Therapeutics: *The Clinical Use of Drugs*. Koda-Kimble MA, Young LY, Kradjan WA, Guglielmo BJ (eds). Lippincott Williams & Wilkins: Philadelphia, 2001

Table 5–5

Oral Antidiabetic Agents: Types and Actions*

Drug Name	Action	Duration of Action	Initial Dosage
Alpha-glucosidase Inhibitors	Inhibit complex carbohydrate digestion and absorption after a meal		
acarbose (Precose)		3 hrs	25 mg with first bite of meal
miglitol (Glyset)		2–3 hrs	25 mg with first bite of meal
Biguanides	Decrease hepatic glucose production and increase peripheral glucose uptake	6–12 hrs	500 mg bid with morning and evening meals
metformin (Glucophage)			850 mg qd with morning meal
Meglitinides	Stimulate insulin secretion		
repaglinide (Prandin)		4–6 hrs	0.5–2 mg, 1–30 min before meals
nateglinide (Starlix)		4 hrs	120 mg, 1–30 min before meals
Thiazolidinediones	Reduce insulin resistance, increase glucose uptake by muscles, decrease hepatic glucose production		
rosiglitazone (Avandia)		24 hrs	4 mg qd
pioglitazone (Actos)		24 hrs	15–30 mg qd
First-Generation Sulfonylureas	Promote insulin secretion and increase insulin uptake by the tissues		
acetohexamide (Dymelor)		12–24 hrs	250 mg qd
chlorpropamide (Diabinese)		24–72 hrs	250 mg qd
tolazamide (Tolinase)		10–24 hrs	100–250 mg qd with breakfast
tolbutamide (Orinase)		6–24 hrs	1–2 g qd
Second-Generation Sulfonylureas	Promote insulin secretion and increase insulin uptake by the tissues		
glimepiride (Amaryl)		24 hrs	1–2 mg qd with breakfast
glipizide (Glucotrol)		12–24 hrs	5 mg qd, 30 min before a meal
glyburide (Diabeta, Micronase)		24 hrs	2.5–5 mg qd with breakfast

*Duration of action can vary according to the individual.

α-glucosidase inhibitors decrease the mean HbA1c levels up to 0.5 to 1.0 percent, these effects occur only when they are taken with a complex carbohydrate meal.[31,46]

The most common adverse effects of α-glucosidase inhibitors are flatulence, diarrhea, and abdominal pain. Because α-glucosidase inhibitors delay carbohydrate digestion in the gastrointestinal (GI) tract, they may affect the absorption of other drugs if taken concurrently. Additionally, acarbose and miglitol are not recommended for individuals with inflammatory bowel disease or intestinal obstruction. As with any antidiabetic agent, α-glucosidase inhibitors may produce hypoglycemia.

■ Biguanides

The biguanide class of oral antidiabetic agents consists of one agent, metformin (Glucophage). Metformin lowers glucose concentration but does not cause hypoglycemia in people who do not have diabetes. Metformin is able to decrease hepatic glucose production, decrease glucose intes-

tinal absorption, and improve insulin sensitivity by increasing peripheral glucose uptake and utilization. The specific mechanism to lower blood glucose is thought to occur by decreasing gluconeogenesis,[11,43] but research is still unclear as to whether this actually occurs.[8] Metformin can reduce HbA_{1c} levels up to 1.7 percent and fasting plasma glucose levels by 50 to 70 mg/dL. Usually metformin is administered with meals two or three times daily.

The biguanides can cause diarrhea, abdominal discomfort, metallic taste, nausea, and anorexia. These GI adverse effects are usually dose related and should subside over time. Individuals with renal impairment, hepatic disease, or a history of lactic acidosis should refrain from therapy.

■ Meglitinides

Meglitinides are a new class of nonsulfonylurea agents that stimulate insulin secretion. Two drugs comprise this class; repaglinide (Prandin) and nateglinide (Starlix). Meglitinides work by closing ATP-sensitive potassium channels in the β cell, leading to depolarization and an influx of Ca++, which stimulates the release of insulin. This class of drugs has a rapid onset of action and a short duration of action, and must be given with meals to enhance postprandial glucose utilization. If used separately, repaglinide decreases fasting plasma glucose levels by 61 mg/dL and HbA$_{1c}$ by 1.7 percent. If it is combined with metformin, fasting blood glucose levels decrease by approximately 40 mg/dL.

Meglitinides can cause mild hypoglycemia, particularly if not taken with food. Weight gain of up to 3 percent can occur in some individuals. In addition, meglitinides should not be used by people with type 1 diabetes and a nonfunctioning pancreas.

■ Thiazolidinediones

Troglitazone (Rezulin) was the first thiazolidinedione approved by the FDA in 1997. Since then, two others have joined this class of drugs, rosiglitazone (Avandia) and pioglitazone (Actos). In 2001, troglitazone was withdrawn from the market because of hepatotoxic effects. Thiazolidinediones are still very effective and are classified as insulin sensitizers, meaning that these drugs decrease insulin resistance in the liver and stimulate glucose uptake by muscle tissues. However, to exert their effects on hyperglycemia, insulin must be present in the body to facilitate glucose uptake. When combined with other antidiabetic agents for poorly controlled type 2 diabetes, thiazolidinediones can decrease HbA1c levels by an average of 1 percent.

Thiazolidinediones can cause hepatotoxicity in some individuals, usually in the first few months of therapy, and caution should be advised. Liver function tests are advised before starting therapy, every 2 months for the first year of therapy, and periodically afterward. Thiazolidinediones may also lower hemoglobin and hematocrit levels.[22] Individuals may exhibit increases in plasma volume, and use in patients with heart failure should be cautious. Patients may see an increase in HDL cholesterol levels and an increase in total and LDL cholesterol levels.

■ Sulfonylureas

There are several types of sulfonylureas available. Categorized by their chemical structure, these include four first-generation sulfonylureas and three second-generation sulfonylureas. Second-generation sulfonylureas are approximately 100 times more potent than first-generation sulfonylureas based on a milligram-for-milligram comparison, but there is no evidence of differences in clinical effectiveness between them. As a group, sulfonylureas decrease fasting plasma glucose levels by 50 to 70 percent and HbA1c levels by 1.5 to 1.7 percent.

Sulfonylureas work by stimulating the release of insulin from the β cell of the pancreas and enhancing β-cell sensitivity to glucose. Sulfonylureas are believed to inhibit the potassium ion channel found on the β cell, lower the membrane potential, and cause depolarization. Calcium channels are then opened, increasing the intracellular calcium concentration. The increase in calcium concentration stimulates the release of insulin.[26,47] This class of drugs can also normalize hepatic glucose production and partially reverse peripheral insulin resistance in persons with type 2 diabetes.[17]

Sulfonylureas primarily produce hypoglycemia and weight gain. It is not uncommon for individuals to gain between 2 and 5 kg during the course of therapy. Other adverse effects of sulfonylurea administration include headache, dizziness, and nausea.

*T*he Athletic Trainer's Responsibility

Early detection and treatment of diabetes is crucial to control the various complications associated with the disease. As allied health-care professionals, athletic trainers must thoroughly understand the type of insulin and oral therapies available and how these therapies affect the individual with diabetes, especially in the athletic setting. Athletes with diabetes normally manage their own condition, but circumstances exist in which the athletic trainer may intervene.

There are several factors that an athletic trainer can follow to assist the athlete with diabetes. The first course of action is to review medical files to determine if any athletes have diabetes and to ensure that proper medical examinations have been conducted. The second step is to discuss with the individual with diabetes his or her specific condition and the primary course of action to take if complications arise, including which equipment is necessary to have readily available at practices and games (glucagon kits, carbohydrates, glucose-monitoring devices, etc) and procedures for contacting medical personnel. The athletic trainer must also recognize the signs and symptoms of emergency complications of diabetes and how to handle and prevent these situations.

The athletic trainer should remind athletes to check their blood glucose levels before and after meals and practices and at other appropriate times. The athlete should also be reminded to eat properly and take proper doses of insulin or oral antidiabetic agents in accordance with their physician's instructions. It is also strongly recommended that the athletic trainer periodically inquire about the athlete's condition during games and practices to determine glucose regulation.

What to Tell the Athlete

As an athletic trainer, you may encounter athletes who have diabetes. Although most of these athletes know how to manage their condition, you may be required to help monitor their blood glucose, especially while they are exercising. What can you do?

- Begin by having the athlete monitor his or her own blood glucose levels regularly, both before and after exercise.
- Inform the athlete of the signs and symptoms of hypoglycemia.
- If an athlete experiences hypoglycemia during exercise (practice, games, etc.) have him or her immediately consume a form of carbohydrate and cease the exercise while symptoms are present.
- Have the athlete record his or her intake of food and insulin or oral antidiabetic medications daily to learn fluctuations.
- If hypoglycemia persists while the athlete is exercising, make modifications to his or her diet or medication therapy.
- Make sure the athlete consumes food after exercise to reduce the possibility of hypoglycemia as a result of glucose uptake from the muscles.

Scenario from the Field

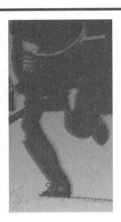

A 23-year-old collegiate tennis player, diagnosed with type 1 diabetes, was placed on a split-mixed method of 8 units of regular and 6 units of NPH insulin before breakfast and the evening meal. Approximately 3 hours after a 1 PM practice, she began developing signs and symptoms of hypoglycemia. What is causing the hypoglycemia, and what actions should be taken to avoid further hypoglycemic episodes?

Her hypoglycemic episode is probably caused by either the insulin regimen (NPH) or a lack of carbohydrate intake before practice. In either case, there are several solutions to avert her hypoglycemic episodes. First, she can adjust the number of NPH insulin units administered to counteract the effects of glucose uptake in the muscles during exercise. NPH has a peak concentration that gradually increases and reaches its highest level in 8 to 14 hours before slowly decreasing. Therefore the athlete can decrease her dose in the morning. Second, she can consume a carbohydrate snack before practice to elevate her glucose levels. Finally, she can avoid practicing during times of peak insulin effects. All three choices would effectively correct her hypoglycemia episodes, but the preferred choice would be a carbohydrate snack before practice.

Diabetes Care Information

For more specific guidelines and recommendations for diabetes care, please refer to:

American Diabetes Association
http://www.diabetes.org
American Medical Association
http://www.ama-assn.org
Diabetes Journals (Diabetes, Diabetes Care, Clinical Diabetes, and Diabetes Spectrum)
http://www.diabetesjournals.org
National Institute of Diabetes & Digestive & Kidney Diseases
http://www.niddk.nih.gov

International Diabetes Federation
http://www.idf.org
American College of Sports Medicine
Position Stand: Exercise and Type 2 Diabetes
http://www.acsm-msse.org/
ADA/ACSM Joint Statement: Diabetes Mellitus and Exercise
*http://www.acsm-msse.org/*Journal Articles (See also References.)
Jimenez, CC: Diabetes and exercise: The role of the athletic trainer. Journal of Athletic Training 32(4): 339–343, 1997.
Guion, WK: Athletes with diabetes: The athletic therapist's role. Athletic Therapy Today 3(3):12–15, 1998.

www.

Discussion Topics

- Is it safe for a person with type 1 diabetes with an insulin pump to participate in contact sports?

- Can weight training be beneficial for persons with diabetes to lower blood glucose?

- Is it the athletic trainer's responsibility to know how to inject insulin for an athlete with type 1 diabetes?

- What are some measures that an athletic trainer can perform to prevent hypoglycemia in a diabetes patient?

Chapter Review

- Approximately 2/3 of all individuals who have diabetes are undiagnosed.

- Insulin, produced by the pancreas, is required by the cells for uptake of glucose.

- Type 1 diabetes is an autoimmune disease that affects the pancreas.

- Type 2 diabetes usually affects older adults.

- Proper monitoring of blood glucose levels is recommended for both types of diabetes.

- The first course of action to manage diabetes is through diet and exercise.

- Insulin needle and syringe, insulin pumps, and insulin pens are three examples of devices to deliver insulin.

- The four types of insulin available are rapid acting, short acting, intermediate acting, and long acting.

- Insulin therapy should take changes in diet and exercise into account to avoid hypoglycemia.

- Diabetic ketoacidosis is the result of using fatty acids instead of glucose for energy.

- Oral antidiabetic agents are prescribed to control hyperglycemia.

- Hypoglycemia can result from oral antidiabetic agent therapy.

References

1. American Diabetes Association: *http://www.diabetes.org/home.jsp.*
2. American Diabetes Association: Economic consequences of diabetes mellitus in the United States in 1997. Diabetes Care 21(2):296–309, 1998.
3. American Diabetes Association Position Statement: Diabetes mellitus and exercise. Diabetes Care 25(suppl. 1):S64–S68, 2002.
4. American Diabetes Association Position Statement: Insulin administration. Diabetes Care 25(Suppl 1):S112–S115, 2002.
5. American Diabetes Association Position Statement: Standards of medical care for patients with diabetes mellitus. Diabetes Care 25(1): S33–S49, 2002.
6. Atkinson, MA, and Maclaren, NK: The pathogenesis of insulin-dependent diabetes. N Engl J Med 331:1428–1436, 1994.
7. Barnett, AH, et al.: Diabetes in identical twins. Diabetologia 20:87–93, 1981.
8. Bell, PM, and Hadden, DR: Metformin. Endocrinol Metab Clin North Am 26:523–537, 1997.
9. Bogardus, C, et al.: Relationship between degree of obesity and in vivo insulin action in man. Am J Physiol 248:E286–E291, 1985.
10. Bunn, HF: Nonenzymatic glycosylation of protein: Relevance to diabetes. Am J Med 70:325–330, 1981.
11. Cusi, K, et al.: Metabolic effects of metformin on glucose and lactate metabolism in non-insulin-dependent diabetes mellitus. J Clin Endocrinol Metab 81:4059–4067, 1996.
12. DeFronzo, R, et al.: Insulin sensitivity and insulin binding to monocytes in maturity-onset diabetes. J Clin Invest 63:939–946, 1979.
13. DeFronzo, RA, et al.: Effect of physical training on insulin action in obesity. Diabetes 36:1379–1385, 1987.
14. Dengel, DR, et al.: Distinct effects of aerobic exercise training and weight loss on glucose homeostasis in obese sedentary men. J Appl Physiol 81:318–325, 1996.
15. Firth, RG, et al.: Effects of tolazamide and exogenous insulin on insulin action in patients with non-insulin-dependent diabetes mellitus. N Engl J Med 314:1280–1286, 1986.
16. Fujimoto, WY, et al.: Prevalence of complications among second-generation Japanese-American men with diabetes, impaired glucose tolerance or normal glucose tolerance. Diabetes 36:730–739, 1987.
17. Groop, LC: Sulfonylureas in NIDDM. Diabetes Care 15(6): 737–754, 1992.
18. Gumbiner, B, et al.: Effects of a monounsaturated fatty acid-enriched hypocaloric diet on cardiovascular risk factors in obese patients with type 2 diabetes. Diabetes Care 21:9–15, 1998.
19. Harris, MI: Classification, diagnostic criteria, and screening for diabetes. National Diabetes Data Group, National Institutes of Health, National Institute of Diabetes & Digestive & Kidney Diseases.
20. Harris, MI, et al. (eds.): Diabetes in America, ed 2. NIH Publication No. 95-1468. Washington, D.C., United States Government. Printing Office, 1995, pp 15–36.
21. Harris, MI: Impaired glucose tolerance in the U.S. population. Diabetes Care 12:464–º474, 1989.
22. Heilbronn, LK, et al.: Effect of energy restriction, weight loss,

and diet composition on plasma lipids and glucose in patients with type 2 diabetes. Diabetes Care 22(6):889–895, 1999.

23. Henry, RR: Thiazolidinediones. Endocrinol Metab Clin North Am 3:553–573, 1997.

24. Henry, RR, et al.: Glycemic effects of intensive caloric restriction and isocaloric refeeding in non-insulin-dependent diabetes mellitus. J Clin Endocrinol Metab 61:917–925, 1985.

25. Henry, RR, Wallace, P, et al.: Effects of weight loss on mechanisms of hyperglycemia in obese non-insulin-dependent diabetics. Diabetes 35:990–998, 1986.

26. Holleman, F, et al.: Reduced frequency of severe hypoglycemia and coma in well-controlled IDDM patients treated with insulin lispro. Diabetes Care 20:1827–1832, 1997.

27. Howey, DC, et al.: {Lys (B28), Pro (B29)-human insulin: A rapidly absorbed analogue of human insulin. Diabetes 43(3):396–402, 1994.

28. Kelley, DE, et al.: Relative effects of calorie restriction and weight loss in non-insulin-dependent diabetes mellitus. J Clin Endocrinol Metab 77:1287–1293, 1993.

29. Koivisto, VA, and Felig, P: Alterations in insulin absorption and in blood glucose control associated with varying insulin injection sites in diabetic patients. Ann Intern Med 92:59–61, 1980.

30. Kolterman, OG, et al.: Receptor and postreceptor defects contribute to the insulin resistance in non-insulin-dependent diabetes mellitus. J Clin Invest 68:957–969,1981.

31. Kumar, O, Miller, L, et al.: Use of dexamethasone in treatment of insulin lipoatrophy. Diabetes 26(4):296–299, 1977.

32. Martin, AE, and Montgomery, PA: Acarbose: An α-glucosidase inhibitor. Am J Health-Syst Pharm 53:2277–2290, 1996.

33. McDonald, MJ: Postexercise late-onset hypoglycemia in insulin-dependent diabetic patients. Diabetes Care. 10:584–588, 1987.

34. Newman, B, et al.: Concordance for type 2 (non-insulin-dependent) diabetes mellitus in male twins. Diabetologia 30:763–738, 1987.

35. Nolte, MS: Insulin therapy in insulin-dependent (type 1) diabetes mellitus. Endocrinol Metab Clin North Amer 21:281, 1992.

36. Olefsky, JM, Kolterman, OG, et al.: Insulin action and resistance in obesity and noninsulin-dependent type II diabetes mellitus. Am J Physiol 243:E15–E30, 1982.

37. Reaven, GM, et al.: Nonketotic diabetes mellitus: Insulin deficiency or insulin resistance? Am J Med 60:80–88, 1976.

38. Rice, B, et al.: Effects of aerobic or resistance exercise and/or diet on glucose tolerance and plasma insulin levels in obese men. Diabetes Care 22(5):684–691, 1999.

39. Ryan, AS, Pratley, RE, et al.: Resistive training increases insulin action in postmenopausal women. J Gerontol 51A: M199–M205, 1996.

40. Scarlett, JA, et al.: Insulin treatment reverses the insulin resistance of type II diabetes mellitus. Diabetes Care 5:353–363, 1982.

41. Simonson, DC, et al.: Mechanism of improvement in glucose metabolism after chronic glyburide therapy. Diabetes 33: 838–845, 1984.

42. Smutok, MA, et al.: Effects of exercise training modality on glucose tolerance in men with abnormal glucose regulation. Int J Sports Med 15:283–289, 1994.

43. Smutok, MA, et al.: Aerobic versus strength training for risk factor intervention in middle-aged men at high risk for coronary heart disease. Metabolism 42:177–184, 1993.

44. Stumvoll, M, et al.: Metabolic effects of metformin in non-insulin-dependent diabetes mellitus. N Engl J Med 333: 550–554, 1995.

45. Turner, RC, et al.: Insulin deficiency and insulin resistance interaction in diabetes: Estimation of their relative contribution by feedback analysis from basal plasma insulin and glucose concentrations. Metabolism 28:1086–1096, 1979.

46. Wing, RR, et al.: Caloric restriction per se is a significant factor in improvements in glycemic control and insulin sensitivity during weight loss in obese NIDDM patients. Diabetes Care 17:30–36, 1994.

47. Yee, HS, and Fong, NT: A review of the safety and efficacy of acarbose in diabetes mellitus. Pharmacotherapy 16:792–805, 1996.

48. Zimmerman, BR: Sulfonylureas. Endocrinol Metab Clin N Amer 26:511–522, 1997.

49. Zimmet, PZ: Kelly West Lecture 1991: Challenges in diabetes epidemiology: From west to the rest. Diabetes Care 15:232–252, 1992.

50. Zimmet, PZ, et al.: Latent autoimmune diabetes mellitus in adults (LADA): The role of antibodies to glutamic acid decarboxylase in diagnosis and prediction of insulin dependency. Diabet Med 11:299–303, 1994.

Chapter Questions

1. Insulin is released from this type of pancreas cell after stimulation from a meal:
   A. Alpha
   B. Beta
   C. Delta
   D. Theta

2. Which of the following is not a cause of type 2 diabetes mellitus?
   A. Insulin deficiency
   B. Hypoglycemia
   C. Glucose intolerance
   D. Insulin resistance

3. Treatment for type 2 diabetes mellitus can include:
   A. Diet and exercise
   B. Oral hypoglycemic agents
   C. Insulin
   D. All of the above
   E. Only 2 of the above

4. An individual with type 1 diabetes mellitus should follow these guidelines when exercising:
   A. Eat carbohydrates during peak insulin levels.
   B. Monitor glucose in the morning and evening only.
   C. Refrain from contact sports.
   D. Exercise only in the early morning when glucose is high.

5. If stored at room temperature, insulin has a shelf-life of:
   A. 1 year
   B. 90 days
   C. 1 week
   D. 30 days

6. Which of the following is the recommended insulin injection site when exercising?
   A. Arms
   B. Thigh
   C. Abdomen
   D. Buttock

7. This type of insulin is usually injected 3–4 times a day to control for postmeal glucose elevations:
   A. NPH
   B. Lantus
   C. Lente
   D. Humalog

8. Which of the following is not a sign and symptom of ketoacidosis?
   A. Hypoglycemia
   B. Hyperglycemia
   C. Excessive urination
   D. Difficulty breathing

9. Which type of oral antidiabetic agent targets the enzyme of the intestinal mucosa to inhibit carbohydrate catabolism?
   A. Biguanides
   B. Meglitinides
   C. Alpha-glucosidase inhibitors
   D. Thiazolidinediones

10. What is the normal preprandial glucose value of whole blood?
    A. <100 mg/dL
    B. 6 percent
    C. <110 mg/dL
    D. <180 mg/dL

11. What is a desired HbA1c level?
    A. <12%
    B. <10%
    C. <8%
    D. <6%

12. Which of the following types of oral antidiabetic agent controls hypoglycemia at the muscle?
    A. Metformin
    B. Meglitinides
    C. Sulfonylureas
    D. Thiazolidinediones

6

Drugs for Cardiovascular Arrhythmias and Hypertension

Chapter Objectives

After reading this chapter, the student should have a working knowledge of the following concepts:

1 Some of the more notable athletes who have experienced cardiovascular problems and related complications, resulting in their death.

2 Possible reasons why cardiovascular arrhythmias and hypertension become more of a problem at the collegiate and professional levels

3 Examples of common cardiac arrhythmia conditions

4 Examples of common hypertension problems

5 Types of drugs used to control cardiac arrhythmias and hypertension problems

6 Side effects of drugs used to control cardiac arrhythmias and hypertension

7 Combined effects of drugs for cardiac arrhythmia and hypertension that can affect athletes

8 Signs of improper use or abuse of these drugs

Chapter Outline

Arrhythmias
    Class I
    Class II
    Class III
    Class IV
    Adverse Effects
    Antiarrhythmic Drug Interactions

Device Therapy
Hypertension
    Medications for Hypertension
    Adverse Effects
What to Tell the Athlete
Scenario from the Field

*O*ver the past 10 to 12 years great progress has been made in the control of cardiac arrhythmias and hypertensive problems. In 1990 the process for starting cardiopulmonary resuscitation (CPR) began with a "precordial thump"[20] Today it begins with early defibrillation. At that time one of the main medications used by physicians during cardiac emergencies was lidocaine to decrease premature ventricular contraction (PVC).[20] Today lidocaine is still used, but there are newer antiarrhythmics that may be used preferentially. Additionally, in the early 1990s there was an awakening of the sports medicine community regarding cardiac problems in athletes as a result of the untimely death of Loyola Marymount University (LMU) basketball player Hank Gathers. At the time of his death, Gathers was playing in a basketball game for LMU. The cause of his death was secondary to presumed hypertrophic cardiomyopathy. Other prominent athletes who have died from cardiac causes include basketball player "Pistol Pete" Maravich (abnormal coronary arteries), U.S. Olympic volleyball star Flo Hyman (ruptured aortic aneurysm associated with Marfan's syndrome), running advocate Jim Fixx (heart attack while running), and baseball pitcher Darryl Kile (atherosclerotic coronary artery disease). The athletic trainer must recognize the importance of broadening his or her knowledge base to include technical information, such as cardiovascular conditions, that affect the health and performance of the athlete. After the passing of Hank Gathers, the immediate care given by the athletic trainer was closely analyzed. Why did this unfortunate consequence occur? The inconsistency exhibited by Gathers in taking the proper amount of the prescribed medication at proper intervals was determined to be a contributing factor to his death. The findings from the Hank Gathers case gave athletic trainers the realization that they must help athletes to better understand the importance of following dosage regimens as prescribed. The athletic trainer must now see that a part of his or her role is to help keep athletes on track with their medication regimens, ensuring that dosing occurs in the appropriate amounts and at the proper times.

In the 1980s and 1990s little, if any, information regarding cardiac and hypertension problems in athletes was published. However, if one were to conduct a review of newspaper and sports magazine articles of those decades regarding cardiovascular disorders and sudden cardiac death in athletes, it would become apparent that many of these problems occurred in collegiate and professional sports settings. Based on current knowledge, it is not proper to state that younger players do not experience cardiovascular problems; it is more appropriate to say that these problems do not receive the same publicity as those in the older athlete. Some exercise physiologists and physicians suggest that younger athletes do not stress the cardiovascular system as much as college or professional athletes. For example, high-school athletes may participate in a number of different sports during the school year, with each sport imposing different cardiovascular demands. High-school athletes spend most of their practice time learning skills and strategies, which does not maximally stress the circulatory system, so their cardiovascular challenges are limited compared to those of college or professional athletes. Because a high-school athlete does not have maximal demands on the cardiovascular system, many potential cardiovascular problems typically go undiscovered until the athlete gets to the college, university, or professional level, where the focus of his or her training changes to the total fitness of the cardiovascular system. However, there are documented cases of high-school athletes collapsing during activity because of cardiovascular difficulty. The American College of Cardiology has developed a sports classification system (Table 6–1) so that physicians can recommend what types of sports an athlete with a cardiac condition may participate in safely. Each physician must make his or her own decisions for athletic participation based on the best interest of the athlete.

New information regarding gender differences in sudden cardiac death and arrhythmias suggests that each gender may be more susceptible to certain types of arrhythmic conditions. Women have a lower incidence of sudden cardiac death and men have a higher incidence of atrial fibrillation.[24] Additionally, the incidence of arrhythmias is increased in pregnant women. Wolbrette et al. reported that atrial fibrillation is generally more difficult to treat in women.[24]

Athletes can experience numerous types of cardiac and vascular problems. Because there are so many types of potential cardiovascular problems and medications, we cannot discuss all of them in this chapter. Franklin and Shepard provide a good review article for athletic trainers regarding many different cardiac problems experienced by athletes.[5]

The most prevalent treatable conditions in the athlete are cardiac arrhythmias and hypertension. In this chapter we first discuss the drugs used to treat cardiac arrhythmias, and then move on to drugs that could be prescribed for hypertension in the athlete.

*A*rrhythmias

Cardiac arrhythmia is defined in *Taber's Cyclopedic Medical Dictionary* as "Irregular heart action caused by physiological or pathological disturbances in the discharge of cardiac impulses from the sinoatrial node or their transmission through conductive tissue of the heart."[25] Cardiac arrhythmias (Table 6–2) can be a result of many different etiologies from severe electrolyte imbalances to hypertrophic cardiomyopathy and various other disease processes.[17]

Cardiac arrhythmias are not considered highly prevalent in the general population because only about 0.4 percent of people, mostly white men, experience atrial fibrillation.[7] This percentage increases slightly in older populations. Often the medications do not repair or correct the problem or disease process that is occurring in the abnormal heart, but instead control arrhythmias and assist the heart in maintaining a natural rhythm. In recent years, physicians have also controlled cardiac arrhythmias with device-based techniques such as implantable pacemakers or defibrillators.[8] For the athletic trainer, it would be wise to understand the implications of both treatment options because athletes with arrhythmias may present to the athletic trainer with either of these treatment plans.

Table 6–1

Classification of Sports (Based on Peak Dynamic and Static Components During Competition)

	A. Low Dynamic	B. Moderate Dynamic	C. High Dynamic
I. Low Static	Billiards Bowling Cricket Curling Golf Riflery	Baseball Softball Table tennis Tennis (doubles) Volleyball	Badminton Cross-country skiing (classic technique) Field hockey* Orienteering Race walking Racquetball Running (long distance) Soccer* Squash Tennis (singles)
II. Moderate Static	Archery Auto racing*† Diving*† Equestrian*† Motorcycling*† Running (sprint) Surfing*† Synchronized swimming†	Fencing Field events (jumping) Figure skating* Football (American)* Rodeoing*† Rugby* Swimming Team handball	Basketball* Ice hockey* Cross-country skiing (skating technique) Football (Australian rules)* Lacrosse*
III. High Static	Bobsledding*† Field events (throwing) Gymnastics*† Karate/judo* Luge*† Sailing Rock climbing*† Waterskiing*† Weight lifting*† Windsurfing*†	Body building*† Downhill skiing*† Wrestling*	Boxing* Canoeing/kayaking Cycling*† Decathlon Rowing Speed skating

*Danger of bodily collision.
†Increased risk if syncope occurs.
Source: Mitchell, JH, et al.: Classification of sports. JACC, 24:845, 1994, with permission.

Interestingly, arrhythmias may be present and then disappear for unknown reasons.[26] This phenomenon can certainly cause problems for the active athlete and the healthcare provider. Arrhythmias can result in syncope, which can be fatal in certain sports such as diving, downhill skiing, and gymnastics. For athletes participating in sports in which a sudden loss of consciousness can result in death, closely monitored drug therapy becomes more significant. Additionally, certain illegal drugs such as cocaine can also cause arrhythmias and result in death, as in the case of in Maryland basketball player and Boston Celtic draftee Len Bias.

Zipes recommends that all athletes with a diagnosed arrhythmia who are deemed fit to participate in athletics should be reevaluated after they have participated in a conditioning program for their sport to determine if any conditioning effects are noted in the athlete's arrhythmia.[26] Athletic trainers should also be vigilant in encouraging the athlete to maintain compliance in taking their prescribed medication. Too often athletes think that they are feeling better or want to reduce an adverse effect of a drug by discontinuing its use, leading to potentially lethal consequences.

To understand which drugs are used in differing situations, a basic understanding of the different types of cardiac arrhythmias is necessary. Some of these are benign changes in cardiac rhythm requiring no treatment. Others are life threatening.

Irregular heart rhythms are common in the developing hearts of children and adolescents. Sinus arrhythmia, the most common type, produces changes in heart rate with normal respiration. It requires no treatment.

Irregular beats can occur in the atria or atrioventricular junction (premature atrial contraction [PACs]) or supraventricular premature beats) or from the ventricle (PVCs).

Table 6–2	
Common Forms of Arrhythmias	
Classification	**Characteristic Rhythm**
Sinus Arrhythmias	
Sinus tachycardia	>100 beats/min
Sinus bradycardia	<60 beats/min
Sick sinus syndrome	Severe bradycardia (<50 beats/min); periods of sinus arrest
Supraventricular Arrhythmias	
Atrial fibrillation and flutter	Atrial rate >300 beats/min
Atrial tachycardia	Atrial rate >140–200 beats/min
Premature atrial contractions	Variable
Atrioventricular Junctional Arrhythmias	
Junctional rhythm	40–55 beats/min
Junctional tachycardia	100–200 beats/min
Conduction Disturbances	
Atrioventricular block	Variable
Bundle branch block	Variable
Fascicular block	Variable
Ventricular Arrhythmias	
Premature ventricular contractions	Variable
Ventricular tachycardia	140–200 beats/min
Ventricular fibrillation	Irregular, totally uncoordinated rhythm

Source: Ciccone, CD: Pharmacology in Rehabilitation, ed 3. FA Davis, Philadelphia, 2002. Used with permission.

The diagnosis of these rhythms cannot be made by simple auscultation; it requires an electrocardiogram.

Premature atrial contractions are usually of little hemodynamic significance and often resolve spontaneously or require no treatment. Occasionally they become more common with caffeine or sympathomimetic medications (e.g, cold-care preparations). Rarely are they associated with structural heart abnormalities. At times, irregular atrial rhythms such as atrial flutter or atrial fibrillation occur in older individuals and may require treatment.

Abnormal rhythms in the ventricles are also common. Some medication treatments may actually worsen ventricular ectopy. Premature ventricular contractions increase with age and may be benign in several instances: (1) isolated contractions, (2) when they are uniform and associated with a normal corrected QT interval, (3) when the cardiac physical examination is normal, (4) when the family history is negative for sudden cardiac death, and (5) when they disappear with exercise.[11] A person may feel the heart pound or beat when these extra beats occur. This sensation does not worsen the prognosis, and reassurance can be given.

Implications for Activity

Athletes with arrhythmias who have been cleared for athletic participation could still have complications. The use of medications to control the arrhythmia must be taken in the proper dosages, at the correct time(s), and will produce some adverse effects. Additionally, the athlete may be taking other over-the-counter (OTC) drugs or supplements that could affect the overall efficacy of the anti-arrhythmic drug. This could lead to complications or even death if not monitored by the treating physician. Athletic trainers should also be vigilant in encouraging athletes to maintain compliance in taking their prescribed medication.

If the rhythm is determined to be significant by cardiac evaluation and appropriate studies, the cardiologist may recommend antiarrhythmic medication.

The drugs discussed in this chapter as being indicated for cardiac arrhythmias often do not repair cardiac tissue that has fallen into a diseased state, but instead alter the dysfunctional rhythm and allow the heart an improved functional capacity. The medications prescribed for arrhythmia are divided into four basic classifications.

Class I   Sodium channel blockers
Class II   β-adrenergic blockers
Class III   Potassium channel blockers
Class IV   Calcium channel blockers

Class I

The sodium channel-blocking drugs are typically divided into three subclassifications. However, for the athletic trainer, it is more important to understand the mechanism of action of this entire classification rather than the technical aspects of how each subclass alters the heart rhythm. The sodium channel blockers inhibit sodium channel activity, which, in turn, retards cell membrane excitability. For a more detailed explanation of the Class I arrhythmic medications, one can read Ciccone or Smith and Reynard.[4,22]

Class II

Beta-adrenergic blocking agents make up this class of drugs that work to control arrhythmias by antagonizing the stimulation of the heart via the sympathetic system. The beta blockers were the first antiarrhythmic drugs produced to assist people with tachycardia. Originally, when cardiac responses were determined, they were divided into the "alpha effects," which were excitatory in nature, and the "beta effects," which were inhibitory in nature. The beta blockers come by their name because of their inhibitory role in the control of arrhythmias.

The mechanism of action of these drugs is not clear, but it may involve potassium and sodium exchange. In any event, they stabilize cell membrane excitability to control heart rhythm.

Beta blockers have been used as performance-enhancing aids to control heart rhythm, breathing, and muscular movement in biathlons, riflery, archery, shooting, and synchronized swimming. These agents are banned as performance aids, and the athlete must be aware of the regulations of the relevant sports organizations' governing bodies.

When athletes use beta blockers, they must understand that they may have difficulty in achieving their maximal heart rate. This can affect performance and endurance. Athletes who take beta blockers need to understand the ramifications of reducing their maximum heart rate, which is what happens when they take these drugs as prescribed. Beta blockers do not allow the athlete's heart rate to reach maximum, so the athlete must use a perceived exertion protocol (such as that utilized in the graded treadmill test in exercise physiology laboratories.)

Class III

The drugs in this classification direct their effect by delaying repolarization. They do this by blocking the potassium channels of the cardiac muscle. These drugs may also have an effect on the sympathetic control of the heart rhythm.

Class IV

The drugs in this classification control heart rhythm by slowing the calcium activity of the sinus and atrioventricular (AV) nodes. These drugs slow conduction velocity, mainly at the AV node, and thus slow the heart rate.

Adverse Effects

The recognized and expected adverse effects of this class of drugs are lethargy, fatigue, bradycardia, hypotension (orthostatic), and sometimes a feeling of cold in the extremities. Some people experience additional adverse effects such as rashes, pruritus, headache, nausea, diarrhea, swelling, behavioral disturbances, disorientation, and other problems. If the athlete is experiencing any of these additional adverse effects, he or she should consult his or her physician immediately. Despite their purpose—reducing arrhythmia—one of the most common adverse effects of the anti arrhythmic drugs is an increase in rhythm disturbances. Because they work to control a single type of arrhythmic activity, these drugs can result in other types of cardiac arrhythmias.[8]

Antiarrhythmic Drug Interactions

It appears that there are numerous drug interactions involving antiarrhythmic drugs, and the physician should discuss with the athlete and athletic trainer any drug interactions that can occur. We have organized a short table of drug interactions (Table 6–3) so that the athletic trainer can get an idea of the interaction possibilities with this class of drugs.

Device Therapy

Pacemakers were first implanted in 1958 and since that time have undergone dramatic improvements in design

Table 6–3

Examples of Antiarrhythmic Drug Interactions

Antiarrhythmic Drug (Trade Name)	Combined with	Result
Flecainide (Tambocor)	Cigarette smoking	Decreased plasma concentration of flecainide
	Cimetidine (Tagamet), SSRIs (Prozac, Paxil)	Increased plasma concentration of flecainide
Propafenone (Rythmol)	Cimetidine (Tagamet), SSRIs (Prozac, Paxil)	Increase in propafenone concentration

Source: Information collated from Trujillo, TC, and Nolan, PE: Antiarrhythmic agents: Drug interactions of clinical significance. Drug Safety 23:509–532, 2000.

and function. Implantable cardioverter defibrillators (ICDs) were first used in 1980 to control life-threatening ventricular arrhythmias. These, too, have progressed in design and function since inception. In recent years a number of clinical trials were completed demonstrating the effectiveness of both types of devices for control of cardiac arrhythmias.[2,10,21] The athletic trainer should be aware of the types of device therapy available to control cardiac arrhythmias and any precautions to follow to make sure that the athlete is safe as he or she participates in a sport.

The purposes of these devices are to detect the heart rhythm and treat abnormalities. They can be set to treat bradycardia, tachycardia, or ventricular fibrillation by either pacing or synchronized cardioversion.[9] Implantation can be performed transvenously and no longer requires hospitalization or open-heart surgery. The use of ICDs to prevent sudden cardiac death is currently being evaluated.[16]

The ICD is not a common treatment in competitive athletics. In the rare case when an athlete requires an ICD, clearance for participation should be given by the prescribing cardiac electrophysiologist. The athletic trainer will want to discuss with the athlete's physician any special precautions or arrangements that should be made to ensure the safety of the athlete.

*H*ypertension

Systemic hypertension is the most common cardiovascular condition observed in competitive athletes.[14] For an adult athlete to be diagnosed with hypertension, he or she must have his or her blood pressure measured by sphygmomanometry on at least three separate occasions (Table 6–4). On all three occasions, the systolic readings must be above 140 mm Hg.[25]

Internet Resource Box

The American Society of Hypertension has a very user-friendly Website that can provide the athletic trainer with some practical information to assist the athlete who has recently been diagnosed with hypertension:
www.ash-us.org

The American Society of Hypertension (ASH) estimates that about 24 percent of the population suffers from hypertension, with women comprising slightly more than 50 percent of the total. The ASH also estimates that over 90 percent of the population suffers from hypertension without an identified cause, a condition also known as "essential hypertension."[4] In contrast, there is also secondary hypertension, which does have an underlying or diagnosable cause. It develops in fewer than 5 percent of physically active patients and is most commonly related to vascular or parenchymal renal disease.

Blood pressure abnormalities can be subdivided into multiple classifications as outlined in Table 6–5.[9]

Normal blood pressure measurements carry the recommendation of allowing full sports participation if there is no concomitant heart disease.

Prehypertensive measurements mean that the physician is going to have to make a decision based on the signs and symptoms exhibited. In some situations the athlete could have an antihypertensive medication prescribed based on the type of sport he or she is participating in and the intensity of participation. However, if the physician determines the intensity of the sport to be low or the athlete does not have severe symptoms, the athlete may not be required to take any medication to continue participation. There is evidence that exercise can assist with the reduction of mild hypertension, and the athlete may be exercising per his or her physician's orders.

Table 6–4

Guidelines for Measurement of Blood Pressure

Posture

Blood pressure obtained in the sitting position is recommended. The subject should sit quietly for 5 minutes, with the back supported and the arm supported at the level of the heart, before recording blood pressure.

Circumstances

- No caffeine during the hour preceding the reading
- No smoking for 30 minutes preceding the reading
- A quiet, warm setting

Equipment

- Cuff size
- The bladder should encircle and cover two-thirds of the length of the arm; if it does not, place the bladder over the brachial artery.
- If bladder is too short, misleadingly high readings may result

Manometer

- Aneroid gauges should be calibrated every 6 mo against mercury manometer

Technique

- Number of readings: On each occasion, take at least two readings, separated by as much time as practical. If readings vary by >5 mm Hg, take additional readings until two consecutive readings are close.
- If the initial values are elevated, obtain two other sets of readings at least 1 week apart.
- Initially, take pressure in both arms; if the pressures differ, use the arm with the higher pressure.
- If the arm pressure is elevated, take the pressure in one leg (particularly in patients <30 yrs old).

Performance

- Inflate the bladder quickly to a pressure 20 mm Hg above the systolic pressure, as recognized by disappearance of the radial pulse.
- Deflate the bladder 3 mm Hg/s.
- Record the Korotkoff phase V (disappearance), except in children, in whom use of phase IV (muffling) may be preferable when disappearance of the sounds is not perceived.
- If the Korotkoff sounds are weak, have the patient raise the arm and open and close the hand 5 to 10 times, and then reinflate the bladder quickly.

Recordings

- Record blood pressure, patient position, and arm and cuff size.

Reproduced with permission from Kaplan et al.: Task Force 4, 26th Bethesda Conference, J Am Coll Cardiol 1994;24:845–899, 1994.

Hypertension, once diagnosed by a physician, is further subdivided into two stages:

- Stage 1 hypertension should be monitored closely by the athlete and the athletic trainer. Be sure to check with the athlete's physician regularly to report any changes in blood pressure measurements in the hypertensive athlete.
- Depending on the physician's examination, testing, and final decision, the athlete with Stage 2 hypertension could be restricted from sports participation requiring a high dynamic output. Once the athlete is on medication and has the hypertension under control, the physician may allow him or her to participate in sports requiring high static capabilities. If the athlete is determined to participate in sports, the athletic trainer must be vigilant in monitoring his or her compliance in taking the medication (Table 6–5).

The athletic trainer or physician should obtain a clinical history of the athlete. This should include inquiring about behaviors that affect blood pressure, such as the use of smoking or chewing tobacco, alcohol or drugs (including OTC stimulants such as caffeine and cold-care medication, diet pills, cocaine, and anabolic steroids), and diet. Specific questions regarding use of salt and intake of high-sodium and high-fat foods should be determined. Additionally, ask the athlete about the use of dietary supplements, particularly ma huang and other supplements containing any amount of ephedra. Increased stress, although difficult to quantify, increases circulating catecholamines and may also be a precursor to high blood pressure.

Implications for Activity

For some athletes, the physician may encourage exercise to help reduce mild hypertension. If the physician makes this decision, the athletic trainer must monitor the athlete's blood pressure on a daily basis. The athletic trainer has to follow the directives of the physician regarding when to reduce the athlete's activity level based on increased blood pressure. Keeping a log of the athlete's blood pressure readings and reporting them to the physician will facilitate the athlete's continuing participation in sports.

Nondrug treatment should be initiated after the athlete has been diagnosed with hypertension. These methods include changing the diet to include less processed food and more fruits, vegetables, and fiber. Regular aerobic exercise and weight loss can improve lifestyle and con-

Table 6–5

Classification of Blood Pressure		
Class	Systolic Blood Pressure (mm Hg)	Diastolic Blood Pressure (mm Hg)
Normal	<120	<80
Prehypertension	120–139	80–89
Hypertension		
Stage 1	140–159	90–99
Stage 2	≥160	≥100

Source: United States Department of Health and Human Services, Joint National Committee on Prevention, Detection, Evaluation, and Treatment of High Blood Pressure. Seventh Report. 2003.

tribute to lower blood pressure. Limiting alcohol use and managing stress by biofeedback or relaxation techniques is also recommended.

▓ Medications for Hypertension

There are several "families" of antihypertensive medications that lower blood pressure. Depending on the clinical case, one family of medication may be more suitable than another. The physician may also elect to use a combination of medications to control hypertension.[12]

Diuretics are drugs with a net effect of promoting salt and water loss, which decreases systemic vascular pressure. This is accomplished by reducing sodium chloride and water reabsorption.

Calcium channel blockers are vasodilators because they block the movement of calcium into smooth muscle cells. Vasodilators inhibit the contractile mechanism of the cells. The blood vessels become less constricted, allowing uninhibited blood flow.

Angiotensin-converting enzyme (ACE) inhibitors act on the renin-angiotensin system. When blood pressure falls, renin is released from the kidneys and joins with angiotensinogen enzyme, released by the liver, to become angiotensin I. A converting enzyme creates angiotensin II, a very potent vasoconstrictor, which results in increased blood pressure. To inhibit this type of blood pressure increase, ACE inhibitors prevent conversion of angiotensin I to angiotensin II.

The newest entrants in this renin-angiotensin strategy are the angiotensin II blockers. These drugs block the angiotensin II receptors at the cellular level, thus stopping the angiotensin II from causing an increase in blood pressure.[15]

Beta blockers are medications that inhibit sympathetic activity in the body. They reduce blood pressure by decreasing heart rate, the force of myocardial contraction, and cardiac output. This concomitantly reduces peripheral vascular resistance.

Alpha blockers block alpha-1 adrenergic receptors in the smooth muscles of the peripheral vasculature, which leads to vasodilation and lowering of blood pressure.[3,6]

Table 6–6 provides an overview of the general categories of activity that an athlete with hypertension might be able to participate in while being monitored by the physician and athletic trainer. It should always be remembered that athletes with hypertension must be checked and rechecked regularly to be sure their medication is controlling their known cardiovascular problem.

▓ Adverse Effects

There are potential adverse effects with all of these classes of antihypertensive medications. Diuretics may lead to fluid depletion, which in turn leads to dehydration, orthostatic hypotension, or electrolyte imbalances. Orthostatic hypotension can be the result of fluid depletion, so the athletic trainer should continually remind athletes taking diuretics—and, for that matter, all athletes—to rehydrate when losing a great deal of water volume during activity. ACE inhibitors often cause an annoying dry cough, which may lead to their discontinuance. Beta blockers may significantly decrease heart rate, leading to bradycardia, dizziness, or fatigue. Another common adverse effect is bronchoconstriction. Therefore beta blockers should be used with caution in asthmatics. Alpha blockers can cause reflex tachycardia or orthostatic hypotension.

Table 6–6	

Hypertension in the Athlete/Active Population

Participation in Athletics

Controlled blood pressure is important because of the increase in pressure resulting from all types of exercise.

Blood Pressure	Restriction Recommendations
High normal	No restrictions
Controlled	
Mild to moderate	Limit isometric training or sports in athletes with end-organ damage
	Limit to low-intensity dynamic sports
	No isometric activity
Uncontrolled	
Mild to moderate	Limit to low-intensity dynamic sports
	No isometric activity
Severe	
No end-organ damage	Limit to low-intensity dynamic sports
Secondary hypertension (renal origin)	Limit to low-intensity dynamic sports
	(collision sports could result in further kidney damage)

Source: Joint National Committee on Prevention, Detection, Evaluation, and Treatment of High Blood Pressure. Seventh report. United States Department of Health and Human Services. NIH Publication No. 03-5233, May 2003.

The story of Hank Gathers is much like the above situation. Hank Gathers suffered from an abnormal heart rate and was put on medication to control the heart rhythm. He had been experimenting with his medication dosage because the dosage prescribed by his physician was causing lethargy and other adverse effects that he did not like and that prevented him, he thought, from performing at his top level. In the video of his last basketball game, it is apparent that he was playing with a decreased cardiac output, as evidenced by his stumbling and weaving as he tried to run down the basketball court. His last minutes played out in severe circulatory distress as he collapsed in the middle of the court. Unfortunately, neither the athletic trainer who was summoned nor the emergency services provided could save his life.

What to Tell the Athlete

The athletic trainer should be supportive of the athlete, encouraging him or her to keep follow-up physician visits to check status or repeat regular blood work. Here are some tips for the athletic trainer when educating the athlete about these drugs:

▪ The athlete should not modify dosing recommendations by taking only half of the prescribed dose or taking a full dose every other day to reduce potential adverse effects

▪ The athletic trainer should encourage the athlete to report any adverse effects to the physician immediately.

▪ The athlete must be cautioned not to take some type of natural supplement or other drug for an energy boost that interferes with the prescribed medication.

▪ The athlete needs to understand that he or she must take the medication as directed and should not be embarrassed or uncomfortable that he or she needs this type of therapy.

Scenario from the Field

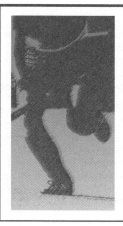

A physician told a high-school football player with a diagnosis of tachycardia that when he felt his heart rate getting too high, he should sit out until his heart rate returned to normal. Not all physicians would offer this exact advice to the player, but this physician obviously did not feel that the player's condition warranted medication or further intervention. However, it is frightening that a player with a condition such as tachycardia would be allowed to monitor his own physical symptoms and make the determination of whether he should continue to participate. It would be surprising if the athlete did not stop participation when his heart rate was abnormal and suffered severe consequences.

Discussion Topics

- How do cardiac arrhythmias differ from hypertension?

- What are some of the adverse effects that an athletic trainer should look for when an athlete is taking a cardiovascular medication?

- Why would an athlete take a cardiovascular medication for ergogenic purposes?

Chapter Review

- Cardiovascular risks are as much part of the athlete trainer's concerns as are other disorders the athlete may experience.

- There are numerous cardiovascular conditions that the athlete might experience. The two most common types are arrhythmias and hypertension.

- Cardiac arrhythmia is generally defined as an irregular heartbeat.

- Cardiac arrhythmias can have a number of etiologies, from genetic predisposition to nutritional factors.

- Antiarrhythmic medications, like any other drugs, can produce adverse effects. Additionally, this class of drug can produce arrhythmic activities as an adverse effect.

- Antiarrhythmic medications are classified into four basic categories: sodium channel blockers, beta-adrenergic blockers, drugs that prolong repolarization, and calcium channel blockers.

- Implantable devices are becoming more common for the treatment of cardiovascular arrhythmias.

- Hypertension can also be a problem experienced by competitive athletes.

- Hypertension can be classified into two stages: stage 1 (physician oversight) and stage 2 (physician monitoring and prescription medication).

- Hypertension medications include diuretics, calcium channel blockers, ACE inhibitors, angiotensin II blockers, beta blockers, and alpha blockers.

- The adverse effects associated with medications for hypertension are varied and sometimes individual to the athlete.

References

1. American College of Cardiology: 26th Bethesda Conference: Recommendations for determining eligibility for competition in athletes with cardiovascular abnormalities. J Am Coll Cardiol 24:844, 1994.
2. Atle, JL, and Bernstein, AD: Cardiac rhythm management devices: Part 1. Anesthesiology 95:1265, 2001.
3. Cauffield, JS et al.: Alpha blockers: A reassessment of their role in therapy. Am Fam Physician 54:263, 1996
4. Ciccone, CD: Pharmacology in Rehabilitation, ed 3. FA Davis, Philadelphia, 2002, p 303.

5. Franklin, BA, and Shephard, RJ: Avoiding repeat cardiac events. Phys Sportsmed 28:31, 2000.

6. Frishman, WH, and Kotob, F: Alpha-adrenergic blocking drugs in clinical medicine. J Clin Pharmacol 39:7, 1999.

7. Fuster, V, et al.: ACC/AHA/ESC guidelines for the management of patients with atrial fibrillation: Executive summary. J Am Coll Cardiol, 38:1231, 2001.

8. Gold, MR, and Josephson, ME: Cardiac arrhythmia: current therapy. Hospital Practice 34:27, 1999.

9. Groh, WJ, et al.: Advances in the treatment of arrhythmias: Implantable cardioverter-defibrillators. Am Fam Phys 57:297, 1998.

10. Gregoratos, G, et al: ACC/AHA guidelines for implantation of cardiac pacemakers and antiarrhythmia devices: A report of the American College of Cardiology/American Heart Association Task Force on practice guidelines (Committee on pacemaker implantation). J Am Coll Cardiol 5:1175, 1998.

11. Gutgesell, HP, Barst, RJ, Humes, RA, et al.: Common cardiovascular problems in the young, part I: Murmurs, chest pain, syncope, and irregular rhythms. Am Fam Phys 56:1825, 1997.

12. Houston, MC: Alpha 1-blocker combination therapy for hypertension. Postgrad Med 104:167, 1998.

13. Joint National Committee on Prevention, Detection, Evaluation, and Treatment of High Blood Pressure. Seventh report. U.S. Dept. of Health and Human Services. NIH Publication No. 03-5233, May 2003.

14. Kaplan, NM, et al.: Systemic hypertension. J Am Coll Cardiol 24:845, 1994.

15. Kaplan, NM: Angiotensin II receptor antagonists in the treatment of hypertension. Am Fam Physician 60:1185, 1999.

16. Kusumoto, FM, and Goldschlager, N: Device therapy for cardiac arrhythmias. JAMA 287:1848, 2002.

17. Maron, B. Hypertrophic cardiomyopathy. Phys Sportsmed 30(1):19, 2002.

18. Mitchell, JH, et al.: Classification of sports. J Am Coll Cardiol 24:845, 1994.

19. Niedfeldt, MW: Managing hypertension in athletes and physically active patients. Am Fam Physician 66(3):445, 2002.

20. Rund, DA: Cardiac Arrest. Phys Sportsmed 18(3):97, 1990.

21. Sanders, GD, et al: Potential cost effectiveness of prophylactic use of the implantable cardioverter defibrillator or amiodarone after myocardial infarction. Ann Intern Med 135:870, 2001.

22. Smith, CM, and Reynard, AM: Essentials of Pharmacology. WB Saunders Co., Philadelphia, 1995, p 256.

23. Trujillo, TC, and Nolan, PC: Antiarrhythmic agents: drug interactions of clinical significance. Drug Safety 23:509, 2000.

24. Wolbrette, D, et al: Gender differences in arrhythmias. Clin Cardiol 25:49, 2002.

25. Venes, D (ed.): Taber's Cyclopedic Medical Dictionary. FA Davis, Philadelphia, 2001.

26. Zipes, DP, and Garson, A: Arrhythmias. J Am Coll Cardiol 24:845, 1994.

Chapter Questions

1. It is possible for an athlete taking medication for a cardiac arrhythmia to experience increased arrhythmias.

   True   False

2. How many categories of antiarrhythmia drugs were discussed in this chapter?
   A. 1
   B. 2
   C. 3
   D. 4

3. Beta blocker medication can be prescribed by a physician for which of the following disorders?
   A. Hypertension and inflammation
   B. Arrhythmias and balance disorders
   C. Hypertension and arrhythmias
   D. Inflammation and arrhythmias

4. Implantable devices are now more commonly used to control which disorder?
   A. Cardiac arrhythmias
   B. Respiratory dysfunction
   C. Balance disorders
   D. Joint inflammation

5. Hypertension is divided into multiple categories in this chapter. Which activity is contraindicated in *all* categories?
   A. Collision sports
   B. Isotonics
   C. Plyometrics
   D. Isometrics

6. Athletes who are fit and competing at high levels will not experience hypertension.

   True   False

7. An athlete must be referred to a physician when the athlete's blood pressure reading reaches which of the following measurements:
   A. 135/85
   B. 140/90
   C. 120/80
   D. 125/85

8. Diuretics are usually prescribed by a physician for which of the following disorders?
   A. Hypertension
   B. Inflammation
   C. Weight loss
   D. Asthma

9. Sinus tachycardia is generally defined as which of the following:
   A. Greater than 80 beats per minute
   B. Greater than 90 beats per minute
   C. Greater than 100 beats per minute
   D. Greater than 200 beats per minute

10. Sinus bradycardia is generally defined as which of the following?
    A. Less than 70 beats per minute
    B. Less than 60 beats per minute
    C. Less than 50 beats per minute
    D. Less than 40 beats per minute

7 *Respiratory Drugs*

Chapter Objectives

After reading this chapter, the student will:

1 Understand the general mechanisms whereby respiratory drugs affect breathing difficulties.
2 Understand the pathology, signs, and symptoms of asthma.
3 Understand the different types of asthma and bronchoconstriction.
4 Understand the general classes of medications used in treating the respiratory conditions most commonly associated with athletic activities.
5 Understand the difference between medications that promote bronchodilation and those that affect respiratory inflammation.
6 Understand the different types of drugs used to treat the common cold and allergic conditions.

Chapter Outline

*A*thletic trainers and athletes can both benefit from a comprehensive understanding of the medications used to treat conditions affecting the respiratory system. The athletic trainer and, to some extent, the affected athlete need to be aware of drug classes and their actions for a variety of reasons. Some of the drugs discussed in this chapter are banned for use during competition by organizations such as the International Olympic Committee and the National Collegiate Athletic Association. In addition, the athletic trainer will probably have to answer questions, provide suggestions, and dispel myths associated with the pharmacological treatment of conditions such as asthma, allergies, and the common cold. This chapter provides basic information about the chemical receptors activated by drugs used to treat respiratory conditions. Additionally, it discusses many of the drugs used for the treatment of specific conditions affecting the respiratory system.

Respiration and Ventilation

The human respiratory system has two primary functions: cellular respiration and ventilation. Cellular respiration refers to the exchange of gases at the cellular level within the alveoli in the lungs. Ventilation refers to the movement of air in and out of the lungs through a series of air passages. The structures of the respiratory system involved in ventilation include the: nose, mouth, trachea, bronchial tree, and diaphragm.

The upper portion of the respiratory system is mainly responsible for conditioning inhaled air from the environment. To maintain normal ventilatory function, it is critical that the upper respiratory system adjust the temperature and humidify the inhaled air, as well as provide filtration of the contaminants in the ambient air. These functions ensure that inhaled particulate matter from the environment does not pass through and damage the lungs. Filtration of inspired air occurs mainly as the inhaled air passes over the mucus-lined epithelium of the trachea. The branches of the bronchial tree are lined with smooth muscle, which adjusts the constriction and dilation of the airways in response to the needs of the body. For example, if exercise becomes intense, the bronchial tree dilates to allow more air to pass into the lungs.

There are times when this physiological function is inhibited in the athlete and some type of drug therapy is necessary for the athlete to perform at an unrestricted level. The drugs discussed in this chapter all affect the movement of air through the respiratory system via the receptors on the related tissues.

■ Respiratory System Receptors and Functions

As discussed in Chapter 2, drugs work through their actions on chemical receptors located in various tissues. In most cases, the goal of using a drug is to affect the target tissue with little or no effect on tissues unrelated to the condition for which the drug is being used. In the respiratory system, receptor specificity is a very important issue and has prompted continued development in many of the agents discussed in this chapter.

One of the major systems regulating the respiratory system is the autonomic nervous system. A main function of the autonomic nervous system is to regulate smooth muscle tone in the respiratory system and thereby maintain the balance between bronchoconstriction and bronchodilation. Two significant neurotransmitters mediate the action of the autonomic nervous system: acetylcholine and norepinephrine. Specific receptors for each of these neurotransmitters—cholinergic receptors for acetylcholine and adrenergic receptors for norepinephrine—are located at the postsynaptic terminals of the neurons through the autonomic nervous system.

The cholinergic receptors are subdivided in to muscarinic and nicotinic types. Medications that block the activity of the cholinergic receptors (anticholinergics) are used in the treatment of allergies, colds, and some chronic obstructive pulmonary diseases. In general, anticholinergics cause decreased salivation, dry mouth, and gastric activity.

Adrenergic receptors are also divided into two subtypes: alpha and beta. Both of these subtypes are further subdivided into two groups: alpha-1 and alpha-2 and beta-1 and beta-2. Adrenergic receptors vary in their effects on a continuum from relaxation to excitation. In general, the alpha-1 and beta-1 receptors excite tissues and the alpha-2 and beta-2 receptors relax tissues.[10]

The alpha receptors, alpha-1 and alpha-2, are located in different tissues of the body. The alpha-receptors are located primarily in peripheral blood vessels and cause vasodilation. The alpha-2 receptors are considered autoreceptors and have a small role in the regulation of respiratory function. The alpha-1 receptors are not discussed in this chapter in as much detail as the beta-2 receptors because they have less of an effect on athletes with respiratory problems.

In contrast to the alpha receptors, the beta receptors, specifically the beta-2 receptors, are critical in the regulation of respiratory function. The division of the beta-adrenergic receptors is based on their location and function. Beta-1 receptors, located in cardiac muscle, increase the rate and strength of heart contraction, and beta-2 receptors are located in the smooth muscles of the respiratory tract. The concentration of the beta-2 receptors varies according to the airway size, with the highest concentration found at the smallest airways at the end of the system.[10] Therefore, in this chapter we focus on the drugs that effect the beta-2 receptors.

Histamine is an endogenous chemical that plays a major role in regulating localized inflammation. The receptors activated by histamine affect the regulation of physiological functions such as gastric function, nerve activation, and the inflammatory process. Three subtypes of histamine receptors are found in the body: H1, H2, and H3. However, only H1 and H2 are targeted by specific drug types. In general, activation of these receptors by histamine can cause increased capillary permeability, increased capillary dilation, itching, smooth muscle constriction, and pain.[10]

The H1 receptors are found on smooth muscle and nerve endings. Specific activation of these receptors causes allergic reactions, inflammation, bronchoconstriction, increased mucus secretions, and nasal congestion. It is the H1 receptors that are targeted by classic antihistamine medications. H2 receptors are located in the gastrointestinal tract and assist in the regulation of stomach acid regulation. (This topic is discussed in Chapter 8.) With this general background on the structure and function of the respiratory system, we can proceed to the discussion of specific respiratory disorders.

Asthma

Millions of people in the United States have asthma, and billions of dollars are spent annually on their care. Asthma is a condition of the respiratory system involving narrowing (bronchoconstriction) and inflammation of the small air passages of the lower respiratory system. Not only is asthma a serious condition affecting the general health of people, but it also affects their ability to be physically active and participate in sports at maximal levels.

Technically, asthma, exercise-induced asthma (EIA), and exercise-induced bronchoconstriction (EIB) are separate conditions and are treated differently. True asthma is characterized by both bronchoconstriction and inflammation in the respiratory tract. Triggers that irritate the airways cause an asthma attack, now referred to as an exacerbation. Some athletes may have triggers such as chemicals or air pollutants that, when breathed into the lower respiratory system, start the inflammatory cascade of events. When asthma is triggered by exercise, it is classified as EIA. Unfortunately, exercise triggers symptoms in some people. The increased airflow into the lungs from the physiologic demands of exercise irritates the airway, initiating an inflammatory process in the airways. Exercise is a trigger for approximately 80 to 90 percent of individuals with asthma.[3] Those with EIA must have excellent control of their underlying asthma to be able to prevent asthma exacerbations during physical activity.

EIB without active inflammation is technically not exercise-induced asthma because the bronchoconstriction and inflammatory components are not both present, and therefore it is classified as EIB. It occurs in approximately 11 percent of individuals who do not have asthma,[3] and its occurrence may be as high as 50 percent in elite athletes.[11]

As mentioned earlier, acute asthma attacks involve both an inflammatory and a bronchoconstriction component. The inflammatory process initiates increased mucus production along the airway lining and bronchoconstriction results from contraction of the smooth muscles of the airways.

In an asthmatic reaction, the most significant event that occurs as a result of the inflammatory response is the increase in mucus production by the body. This is a protective mechanism used by the body to coat the airway and protect it from exposure to the incoming irritant. Under normal circumstances, this is a good protective approach adopted by the body, which produces a thick, sticky substance and spreads it over the sensitive tissues of the lower respiratory system to limit tissue damage from the irritant.

Obviously, however, this can become problematic if the source of irritation is not decreased or removed and mucus production continues in individuals who are sensitive to that particular irritant. For example, some people can be exposed to a smoke-filled environment for an extended period of time and never have an asthma exacerbation. On the other hand, for some people, a brief exposure to the same environment may be significant enough to start the cascade of events that is an asthma exacerbation. In these individuals, if the system continues to be irritated, the airways become excessively coated with mucus, resulting in airflow resistance.

Another mechanism used by the body to protect the airway from exposure to an irritant is to simply constrict the size of the airway. Like mucus coating the airway, this is also an effective protective mechanism by the body. However, excessive bronchoconstriction can also be problematic to the athlete because of the dramatic decrease in the volume of air that can be exchanged between the lungs and the outside environment. Both of these protective mechanisms result in increased respiratory effort.

The classic signs associated with an acute asthma exacerbation are shortness of breath and wheezing after exercise. However, care must be exercised not to overemphasize the presence or absence of wheezing in determining if a person is having an acute asthma exacerbation. Other signs and symptoms, such as a cough, headache, stomach cramps, pain or tightness in the chest, and nausea can also indicate a potential asthma exacerbation. These signs and symptoms typically start 6 to 8 minutes after the onset of strenuous exercise, but they may not reach maximum severity until up to 15 minutes after the cessation of exercise. Typically, spontaneous return to baseline respiratory function occurs within 20 to 60 minutes after onset of symptoms.

■ Asthma Treatment Options

Athletic trainers often interact with athletes who use an inhaler, more formally known as a metered-dose inhaler (MDI). These athletes are able to maintain adequate control of their asthma symptoms. Unfortunately, athletic trainers may also come into contact with athletes who do not have their asthma under control or who, in many cases, have not yet been given a diagnosis of asthma. For athletic trainers to be ready to deal with the undiagnosed asthmatic athlete, they need to have a basic understanding of asthma from physiological, pharmacological, and management perspectives.

Most true asthma exacerbations have both inflammatory and bronchoconstriction components. Therefore the use of medications to control and treat asthma may address either or both of these problems. Currently, the most widely accepted approach to asthma treatment is to initially control the inflammatory process associated with the trigger and thus prevent bronchoconstriction onset. This approach is reflected in the switch from heavy dependence on "rescue" inhalers to the increased use of controlling agents. With respect to EIA, the athlete typically experiences little or no active inflammatory process and the primary complication is the bronchoconstriction associated with the exercise trigger. Thus, the treatments for asthma and EIA are different. Asthma exacerbations are categorized according to the severity and the frequency of the symptoms. In general, asthma is broken down into four categories: mild intermittent, mild persistent, moderate persistent, and severe persistent (Table 7–1).

■ Commonly Used Drugs for Asthma Control

Numerous pharmacological approaches are used to treat asthma. Some of the factors that influence the chosen approach are the severity and frequency of the exacerbations and the convenience of using the drug. The drugs used to treat asthma can be classified into two groups: bronchodilators and anti-inflammatory agents. Anti-inflammatory agents can be further divided into steroidal and nonsteroidal types.

As their name implies, bronchodilators are used to dilate the bronchioles of the respiratory tract after the onset of bronchoconstriction. A bronchodilating MDI delivers a measured (metered) dose of medication each time it is activated. Historically, bronchodilating MDIs were used to rescue the user from an asthma attack, and therefore are commonly referred to as "rescue inhalers." It should be mentioned that some bronchodilators result in a relaxation of the smooth muscles in the airways, but they have not been demonstrated to be effective as "rescue" inhalers because they may take 1 to 2 hours to reach their maximum effectiveness.

It is generally accepted that anyone with persistent asthma should use a controlling agent for the inflammatory component in conjunction with a "rescue" inhaler for the

Table 7–1

Categories of Asthma

Classification	Characteristics
Mild Intermittent	Symptoms no more than 2 times per week No symptoms between exacerbations Exacerbations last no longer than a few days Symptoms at night less than 2 times per month
Mild Persistent	Symptoms more than 2 times per week but less than once a day. Nighttime symptoms more than 2 times per month
Moderate Persistent	Symptoms daily Daily use of "rescue" inhaler Nighttime symptoms more than once a week
Severe Persistent	Continuous symptoms Activity limited by symptoms Frequent exacerbations and nighttime symptoms

Source: Adapted from National Heart Lung and Blood Institute: Expert panel report 2–Guidelines For the Diagnosis and Management Of Asthma. National Institutes of Health, Bethesda, Md:, 1997 NIH Publication No. 97–4051.

bronchoconstriction. Individuals with mild intermittent asthma are typically treated with a bronchodilator as needed, based on symptoms and activity level.

The role of corticosteroids in asthma and respiratory care in general is to combat inflammation of the airways associated with certain respiratory conditions. Thus, they indirectly prevent inflammation-mediated bronchoconstriction through the inhibition of prostaglandins and leukotrienes. In addition, corticosteroids reverse vascular permeability associated with the inflammation process. Too many times, athletes rely on a corticosteroid MDI to resolve an initial anti-inflammatory asthma exacerbation during practice or competition. As we will discuss, the athlete should focus more on prevention of the exacerbation with the use of controlling drugs.

Oral medications are an attractive alternative to the use of inhaled steroids in the control of asthma. Typically, they are administered orally once or twice a day. In addition, there is no fluctuation in delivery of the medication, which may result from improper use of the MDI. These drugs are used for the control of mild persistent asthma requiring anti-inflammatory treatment and are not effective as a rescuing agent because they do not have a rapid bronchodilating effect. It is important to note that all individuals who use either steroids or nonsteroidal anti-inflammatory medications still need access to a "rescue" inhaler in the event of an asthma exacerbation (Table 7–2).

How Asthma Drugs Work

Understanding the mechanism by which bronchodilators work requires a thorough understanding of the receptors associated with the autonomic nervous system's neurotransmitters and how their action is altered to achieve relaxation of the smooth muscles of the airways. As pointed out earlier in this chapter, the neurotransmitter receptors involved in the autonomic nervous system's respiratory control are adrenergic and cholinergic. The corresponding drug classes used to regulate the function of the respiratory system are adrenergic agonists and anticholinergic drugs. The mechanism of action of these two drug types is different. The adrenergic agonists (as their name implies) actually activate and promote the action of the specific receptor, causing muscle relaxation of the smooth muscle and resulting in bronchodilation. The adrenergic agents currently used for respiratory conditions target the beta-adrenergic receptors and, more specifically in most cases of asthma, the beta-2 receptors.

The anticholinergic drugs work by a different mechanism from that of the adrenergic agonists in that they bind to the receptor site with the intent of blocking the receptor from being activated by impulses transmitted through the autonomic nervous system. The blocking of the receptor reduces bronchoconstriction by preventing the smooth muscle contraction that is generally induced by normal cholinergic receptor activation. Although, to some extent, these drugs do affect the respiratory system, their use in asthma treatment is typically limited. As will be discussed later in this chapter, anticholinergic drugs play a greater role in the mechanism by which some of the antihistamines work in the reduction of cold symptoms.

Beta-Adrenergic Bronchodilators

Beta-adrenergic bronchodilators ideally target specifically the beta-2 adrenergic receptors. When these agents are administered, they bind to the beta-2 adrenergic receptors of the smooth muscles in the lower respiratory system. When they attach to the beta-2 receptors, they cause relaxation of the bronchial muscles and, in turn, the bronchioles dilate, allowing increased air flow. These drugs are agonists in their actions and therefore cause dilation of the bronchioles, even though they do not affect the inflammatory process that is occurring.

In general, beta-2 agonists can be classified according to the length of time they are effective after administration. Their classification is based on a continuum from short acting to long acting. The chemical structure of the beta-2 agonist is the primary factor that determines the length of time it will work. Specifically, the longer the length of the chemical side chain on the base molecule, the longer the effects will last. A molecule with a relatively long side chain will become embedded in the cell membrane adjacent to the receptor and remain attached to the receptor site for a longer period of time than will a molecule with a short chemical side chain. The beta-2 agonists are specifically targeted to the bronchial smooth muscle and do not affect the cardiac muscle, which contains both beta-1 and beta-2 receptors. Over-the-counter (OTC) asthma preparations are generally nonselective agonists that can affect the cardiac muscle, resulting in an increase in heart function. They are disallowed for use during competition by many organizations.

Historically, beta-2 agonists have been used as rescue and prophylactic drugs to control asthma and treat bronchitis and emphysema by means of their long duration of action. Therefore, the short-lasting beta-2 agonists such as albuterol (Proventil, Ventolin) are used for two specific reasons in the management of asthma symptoms: as "rescue" drugs for rapid bronchodilation when an asthma attack has started, and as a prophylactic treatment to prevent respiratory com-

Table 7–2

Rescue Inhalers

Category	Medication	Timeline/Delivery	Examples	Function
Bronchodilators	Beta agonists	Short acting	Albuterol	Rescue
		Long acting	Serevent	Control
Anti-inflammatory agents	Steroidal	MDI	Flovent, Azmacort	Control
		Oral drugs	Prednisone	Control
	Nonsteroidal	MDI	Intal, Tilade	Control
		Oral drugs	Singulair, Accolate	Control

plications caused by exercise.[12] The long-acting bronchodilators (e.g., Serevent) are more commonly used as controlling drugs because of their longer-lasting effects on airway relaxation.

Specificity of Bronchodilators

Historically, the progression of bronchodilator use has evolved from agents that stimulate both the beta-1 and beta-2 adrenergic receptors to the specific drug that activates only the beta-2 receptors of the respiratory system. This transition has encouraged the prescription of beta-2 agonists by physicians because the negative cardiac effects, such as tachycardia, are eliminated with the use of the beta-2 agonists. The longer-acting beta-2 agonist agents such as salmeterol (Serevent) are particularly useful because these sustained-release formulations can be effective up to 12 hours. These long-lasting agents are not typically the first line of treatment and are often added to the treatment plan in individuals who are already using inhaled steroids.[6] One common reason for adding these to the treatment plan is to assist in the control of nighttime symptoms. In addition, the long-acting beta-2 agonists may be used in people who need additional asthma control, but it is not desirable to increase their steroid dose. These long-acting agents are not without drawbacks. They should not be used as rescue agents because of their extended onset of action.

Implications for Activity

It is important for the athlete and the athletic trainer to understand the athlete's specific "triggers" so that the athlete can continue participating in activity. If the athlete knows what is likely to trigger an asthmatic exacerbation, he or she can try to avoid that trigger. This will add to the effectiveness of the management of the disorder.

Some short-acting bronchodilators include albuterol (the most common), levalbuterol, and pirbuterol. These drugs are classified as short-acting agents and are most commonly prescribed and used as "rescue" medications. In athletics these drugs can also be used as "preventive" agents if administered before exposure to the asthma trigger. In individuals for whom exercise is a trigger for their symptoms, administration of a short-acting beta-2 agonist before activity may prevent the onset of symptoms (Box 7–1). This preventive approach is typically used in people who either do not have underlying chronic asthma or who have good control over their underlying asthma.

Anticholinergic Bronchodilators

Anticholinergic bronchodilators reduce airway constriction and inhibit cholinergic stimulation by blocking the acetylcholine activation of the receptor. Because the anticholinergic drugs attach to receptors on the parasympathetic system, they create adverse effects such as sedation through the central nervous system.[7] The anticholinergic agents are classified according to the receptors they block: either muscarinic or nicotinic. In general, anticholinergic bronchodilators are more commonly used for chronic respiratory conditions such as chronic obstructive pulmonary disease (COPD) or chronic bronchitis, but some athletes may have these medications prescribed to treat their asthma. Anticholinergic medications do not have labeled indications for use in asthma in the United States because they have more potential adverse effects (mainly as a result of muscarinic receptor activation) and are clearly not superior to beta-2 agonists.[10]

Anti-inflammatory Asthma Medications

Most physicians view asthma as a chronic disease that produces an inflammatory response in the tracheobronchial tree. Therefore, an anti-inflammatory medication is warranted for proper treatment. Anti-inflammatory drugs are effective in controlling the inflammatory response stimulated by the trigger and prevent exacerbations. The inflammatory response is discussed in detail in Chapter 3. The use of both steroidal and nonsteroidal medications for asthma control is discussed here.

Corticosteroids

Corticosteroids, which are secreted naturally by the adrenal cortex, are classified as glucocorticoids, mineralocorticoids, and sex hormones (androgens and estrogens). Mineralocorticoids assist in the regulation of fluid reabsorption and will

---

BOX 7–1

Suggested Protocol for Medication and Warm-up Before Activity

30 minutes before exercise: Beta-2 agonist
20 minutes before exercise: Mast cell stabilizer
15 minutes before exercise: Warm up

These are suggested timelines that should be fine-tuned by the athlete according to individual need.

not be discussed here. The sex hormones play little, if any, role in the regulation of respiratory function and thus will not be included in the following discussion. The focus will be on the glucocorticoids, the most important of which is cortisol, commonly known as hydrocortisone. These drugs retard inflammation by inhibiting the formation of some of the proteins associated with the inflammatory process.

Corticosteroid synthesis is regulated by the complex interaction among the adrenal cortex, pituitary gland, and the hypothalamus. The body is unable to differentiate between naturally occurring corticosteroids and those administered as medications. Oral administration of exogenous steroids may result in suppression of the body's own cortisone production because the body perceives no need to produce cortisone. Oral corticosteroids are typically administered in a tapering dose that prevents suppression of natural cortisol production. This issue of cortisone production suppression is not a serious complication of inhaled administration because the drugs are delivered directly to the respiratory tissue and have little or no effect on the three structures responsible for corticosteroid synthesis.

Nonsteroidal Asthma Medications

The mechanism by which nonsteroidal asthma medications work differs from that of corticosteroids. Specifically, the nonsteroidal asthma medications either stabilize mast cells (inhaled drugs) or modify leukotriene productions (oral drugs). Like the steroid drugs used for asthma, the nonsteroidal drugs are not effective as rescue medications.

Mast cell stabilizers prevent mast cells from releasing inflammatory mediators. Specifically, the stabilizing agent prevents the antibody and antigen complex from causing the mast cell to rupture and release inflammatory mediators. The blocking of this cascade of events results in the prevention of bronchoconstriction. Cromolyn sodium is a commonly used mast cell stabilizer and is available in an MDI.

Leukotriene modifiers (antileukotrienes), as the name implies, modify the activity of leukotrienes in the inflammatory process. Specifically, arachidonic acid is converted to leukotrienes, which causes increased airway reactivity and vascular permeability. Leukotriene modifiers, like mast cell stabilizers, indirectly prevent bronchodilation and are available under common brand names such as Accolate and Singulair.

■ Exercise-induced Asthma

As discussed earlier in this chapter, EIA is a result of an underlying asthma condition that is triggered by exercise. There are numerous theories regarding the cause of EIA. Water loss, heat exchange cooling the airways, and, most recently, increased sodium intake have all been implicated in EIA exacerbations.[8,9] The athlete must first have a formal diagnosis by a physician. Treatment usually follows the same preventive path as that outlined for other asthmatic conditions. It is suggested that an athlete experiencing EIA closely follow a pre-exercise routine that includes both medication and proper warm-up before engaging in practice or competition[8] (See Box 7–1).

Refractory Period

There is also a phenomenon known as the *refractory period* that affects some athletes who experience EIA on a regular basis. This phenomenon is poorly understood, and not all people with EIA experience this refractory period. Little science is available to explain why some people experience it and others do not. Much of the understanding of the refractory period comes from subjective patient observations. Each athlete needs to determine if he or she is able to use this period to his or her benefit.

Approximately 50 percent of athletes with EIA have found that they experience a symptom-free refractory period shortly after an asthma exacerbation. After the attack is over and all symptoms have resolved, they can return to activity with little or no restrictions for 1 to 2 hours.

Individuals who are capable of taking advantage of this refractory period follow a very specific routine. Before using their beta-2 agonist inhaler, they warm up and bring their system close to the threshold where symptoms would begin. At this point, they stop activity and use their inhaler. Within a few minutes of the use of the inhaler, they are able to return to activity, and many times remain symptom free.

As mentioned previously, the difficulty with this approach is that not all individuals who have EIA experience a refractory period, and not everyone who experiences it has consistent results with its use. For these reasons, it is highly recommended that, if someone is going to use this refractory period approach, he or she should experiment extensively with its personal implications before relying on it for use during competition.

■ Adverse Effects of Asthma Medications

The range of adverse effects of asthma medications varies greatly, depending mainly on the class of medication. Asthma medications delivered via MDI generally have less serious adverse effects than oral medications because of the localized delivery of the medication via MDI in comparison to the systemic effects of oral asthma medications.

The adverse effects of beta-2 agonists are relatively minor because of the specificity of receptors in the respiratory system. Common adverse effects include nervousness, restlessness, trembling, throat irritation, and potential airway hypersensitivity. There is some evidence that the use of beta-2 agonists for the daily treatment of asthma may cause airway hypersensitivity and decrease their effects as a rescue drug.[6]

Inhaled steroids, like other inhaled medications, have relatively minor adverse effects, none of which are systematic. The localized adverse effects are throat irritation and hoarseness. The inhaled steroid residue that remains in the mouth alters its bacterial environment, allowing opportunistic yeast infections to develop in the mouth. To limit this problem, users are encouraged to rinse the mouth and brush the teeth after each use of an inhaler.

The use of oral steroids in the treatment of respiratory conditions has the potential for both short-term and long-term adverse effects. In the short term, the patient may experience increased appetite, acne, poor wound healing, fluid retention, and insomnia. More severe are the known potential adverse effects of long-term use, such as avascular necrosis, osteoporosis, glaucoma, and decreased muscle mass. As mentioned previously, most inhaled medications have fewer adverse effects than oral preparations because of their localized delivery and receptor specificity.

Adverse effects of the inhaled nonsteroidal asthma medications are a bitter taste in the mouth after administration, throat irritation, and dry mouth. For some athletes, the bitter taste can be so significant that they refuse to use the drug. Additionally, oral nonsteroidal asthma medications produce some of the same adverse effects as the inhaled preparations, such as dry mouth and sore throat. The oral nonsteroidal asthma medications may also cause the athlete to experience headache and skin rash.

*A*llergies

An allergic reaction is generally the result of some adverse environmental stimulus. Depending on the season of the year, the geographical location, or other environmental conditions, allergies may present problems for the athlete and, secondarily, the athletic trainer. In general, two classes of drugs are used for the treatment of allergies: antihistamines and corticosteroids (nasal sprays).

■ Antihistamines

Histamine is a substance that exists naturally in human mast cells and the basophilic type of white blood cell. It causes blood vessel dilation and subsequently an inflammatory response in the area affected. When histamine receptors are activated, they cause an inflammatory response characterized by the classic allergy symptoms: runny nose, itchy and watery eyes, and sneezing. Most antihistamine agents are antagonists to these histamine receptors. Specifically, they bind to the receptor site and prevent it from being activated. Antihistamines produce three general effects on the body: alteration of histamine action, sedation, and anticholinergic activity (decreased salivation, dry mouth, and constipation).[10]

Like other classes of drugs, antihistamines have been grouped into generations as they have continued to be discovered and developed. Currently there are first- and second-generation antihistamines. The major differences between the two generations are the amount of time in which they stay active in the body and the extent to which they promote drowsiness. Essentially, improvements have been made so that the second-generation agents last longer and cause less drowsiness. The first-generation medications are effective for 4 to 6 hours and the second-generation medications can provide up to 12 hours of symptom relief. The second-generation antihistamines, because of their structure and receptor specificity, have fewer anticholinergic effects as well as a decreased sedative effect.

When histamine action is blocked through the use of an antihistamine drug, two changes occur in the body: the increased vascular permeability caused by histamine release is halted and smooth-muscle constriction of the airways is decreased. This decrease in vascular permeability effectively decreases the magnitude of the allergic response by not allowing histamine to escape from the vascular network and produce an inflammatory response in the surrounding cells. At the same time, the decrease in smooth-muscle constriction eases respiration because dilation occurs as an effect of the drug-imposed relaxation of the airways.

Many first-generation antihistamines have a sedative effect. The mechanism of this effect is a result of the antihistamine crossing the blood-brain barrier and acting as an antagonist to both serotonin and acetylcholine. Some practitioners suggest that athletes use a first-generation antihistamine during the evening and night and switch to a second-generation antihistamine during the day. Caution should be exercised when prescribing this approach because the sedative effect of a first-generation antihistamine may produce some sedating carryover effects in the daytime hours.

BOX 7–2

Adverse Effects of Antihistamines

Mucous membrane dryness
Cardiac stimulation
Blurred vision
Decreased gastrointestinal motility
Urinary retention

Although the use of antihistamines results in decreased symptoms and increased patient comfort, as with many medications, their use is sometimes questioned. Impeding these effects is not always a good thing. The body produces mucus in an effort to protect the linings of the airways, promote the removal of particulate matter, and facilitate the expectoration of infectious agents from the respiratory system. If the body's normal response of mucus production is halted, the body may be less able to perform these functions, leading to other problems. Antihistamines are not without their adverse effects (Box 7–2). It is important to keep abreast of any complications that may occur as a result of antihistamine use and recommend that the athlete report any problems to the physician.

One difficulty with the use of antihistamines in the treatment of allergies is that they may not be effective in decreasing nasal blockage, a particularly uncomfortable symptom experienced by many allergy sufferers. The type of drug known to work best at decreasing nasal congestion is known as a decongestant. Many of the second-generation antihistamines, such as Claritin-D (loratadine-D) and Allegra-D (fexofenadine-D), are available in preparations that include a decongestant. After the antihistamine blocks the advancement of allergic symptoms, the decongestant assists with the resolution of the runny nose and head congestion. If an athlete is taking only an antihistamine, it will take longer for the symptoms to resolve. However, the body's inherent protective mechanism will catch up as long as future histamine release is controlled. Simply put, taking an antihistamine alone will actually extend the time during which the athlete experiences allergy symptoms (Table 7–3).

■ Steroidal Nasal Sprays

Nasal steroid medications are specifically used for allergic rhinitis. They are not used for symptoms of the common cold because they are ineffective in treating viral conditions. They are effective in decreasing nasal congestion, sneezing, and rhinorrhea. Because of their local application, they have essentially no systemic effects as are seen with oral steroid treatments. Because these drugs are delivered locally, there is a potential for nasal irritation, dryness, and epistaxis. In rare cases, septal perforations may develop, and therefore users of these agents are instructed to direct the flow of the spray away from the nasal septum (Table 7–4).

*C*oughs and Colds

The athletic trainer often assists athletes in dealing with symptoms of allergies or the common cold. Many symptoms of the common cold are similar to those of allergies, and it is sometimes difficult to distinguish between them. Symptoms such as runny nose, mild sore throat, and watery eyes are seen in both the common cold and allergic reactions. In general, the common cold refers to a nonbacterial (viral) infection of the upper respiratory system.

Table 7–3			
Common Antihistamines			
First Generation		**Second Generation (Nonsedating)**	
Drug	*Brand Name*	*Drug*	*Brand Name*
Diphenhydramine	Benadryl	Loratadine	Claritin
Chlorpheniramine	Chlor-Trimeton	Fexofenadine	Allegra
Triprolidine	Actifed Cold & Sinus*	Cetirizine	Zyrtec
*Commonly found in preparations containing other active ingredients			

Table 7–4	
Over-the-Counter Nasal Decongestant Sprays	
Brand Name	**Active Ingredient**
Afrin	Oxymetazoline hydrochloride 0.05%
Neo-Synephrine	Phenylephrine hydrochloride 0.5%

■ Cough and Cold Medications

Four classes of medications are used to treat the symptoms of the common cold: decongestants, antihistamines, expectorants, and antitussives. All four of these classes are available in prescription and OTC forms. The vast majority of all cold medications used by patients are OTC preparations. *Decongestants* trigger vasoconstriction, resulting in mucosal drying. *Antihistamines* combat the effects of increased histamine, including nasal congestion and mucosal irritation. *Expectorants* facilitate the removal of mucus from the respiratory system and *antitussives* suppress coughing. It is important to note that many of these medications may contain a combination of decongestant, antihistamine, expectorant, antitussive, and other agents. For example, an OTC medication such as Vicks NyQuil contains acetaminophen, an analgesic used for pain relief and fever reduction; pseudoephedrine, a decongestant; dextromethorphan, a cough suppressant; and doxylamine succinate, an antihistamine.

Implications for Activity

Many cough and cold medications contain multiple agents. A common agent in cold medications is antihistamine. The use of antihistamines by an athlete with a cold may cause the athlete to be tired and lethargic, reducing the energy level he or she is able to produce in practice or competition. An athlete who needs to clear up a runny nose should use a cold medicine containing a decongestant. The decongestant will help to dry the nose and sinuses without producing drowsiness.

Decongestants

As their name implies, decongestants are used to decrease congestion of the upper airways. Congestion is essentially a result of inflammation of the mucosa lining the upper air-

way. The main reason for decongestants is to reduce the discomfort associated with sinus and ear pain from pressure. Although decongestants may lead to some drying of the mucosa as a result of localized vasoconstriction, their effectiveness in drying an area can sometimes be limited. When a decongestant is not effective in drying the nasal discharge, an antihistamine can be used to help stop a runny nose.

Decongestants used to treat the common cold and allergies are typically alpha-1 agonists. This means that they bind to the alpha-1 receptors located on blood vessels in the mucosa. Their binding promotes vasoconstriction, resulting in decongestant effects and drying of secretions. They may be administered via a nasal spray, eye drops, or oral preparations. There are potential adverse effects from prolonged use of decongestants: headache, nausea, dry mouth and nose, dizziness, and nervousness. In addition, prolonged application of nasal spray (topical) decongestants can cause a rebound-effect vasodilation after the initial vasoconstriction decreases. This can lead to vascular engorgement of the surrounding mucosa and return or exacerbation of symptoms.

Some of the most commonly used decongestants are orally administered pseudoephedrine (Sudafed), the ophthalmic-preparation of tetrahydrozoline (Visine) and the nasal preparation of oxymetazoline (Afrin).

Antihistamines

Some practitioners use antihistamines as a first-line treatment for the symptoms of the common cold. This approach is sometimes questioned because of the limited role of histamine in the pathology of the virus associated with the common cold. When antihistamines are effective in the treatment of common cold symptoms, it is likely the result of anticholinergic effect, resulting in upper-respiratory drying. This is extremely relieving to the cold sufferer. In addition to reducing upper respiratory secretions, the ability of first-generation antihistamines to induce drowsiness and promote a restful night's sleep may also be beneficial. As will be discussed with regard to expectorants, a question remains as to the beneficial effects of reducing upper respiratory secretions because they are an inherent defense mechanism by the body to fight the virus that causes the symptoms associated with the common cold.

Expectorants

Athletes might decide or be instructed to use a cough syrup to relieve the coughing linked with their cold symp-

BOX 7–3

MDI Use and Technique

An estimated 46 to 59 percent of individuals using MDIs use them ineffectively.[2] Patient education is critical, and the patient should be strongly encouraged to use a spacing device to enhance drug delivery to the lungs.

Directions for Inhaler Use

Always shake the inhaler before use

Hold the inhaler up to the mouth (1–2 inches away from the lips)

[Use of a spacer is recommended]*

Tilt the head back and open the mouth wide

Start to slowly inhale and depress the MDI at the same time

Continue to breathe in until the breath is complete

Hold the breath for approximately 10 seconds

---

*The use of a spacing device between the MDI and the patient promotes optimal medication delivery. A spacing device provides a chamber that allows the medication to be mixed with air before the patient inhales the mixture. Without a spacing device, the mixing of the medication must take place just outside the mouth or inside the mouth. Often the medication does not become mixed and is delivered mainly to the inside of the mouth so that delivery to the lungs is minimal.

toms. There are dozens of cough syrups on the market, most of them OTC products. Cough syrups can contain either an antitussive (cough suppressant) or an expectorant (substance that promotes mucus clearance). Although the athlete many not know this, one of the main reasons for using a cough syrup containing an expectorant is to promote the removal of mucus from the airways by increasing the productivity of the cough. If the coughing linked with a cold is "nonproductive" (dry) and is a hindrance to sleep and rest, it is important to try to eliminate it. A cough suppressant (antitussive) will assist the athlete in getting the needed rest so that the body can battle the cold virus.

Excess mucus produced by the body during the common cold needs to be thin and mobile enough for the coughing mechanism to be effective. Expectorants are a class of drugs used for this purpose. Expectorants facilitate the removal of mucus by increasing its water content. Once it is thinner, it is more mobile, and the coughing mechanism can move the mucus out of the lungs. Guaifenesin is an example of an expectorant that reduces the sur-

face tension and viscosity of the mucus so that it can be coughed up and expelled.

Antitussives

Antitussive agents can suppress the cough from either a central or a local mechanism. It is generally accepted that antitussives should be used for short periods of time for the suppression of coughs caused by irritation of the throat or the common cold. The most common way to inhibit a cough is via a central mechanism—the "cough center," located in the medulla. Dextromethorphan (DM) is the most common ingredient in OTC cough suppressants. It is found in families of OTC preparations such as Robitussin, Tylenol cold products, and NyQuil.

When DM is not effective in controlling a nonproductive cough, an alternative for the physician is to prescribe a narcotic antitussive. Codeine and hydrocodone are common ingredients in prescription cough medicines and work very well in controlling a cough. However, this approach is not without limitations because of the addictive property of narcotics. In most cases when a narcotic cough syrup is prescribed, the duration of the prescription does not exceed 1 week.

An alternative to centrally suppressing the cough is to administer a drug such as Tessalon (benzonatate), which has a local anesthetic effect on the respiratory epithelium.[1] The use of these drugs is a physician's decision and must come through a prescription.

■ Adverse Effects of Cold and Allergy Medications

The use of OTC cold and allergy medications has relatively few serious adverse effects on the body. However, using some of these drugs while participating in sports that require one to react quickly can cause drowsiness and lead to injury. Antihistamines, especially the first-generation drugs, can result in significant drowsiness, even after the drug's half-life is complete. In addition, antihistamines may cause anticholinergic effects such as mucous membrane dryness, cardiac stimulation, decreased gastrointestinal activity, and urinary retention. Decongestants can promote excessive drying of the nose and throat, tachycardia, and restlessness. Individuals using cough syrups that contain guaifenesin may experience dizziness, headache, and nausea. Similarly, the use of antitussives such as dextromethorphan may cause the user to experience mild dizziness, drowsiness, nausea, and stomach cramps.[4]

What to Tell the Athlete

If an athlete is has been diagnosed with asthma and a certain medication has been prescribed to control or alleviate the symptoms, he or she should be counseled and encouraged to be extremely proactive in the use of the medication. Here are some tips for the athletic trainer when educating the athlete about these drugs:

■ For emergency purposes, the athletic trainer can keep an extra short-acting beta2 MDI at the activity site if an athlete cannot locate his or her inhaler when an emergency arises.

■ The athletic trainer should work closely with the athlete to determine whether he or she is experiencing allergies or the common cold.

■ If an athlete is experiencing allergy-like symptoms, he or she can use OTC antihistamines, which may produce a generalized sedation.

■ Prescription antihistamines typically do not cause the drowsiness associated with the OTC medications. However, their cost is much greater. If an athlete is exhibiting the signs and symptoms of the common cold, he or she should first attempt to use OTC medications to alleviate the symptoms before requesting a prescription.

■ The use of nasal sprays for decongestant purposes can result in a rebound effect and create a long-term dependence on the use of nasal spray.

■ Nasal sprays and prescription antitussives should be used for only 1 week. If the symptoms do not subside after 1 week, the athlete should consult the physician for the next step in overcoming the problem.

Scenario from the Field

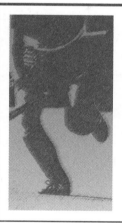

A 15-year-old football player was experiencing a great deal of difficulty breathing when he came to fall football camp for his first year of high-school football. During a practice the first week, he experienced a significant episode of dyspnea and was pulled out of practice. The athletic trainer suggested that his parents take him to his family physician for a thorough examination. After an examination and some testing, the family physician diagnosed the young man with asthma and prescribed both an oral nonsteroidal asthma medication and an inhaler. The high-school athletic trainer helped to educate the athlete about his asthma, and counseled and encouraged compliance with his oral medication regimen. She also assisted the boy with the proper use of the inhaler (with a spacer). The boy was relatively free from asthma symptoms for the remainder of the football season.

Internet Resource Box

For more information on topics discussed in this chapter, please visit the following online sources:

Banned Substances
http:www.ncaa.org/
Drug Resource

http:www.rxlist.com/
Asthma Information
http:jama.ama-assn.org/
http:www.lungusa.org/asthma/
http:www.nlm.nih.gov/medlineplus/druginformation.html

www.

Discussion Topics

- An athlete who has been diagnosed with asthma has given you, her athletic trainer, a rescue inhaler to keep on the field in case she has an exacerbation. Another athlete who has not been diagnosed with asthma approaches you with the signs and symptoms of an asthma exacerbation. Would you consider giving the second athlete, who is having difficulty breathing, a puff or two of the first athlete's rescue inhaler?

- If an athlete has a cold with a runny nose, cough, and sore throat, what type of cold medications would you suggest he or she purchase at the drugstore to minimize the symptoms?

- If an athlete is allergic to a type of grass and notices after practice that he or she is experiencing a moderate skin reaction where his or her skin contacted the grass, what type of medication would you recommend he or she purchase at the drugstore to control this skin reaction? What would be the side effects of any medications used for this problem?

References

1. Ciccone, CD: Pharmacology in Rehabilitation, ed. 3. FA Davis, Philadelphia, 2002.
2. Cochrane, MG, et al.: Inhaled corticosteroids for asthma therapy: Patient compliance, devices, and inhalation technique. Chest 117:542, 2000.
3. Gotshall, RW: Exercise-induced bronchoconstriction. Drugs 62:1725, 2002.
4. Griffith, HWDG: Complete Guide to Prescription and Nonprescription Drugs. Berkley, New York, 2002.
5. Hancox, RJ, et al.: Beta-2 agonist tolerance and exercise-induced bronchospasm. Am J Respir Crit Care Med 165:1068, 2002.
6. Hancox, RJ, and Taylor, DR: Long-acting beta agonist treatment in patients with persistent asthma already receiving inhaled corticosteroids. BioDrugs 15:11–24, 2001.
7. Houglum, JE: Asthma medications: Basic pharmacology and use in the athlete. J Ath Trng, 35:179, 2000.
8. Lacroix, V: Exercise-induced asthma. Phys Sports Med 27:75, 1999.
9. Mickleborough, TD, et al.: A low sodium diet improves indices of pulmonary function in exercise-induced asthma. J Ex Phys Online, 2000:[cited 2002 Sept 27]. Available from *URL:http://www.css.edu/users/tboone2/asep/JEPMickleborough.html.*
10. Rau, JLJ: Respiratory Care Pharmacology, ed. 6. Mosby, St Louis, 2002.
11. Rundell, KW, et al.: Self-reported symptoms and exercise-induced asthma in the elite athlete. Med Sci Sports Exerc 33:208, 2001.
12. Sears, MR: The evolution of beta-2 agonists. Respir Med 95 Suppl B, S2, 2001.

Chapter Questions

1. Can you explain the difference between respiration and ventilation?

2. Can you explain the difference between the types of receptors used by the body in respiration?

3. Can you explain the difference between asthma, exercise-induced asthma, and exercise-induced bronchoconstriction?

4. Explain the physiological reaction of the body during an asthma exacerbation.

5. Explain the EIA refractory period.

6. Explain the differences among antihistamines, decongestants, antitussives, and expectorants.

7. Explain the rebound effect associated with nasal decongestant sprays.

8. Explain the difference between the common cold and allergies.

9. What are the adverse effects of asthma medications?

10. What are the adverse effects of OTC antihistamines and decongestants?

11. What side effects should the athletic trainer look for in an athlete taking medication for asthma?

12. How long should an athlete take a prescription antitussive medication?

8 Drugs for Gastrointestinal Disorders

Chapter Objectives

After reading this chapter, the student will:

1 Be able to recognize the signs, symptoms, and causes of peptic ulcer disease.

2 Be able to recognize the signs, symptoms, and causes of gastroesophageal reflux disease.

3 Understand the pharmacological treatment and adverse effects of drug therapy for peptic ulcer disease and gastroesophageal reflux disease.

4 Understand the etiology, pharmacological treatment, and adverse effects of drug therapy for diarrhea.

5 Understand the etiology, pharmacological treatment, and adverse effects of drug therapy for constipation and intestinal gas.

Chapter Outline

Peptic Ulcer Disease
>   *Helicobacter pylori*
>   Nonsteroidal Anti-inflammatory Drugs
>   Gastric Acid Hypersecretion
>   Peptic Ulcer Disease Drug Treatment and Adverse Effects

Gastroesophageal Reflux Disease
>   Gastroesophageal Reflux Disease Drug Treatment and Adverse Effects

Diarrhea

Diarrhea Drug Treatment and Adverse Effects

Constipation
>   Constipation Drug Treatment and Adverse Effects

Intestinal Gas
>   Intestinal Gas Drug Treatment

The Athletic Trainer's Responsibility

Scenario from the Field

Discussion Topics

Chapter Review

A vast array of gastrointestinal (GI) disorders can cause discomfort and stomach upset. Some of these disorders are peptic ulcer disease (PUD), gastroesophageal reflux disease (GERD), diarrhea, constipation, and intestinal gas. Most GI disorders, however, are never properly reported because athletes do not like to discuss such conditions. This chapter will focus on the common types of GI disorders; their etiology, signs and symptoms; and treatments that require drug management.

Peptic Ulcer Disease

PUD is classified as a chronic inflammatory disorder resulting in the erosion of the mucosa of the stomach or duodenum. Usually, the erosion is a result of gastric acid and pepsin, which are normally available to hydrolyze protein and food so that they can be absorbed by the intestine. However, sometimes the production of gastric acid and pepsin results in ulcer formation. Ulcers also occur in the esophagus and other areas of the GI tract, but not as frequently as in the stomach and duodenum. Risk for developing ulcers increases with age, smoking, alcohol, a history of peptic ulcer disease or GI bleeding, and increased doses of nonsteroidal anti-inflammatory drugs (NSAIDs).[19,35]

Duodenal ulcers usually occur in the beginning portion of the duodenum and gastric ulcers usually occur in the lower one-third of the stomach, also called the *antrum.* PUD is often asymptomatic, but signs and symptoms can include a slight dull ache, discomfort 2 to 3 hours after meals and during the middle of the night, poor appetite, bloating, burping, nausea, and vomiting. Such discomfort can often be relieved by food and antacid medications.

The cause of PUD is multifactoral, ranging from increased acid secretion to factors that decrease the protective mucosal barrier. Neurologic impulses (sight, smell, or taste) can also trigger the secretion of acid. Damage to the mucosal barriers can occur as a consequence of alcohol abuse, cigarette smoking, or continual use of aspirin and NSAIDs. *Helicobacter pylori (H. pylori)* bacterial infection may also directly inflame and damage the mucosal barrier or alter the regulation of gastric acids. Because there are many factors that can cause ulcers, investigators have divided the etiology into three categories: (1) ulcers associated with *H. pylori;* (2) ulcers caused by NSAID use; and (3) ulcers caused by acid hypersecretion.[14]

■ *Helicobacter pylori*

H. pylori is a bacterium of the helicobacter genus. Its mode of transmission is unknown, but it is thought to be from person to person.[9] *H. pylori* can be found almost anywhere in the stomach but is usually concentrated in the antrum. Inflammation of the antrum is the most common cause of *gastritis,*[2,28,40] and elimination of *H. pylori* from this site usually resolves this condition. The exact cause of gastritis caused by *H. pylori* is unknown, but it is thought to result from either production of a cytotoxin, a breakdown of mucosal defenses, or adhesion to epithelial cells.[6] As a result, the lining of the stomach and duodenum weakens and allows the acid to penetrate, causing an ulcer.

■ Nonsteroidal Anti-inflammatory Drugs

Use of NSAIDs is the most common cause of PUD in patients who are not infected with *H. pylori.*[19] NSAID use can damage the stomach lining through inhibition of prostaglandin synthesis. Prostaglandins stimulate mucus and bicarbonate secretion, maintain mucosal blood flow, and participate in epithelial regeneration and cell growth. Without this process, the stomach lining would be vulnerable to acid.

■ Gastric Acid Hypersecretion

Acid secretion in individuals who suffer from PUD has been found to be close to normal. Only when hypersecretion occurs do most individuals suffer from ulcers. The hypersecretion can cause ulcers either by injuring the cells of the mucosa or by activating pepsin. When hypersecretion is the cause of ulcers, it may be the result of Zollinger-Ellison syndrome. Zollinger-Ellison syndrome is a rare condition in which a tumor activates the secretion of gastrin, which then stimulates gastric acid release. Only approximately 0.1 percent of all duodenal ulcers occur from Zollinger-Ellison syndrome.

■ Peptic Ulcer Disease Drug Treatment and Adverse Effects

Treatment of PUD is directed toward relieving ulcer pain, accelerating ulcer healing, and minimizing ulcer recurrence. The following classes of drugs are used for treatment of PUD: H_2-receptor antagonists, proton pump inhibitors, antacids, sucralfate, bismuth compounds, and antibiotics (Table 8–1). Some of these drug classes are available as over-the-counter (OTC) drugs used to treat PUD. As with all OTC items, it is imperative to follow the doses and indications recommended on the drug label. Not following these recommendations may cause unwanted and perhaps severe adverse effects. Therefore anyone who has any questions about which medication to administer or the proper dose should consult his or her physician or local pharmacist.

H_2 Receptor Antagonists

H_2 receptor antagonists decrease gastric acidity by inhibiting histamine from being released by parietal cells. Histamine activates H_2 receptors along the GI tract to increase acid secretion. Common H_2 receptor antagonists include cimetidine (Tagamet), ranitidine (Zantac), nizatidine (Axid), and famotidine (Pepcid). Multiple dosing has been shown to be more effective than single dosing with respect to suppressing gastric acids.[20, 33] These drugs can also treat gastroesophageal reflux and hypersecretory gastric states by increasing the pH of gastric contents.[3,4,17,27]

Table 8–1

Drugs Used to Treat *H. pylori*, GERD, and PUD

Drug—Generic (Brand)	Classification	Indication	Action
Bismuth (Pepto-Bismol)	Bismuth	*H. pylori*	Destroys *H. pylori* bacteria
Metronidazole (Flagyl) Clarithromycin (Biaxin) Amoxicillin (Amoxil)	Antimicrobial	*H. pylori*	Destroys *H. pylori*
Cimetidine (Tagamet) Famotidine (Pepcid) Ranitidine (Zantac) Nizatidine (Axid)	H_2 antagonist	PUD, GERD, *H. pylori*	Blocks H_2 receptors to suppress acid secretion
Omeprazole (Prilosec) Lansoprazole (Prevacid) Rabeprazole (Aciphex) Pantoprazole (Protonix) Esomeprazole (Nexium)	Proton-pump inhibitor	PUD, GERD, *H. pylori*	Inhibits proton-pump acid secretion
Sucralfate (Carafate)	Mucosal protectant	PUD	Binds to ulcer and forms a protective barrier
Metoclopramide (Reglan)	Prokinetic	GERD	Stimulates gastric motility

H_2 receptor antagonists rarely cause serious adverse effects. However, mild adverse effects can include diarrhea, constipation, headache, stomach cramps, dizziness, and rash. These drugs should be used with caution in patients who have renal failure or liver damage because they are not effectively cleared by the kidney and liver.

Proton-pump Inhibitors

Proton-pump inhibitors inhibit gastric acid secretion by blocking the H^+/K^+ adenosine triphosphatase system found at the surface of gastric parietal cells.[3,4,27,37] Omeprazole (Prilosec), lansoprazole (Prevacid), rabeprazole (Aciphex), esomeprazole (Nexium), and pantoprazole (Protonix) are drugs used to effectively treat PUD by blocking the final step of acid production.[3,4,17,27,37]

The main adverse effects of proton-pump inhibitors are stomach pain and diarrhea. Additional possible adverse effects include abdominal distress, headaches, muscle aches, chest pain, sedation, gas, nausea, vomiting, and rash.[3,4,27,37]

Antacids

Antacids neutralize the acid found in the stomach by buffering it and increasing the stomach's pH. Importantly, antacids have no effect on acid production, unlike the H_2 receptor antagonists and proton-pump inhibitors. Although antacids heal ulcers, they are primarily used for the relief of ulcer pain or dyspepsia when used in combination with other anti-ulcer drugs. Antacids are discussed more thoroughly in this chapter in the context of gastroesophageal reflux disease.

Sucralfate

Sucralfate (Carafate) is an prescription-only agent that, when exposed to acid, forms a viscous paste that adheres to the ulcer crater, forming a protective barrier. The drug binds only to the damaged mucosa and maintains the barrier for up to 6 hours. Sucralfate is effective in the short-term treatment of duodenal ulcers and is comparable to H_2 antagonists. Sucralfate is generally well tolerated; its most frequent adverse effect is constipation.

Bismuth Compounds

Bismuth compounds have been used to treat gastrointestinal disorders for many years. The most common agent used today is bismuth subsalicylate (Pepto-Bismol). The mechanism by which bismuth heals ulcers remains uncertain, but theories include providing a local gastroprotective effect, stimulating endogenous prostaglandins, and suppressing *H. pylori* infection.

Bismuth subsalicylate preparations may contain varying amounts of salicylate and therefore may cause problems for patients taking aspirin or other salicylate-containing drugs. It may cause salicylate toxicity in individuals who are on aspirin therapy. Patients should also be aware that bismuth reacts with hydrogen in the colon to from a compound that blackens the stool.

Antibiotics

Antibiotics are used in the treatment of *H. pylori*. Antibiotic drug therapy is associated with various treatment success rates (on average 80 to 95%). The most common antibiotics used for treatment of *H. pylori* include clarithromycin (Biaxin), metronidazole (Flagyl), and amoxicillin (Amoxil). Adverse effects of these antibiotics are mostly GI symptoms such as diarrhea and nausea. Both clarithromycin and metronidazole are known to cause an abnormal taste in the mouth and headache.

Gastroesophageal Reflux Disease

Gastroesophageal reflux disease (GERD) is a common chronic disorder that must be treated for an extended period of time in most individuals. GERD refers to the retrograde movement of gastric contents into the esophagus, usually after eating, because the lower esophageal sphincter (LES) does not close properly. With repeated exposure to *gastric* reflux, the esophagus can become inflamed.[22] In some cases, reflux can cause esophageal strictures, esophageal ulcers, perforations, hemorrhage, aspiration, and motility disorders.[7,30] Only patients who have tissue damage of the esophagus or who suffer from symptoms are said to have GERD.

The most common symptom for individuals with GERD is heartburn.[39] Heartburn is usually described as pain in the center of the chest, sometimes mimicking angina, and primarily occurs after eating. It is caused by contact of acidic gastric contents with the inflamed esophageal mucosa.[13] Other symptoms such as dysphagia, odynophagia (pain on swallowing), bad breath, dry cough, or nocturnal symptoms can occur.[18] Most individuals suffering from GERD do not seek medical treatment initially but try to self-medicate with OTC products to control their symptoms.

Symptoms of GERD can be aggravated by foods, specific body positions (especially lying down), and certain drugs. Foods high in fat can cause GERD because they decrease the LES pressure. Spices, onions, citrus juices, coffee, and caffeine can also cause direct mucosal irritation.[13] Individuals experience symptoms primarily when they are supine or bending over; however, esophageal reflux can occur in any position. Alcohol and certain drug therapies (verapamil, diazepam, and NSAIDs) can also exacerbate GERD symptoms.[11,32]

Gastroesophageal Reflux Disease Drug Treatment and Adverse Effects

Patients who have frequent reflux episodes need to inhibit or prevent gastric acid secretion to promote and facilitate healing. Hence, the goals of therapy are to: (1) eliminate or alleviate symptoms, (2) limit the frequency and duration of GI reflux, (3) promote healing of the mucosa, and (4) prevent complications. H_2 receptor antagonists and proton pump inhibitors used to treat PUD can also treat GERD (see Table 8–1).

Patients are encouraged to alter factors that can cause reflux.[23] They are encouraged to lose weight and wear loose-fitting clothes to decrease gastroesophageal pressure.[22] To decrease acid secretions, patients should also refrain from cigarette smoking, eliminate from their diet foods that lower esophageal pressure or stimulate acid secretions,[21, 22] avoid lying down after meals, and limit their intake of alcohol.

Antacids

Antacids relieve mild to moderate symptoms of GERD by decreasing gastric acidity, thereby increasing LES pressure.[36] Antacids have a rapid onset of action but a short duration. However, if taken with food, the effects of antacids can last up to 3 hours. Generally, antacids are used to provide daytime symptomatic relief for those who have mild to moderate symptoms.[16]

The primary neutralizing compounds used in antacid preparations are calcium, aluminum, and magnesium salts and sodium bicarbonate (Table 8–2). Calcium carbonate is a widely used antacid that dissolves slowly in the stomach and can be found in products such as Tums and Mylanta lozenges. Aluminum hydroxide reacts with gastric acid to form aluminum chloride and water. An example of an aluminum-containing antacid is Amphojel. Magnesium hydroxide produces a short-acting neutralizing effect and is found in milk of magnesia. There are also a multitude of combination products that contain various salts. Some magnesium and aluminum combination products are Maalox tablets and Mylanta Double Strength Liquid. Finally, sodium bicarbonate is an antacid that is found in Alka-Seltzer and similar effervescent products.

Antacids or antacid combination products may produce several adverse reactions. Diarrhea, constipation, alterations in mineral metabolism, and acid-base imbalances are possible effects of continued antacid exposure. The most frequent adverse effect of aluminum-containing antacids is constipation, whereas that of magnesium antacids is diar-

Table 8–2

Antacid Classifications*

Product	Dosage Form(s)	Active Ingredient(s)
Alka-Seltzer	Effervescent tablet	Sodium bicarbonate
Amphojel	Liquid	Aluminum hydroxide
Gaviscon	Chewable tablet	Aluminum hydroxide Magnesium carbonate
Maalox	Liquid	Aluminum hydroxide Magnesium hydroxide
Mylanta	Chewable tablets	Aluminum hydroxide Magnesium hydroxide Simethicone
Milk of magnesia	Liquid	Magnesium hydroxide
Rolaids Extra Strength	Chewable tablets	Calcium carbonate Magnesium hydroxide
Tums	Chewable tablets	Calcium carbonate

*This table is not exhaustive, but is intended to provide a sample of commonly used antacids. Various manufacturers may alter recommended dosage and active and inert ingredients.

rhea. Antacids may also interact with other drugs to affect solubility and absorption.

Prokinetics

Prokinetic agents decrease the amount of esophageal contact time with gastric acid. This is done by stimulating the motility of the upper GI tract without increasing gastric secretions. Metoclopramide (Reglan) is currently the prokinetic drug of choice. Some adverse effects of metoclopramide include restlessness, somnolence, and dizziness.

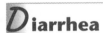iarrhea

Diarrhea is an unpleasant and often embarrassing condition that, if left untreated, usually resolves in a couple of days. It is defined as abnormal frequency and liquidity of fecal discharge compared with normal stools. Diarrhea can be classified as either acute or chronic and may be a result of a GI or non-GI disease.

Acute diarrhea can be of infectious, toxic, drug-induced, or dietary origin. Acute diarrhea occurs with a sudden onset of frequent watery stools accompanied by pain, cramping, flatulence, fever, or vomiting. Most commonly, acute diarrhea is caused by bacterial organisms such as *Shigella, salmonella, campylobacter, staphylococcus.,* and *Escherichia coli.*[1] It can also be caused by food intolerances, viral infections, and parasites.

Chronic diarrhea, lasting more than 2 weeks, is usually of multifactoral etiology and hard to diagnose. Chronic diarrhea is divided into two classifications: organic and functional. Organic diarrhea may be caused by low hemoglobin concentration, low serum albumin, or high erythrocyte sedimentation rate.[5,8,34] Functional diarrhea may be physiological or psychogenic in nature. Causes include stress-related factors, inflammatory bowel disease, and irritable bowel syndrome.

A thorough history of food ingestion during the week before the onset of diarrhea is crucial to help determine the cause. Possible infectious sources include fruits, vegetables, meats, seafood, and water. The toxins in these sources can cause a sudden onset of loose stools, nausea, and possibly fever.

Traveler's diarrhea can occur after ingestion of food or water that is contaminated with bacteria or parasites. Common causes include undercooked meat and seafood, raw vegetables, fruit, and changes in eating habits. The onset of traveler's diarrhea is usually during the first few days of travel in areas of poor hygiene and sanitation, but it can develop at any time during traveling. To prevent traveler's diarrhea, travelers should not drink tap water or unpasteurized dairy products or eat raw meats, fruits, vegetables, or seafood.

■ Diarrhea Drug Treatment and Adverse Effects

There are three primary goals in treating diarrhea: (1) prevent excessive water, electrolyte, and acid-base disturbance, (2) identify and treat the cause, and (3) provide symptomatic relief. Treatments include antiperistaltic agents, adsorbents, and bismuth compounds.

The first priority for an athlete with diarrhea is to control the loss of fluids and dehydration. Fluids with electrolytes such as fruit juices and sport electrolyte drinks should be consumed; carbonated beverages, caffeine, and products with high fructose levels should be avoided. Urine color is probably the easiest way to determine hydration status (yellow = dehydration, clear = hydration).

If the diarrhea persists for several days, if there is blood in the stool, or if the athlete has severe abdominal pain and cramps, he or she should consult a physician to determine its etiology. A thorough medical examination may include stool culture, blood test, or sigmoidoscopy. If the diarrhea is from a bacterial infection, it is not recommended to stop the bowel movements with medication because the bacterial organism will be trapped in the GI tract. Viral infections can be either left alone to run their course or treated with medications (Fig. 8–1).

Antiperistaltic Agents

Antiperistaltic agents are effective in relieving cramps and stool frequency by inhibiting peristalsis and prolonging transition time of the intestinal contents. The most commonly used antiperistaltic is loperamide (Imodium). Loperamide is available OTC and is an effective treatment for nonspecific acute diarrhea, traveler's diarrhea, and chronic diarrhea from inflammatory bowel disease. Loperamide slows intestinal motility and allows water and electrolyte reabsorption from the intestinal lumen to the systemic circulation. Another agent, Lomotil, with a similar mechanism of action is available by prescription.

The most commonly reported adverse affects of antiperistaltic agents are dizziness, dry mouth, and skin rash. These agents can worsen the effects of invasive bacterial infection by not allowing evacuation of the damaging bacteria or toxins. Antiperistaltic agents should be used with caution in individuals who have a fever, a history of antibiotic use, or inflammatory bowel disease (ulcerative colitis or Crohn's disease).

Bismuths

Bismuth compounds are used to treat acute and traveler's diarrhea and stomach upset. Bismuth subsalicylate (Pepto-Bismol) is available OTC to treat diarrhea. Usually, bismuth subsalicylate is prescribed in doses of 30 mL or 2 chewable or dissolvable tablets every 30 to 60 minutes up to 8 times a day.

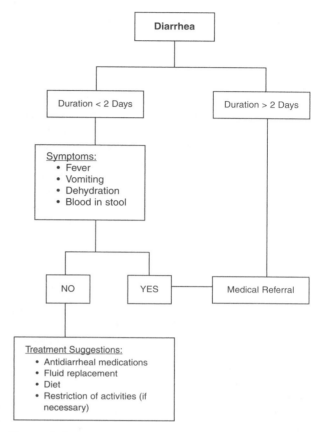

Figure 8–1. Evaluative decisions for treating diarrhea. Adapted from Longe, RL: Antidiarrheal products. In *American Pharmaceutical Association Handbook of Nonprescription Drugs*, ed. 11. Washington, D.C., American Pharmaceutical Association, 1996, p. 253.

*C*onstipation

Constipation is usually described as a decrease in the frequency of fecal elimination and difficulty in passing stool, which is usually hard and dry. Constipation results from an abnormally slow movement of the feces through the colon and an accumulation of feces in the descending colon. Although there are several factors in the etiology of constipation, its most common causes include inappropriate diet (low in fiber), lack of exercise, insufficient fluid intake, excessive intake of foods, and resisting defecation impulses. Other causes of constipation include diabetes, multiple sclerosis, parkinsonism, inflammatory bowel disease, and pregnancy. The use of antidiarrheal agents can also cause constipation and may also cause low back pain, abdominal distention, dull headache, and lower abdominal distress.

■ Constipation Drug Treatment and Adverse Effects

Most nonorganic causes of constipation can be treated by lifestyle modifications. Increasing fiber intake enhances regularity by adding bulk and softening the stool. Increasing fluid intake, especially water intake, helps to alleviate constipation. Aerobic exercise, such as walking, running, or swimming, can decrease the likelihood of constipation. Laxatives and other medications (Table 8–3) can be used in conjunction with lifestyle modification to alleviate constipation. Chronic use of laxatives, referred to as laxative abuse syndrome (LAS) may result in diarrhea, steatorrhea, fluid and electrolyte imbalances, cathartic colon, and liver disease.[31]

Bulk-forming Laxatives

Bulk-forming laxatives, because of their ability to promote fecal evacuation, are the drugs most commonly prescribed for relief of constipation. Bulk-forming laxatives stimulate peristalsis (by distending the bowel) and assist in the passage of the stool. These medications should be taken with plenty of fluids to aid swallowing and to facilitate the drugs' efficacy. These laxatives may also be used to prevent the development of constipation.

The two most common types of bulk-forming laxatives are polycarbophil calcium (Mitrolan, FiberCon) and psyllium (Metamucil, Konsyl). Polycarbophil is normally used for both diarrhea and constipation to restore normal moisture levels and to provide bulk. Psyllium promotes the formation of a soft, water-retaining, gelatinous residue in the bowel.

Bulk-forming laxatives should not be taken by individuals who have intestinal ulcerations, obstruction, or stenosis. Failure to consume adequate water during administration can decrease the drugs' efficacy and may cause esophageal or intestinal obstruction. Abdominal discomfort, diarrhea, and flatulence may also occur.

Fecal Softeners

Orally administered fecal softeners are mainly used to prevent constipation. Softeners increase the wetting efficiency

Table 8–3

Classification and Action of Common Laxatives

Generic Name	Brand Name	Type	Mechanism of Action	Onset of Action
Methylcellulose	Citrucel	Bulk forming	Absorbs water and forms emollient gel that promotes peristalsis	12–72 hrs
Polycarbophil	FiberCon Mitrolan			
Psyllium	Konsyl Metamucil			
Docusate (sodium/calcium)	Colace Surfak	Fecal softener	Facilitates formation of a mixture of fat and water to soften the stool	12–72 hrs
Magnesium citrate	Evac-Q-Kwik	Saline	Draws water into intestine, increases intraluminal pressure, promotes peristalsis	0.5–3 hrs or 12–15 min (rectally)
Magnesium hydroxide	Milk of magnesia			
Magnesium sulfate	Epsom salt			
Sodium phosphate	Fleet Ready-to-use Enema Fleet Phospho-soda			
Glycerin	Glycerin Fleet Babylax	Hyperosmotic	Induces osmosis by retaining fluid in colon; acts as local irritant	0.25–1 hr (rectal)
Lactulose	Cephulac		Retains fluid in colon, increases peristalsis	24–48 hrs
Bisacodyl	Dulcolax Correctol Feen-A-Mint	Stimulant	Increases peristaltic activity	6–10 hrs

of the intestinal fluid and mix the aqueous and fatty substances to soften the fecal mass. The fecal mass usually softens within 1 to 2 days after initiation of therapy; however, it may take as long as 3 to 5 days. Softeners do not stimulate bowel movement unless they are combined with stimulant laxatives. Docusate (Colace, Surfak) is the most commonly used type of medication in this category. Fecal softeners are considered safe and effective agents. Some possible adverse effects include diarrhea and abdominal cramping.

Hyperosmotic Agents

The class of hyperosmotic agents includes glycerin (rectal) and lactulose (oral or rectal). Both agents produce an osmotic effect by causing fluid retention in the colon. Glycerin produces an irritant effect on the colon for quick lower bowel evacuation. Because of this effect, glycerin suppositories are widely used in children. Lactulose is an effective agent that increases the water content of the stool, thereby softening the stool and producing an effect within 24 to 48 hours after administration.

Hyperosmotic agents are relatively safe. Glycerin may cause diarrhea, nausea, or vomiting. The most common adverse effects with lactulose are flatulence, belching, and abdominal discomfort such as cramping, nausea, and vomiting. Excessive doses may lead to diarrhea.

Stimulant Laxatives

Stimulant laxatives increase the propulsive activity of the intestine by local irritation of the mucosa or the intestinal smooth muscle. Most of the stimulant laxatives are of botanical origin, containing active ingredients obtained from seed pods, bark, leaves, and roots of various plant sources. Stimulant laxatives are primarily used for acute constipation; before proctologic, radiologic, and endoscopic examinations; and for preparation of barium enemas. However, they should not be used for more than 3 days because they can alter large intestine function.

There are two categories of stimulant laxatives, diphenylmethane and anthraquinone. Bisacodyl (Dulcolax) is the most commonly used diphenylmethane. Bisacodyl is a nontoxic agent that causes peristalsis on contact with the colon mucosa nerve plexus. Bisacodyl can trigger peristalsis within 15 to 60 minutes of rectal administration or within 6 to 10 hours if taken orally.

The exact mechanism of anthraquinone agents to produce peristalsis is unknown but is thought to primarily affect the colon. Aloe, cascara sagrada, senna, aloin, casanthranol, dan-

thron, frangula, and rhubarb are examples of stimulant laxatives based on anthraquinone agents. Of these, senna is the preferred choice. The compounds in the anthraquinones, after absorption in the GI tract, can be found in human milk and pass their effects to the nursing infant.[15] Therefore caution is advised for breast-feeding mothers.

Most stimulant laxatives can cause severe abdominal cramping, diarrhea, flatulence, electrolyte and fluid deficiencies, and hypokalemia. Individuals may also suffer from allergic reactions, change in heart rate, skin rash, disorientation, and color changes to the urine and feces.

Saline Laxatives

Saline laxatives are composed of soluble salts that draw water from the wall of the small intestine into the feces, then stimulate and increase intestinal motility. Saline laxatives produce stools that are liquid or semi-liquid in nature and are indicated when preparing for GI examinations or when stool specimens are needed. It can also be used for cases of food poisoning and fecal impaction. However, saline salts are not indicated for long-term management of constipation. There are several types of saline salts that are used as laxatives; magnesium sulfate (Epsom salts), magnesium hydroxide (milk of magnesia), magnesium citrate solution, and sodium phosphate (Fleet brand and other premixed enemas). Saline salts have a rapid course of action and should be taken with at least 8 oz of water with oral administration to prevent vomiting.

Long-term use of saline laxatives can cause electrolyte disturbances and may act as a CNS depressants. Individuals with renal impairment can develop toxicity to magnesium ions in saline salts.[29] Up to 20 percent of the magnesium in magnesium salts may be absorbed and produce hypotension, muscle weakness, and electrocardiographic changes.[31] The most common adverse effects include abdominal cramping, nausea, vomiting, and dehydration.

Implications for Activity

The use of laxatives by athletes can be warranted in instances of stress, travel, and other factors that can lead to constipation and GI system dysfunction as outlined. However, some athletes may abuse laxatives for weight loss purposes. When this happens, the adverse effects of dehydration and GI disturbances are increased. This leads to a decrease in performance in many activities. The athletic trainer should educate the athlete regarding the purpose and use of laxatives when short-term use is indicated.

Intestinal Gas

Many individuals complain of belching, abdominal discomfort, bloating, and flatulence, especially after meals. However, the pathogenesis for intestinal gas is largely misunderstood. Gas is thought to arise from three different sources: (1) air swallowing, (2) intraluminal production, and (3) diffusion of gases from the blood.

When we eat, several milliliters of air are deposited into the stomach with every swallow of food or saliva.[26] Over the course of a day, several liters of nitrogen (N_2) found in the air enter the stomach with only approximately 400 mL of N_2 passed as gas. The remaining air is thought to escape into the esophagus or become trapped in the stomach. This trapped air results in a "bloated" feeling for many individuals.

Intraluminal gas (H_2, CH_4, and CO_2) can be produced in the upper gut in various quantities. Carbon dioxide (CO_2) is produced from the interaction of hydrogen ions and bicarbonate. Hydrogen and methane (CH_4) are produced from bacterial metabolism. Methane is not produced by everyone, and individuals who produce methane usually have stools that float. Intraluminal gases produced are eventually released through the rectum.

Most gas production can be the result of malabsorption of carbohydrates and proteins. Fruits and vegetables that contain oligosaccharides and polysaccharides cannot be digested by the enzymes of the bowel; resulting in the production of gas.[38] Individuals with low levels of lactase, which is used to digest lactose, can develop gas. Other sources of food that can produce gas include specific flours, oats, corn, and potatoes.[24] Rice is the only starch that does not produce gas.

Because gases are soluble in lipid and water, diffusion between the lumen and the blood occurs easily. Pressure gradients create the movements of the gases. Most notably, air that is swallowed diffuses into the blood stream of the stomach. Carbon dioxide (CO_2) is extracted into the blood, whereas N_2 diffuses into the lumen. Bacteria in the colon produce CO_2, H_2 and CH_4, which enter the blood, whereas at the same time N_2 diffuses into the colon. The whole process results in gas production in different parts of the GI tract.

■ Intestinal Gas Drug Treatment and Adverse Affects

There are two classes of antiflatulent products available for intestinal gas; simethicone and alpha-galactosidase. Simethicone (Gas-X, Phazyme) is used as a defoaming agent to relieve gas by reducing the surface tension of gas bubbles found in the GI tract. As the surface tension is reduced, gas bubbles are broken and can be released through belching or flatus.[31]

Beano, an alpha-galactoside, is a relatively new drug used to relieve intestinal gas. Beano has an enzyme that breaks down oligosaccharides (a component of beans, whole grains, peas, and lentils) before they are metabolized by colonic bacteria.[10] Beano should be administered with the first bite of the food to be effective.

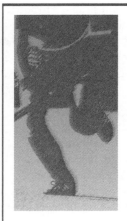

Scenario from the Field

A 22-year-old male baseball player approaches you during practice. He started having diarrhea in the morning and its frequency has been constant throughout the day. He states that he has bowel movements approximately every 40 to 50 minutes. What should you do?

Inquire about the possible cause of the diarrhea. If it is from an infectious source, the diarrhea is needed to help remove the causative bacteria or toxin. If it becomes severe or persists for more than 24 hours, control of the frequency of bowel movements may be needed.

Several OTC medications can be prescribed for this condition. Either Imodium A-D or Pepto-Bismol can be used initially. Make sure you read the label with the athlete and answer any questions about the directions for use. In addition, because the athlete has lost fluid during his diarrhea episodes, make sure that he drinks plenty of fluids. Individuals who have diarrhea often become dehydrated because of the loss of water and electrolytes. Following fluid replacement guidelines for activity and sports will ensure that he receives adequate hydration. Most diarrhea episodes should resolve within 24 to 36 hours with medication. If the athlete reports additional symptoms or the bout continues for a longer duration, please seek medical attention (see Figure 8–1).

*T*he Athletic Trainer's Responsibility

In most instances, PUD and GERD sufferers will not seek medical treatment from athletic trainers. However, some individuals might inform the athletic trainer of their signs and symptoms and ask for an opinion. The responsibility of the athletic trainer is to recognize the condition and refer the athlete to the appropriate medical specialist.

Nearly everyone experiences diarrhea and constipation at some point. Because these conditions are often embarrassing to discuss, it is important for the athletic trainer to have a good relationship with the athlete. A trusting relationship will allow the athlete to discuss the condition openly so that a proper medical evaluation can be made. The athletic trainer must be able to properly determine which OTC medication is appropriate for their athlete's signs and symptoms and how to properly administer the doses. As discussed in Chapter 1, the athletic trainer should document all relevant drug information and distribution.

Internet Resource Box

U.S. National Institute of Diabetes & Digestive & Kidney Diseases
www.niddk.nih.gov

U.S. Department of Health and Human Services, National Institutes of Health
Phone: (301) 496-4000
www.nih.gov

Centers for Disease Control and Prevention
Phone: (800) 311-3435
www.coc.gov

International Foundation for Functional Gastrointestinal Disorders
Phone: (888)964-2001 or (414) 9641799
www.iffgd.org

Discussion Topics

1. What should be your course of action if an athlete has diarrhea during a game?

2. What should you do if an athlete constantly complains of heartburn?

3. What are some foods that can cause intestinal gas if eaten before a game?

4. If your travel kit only could contain two medications for GI disorders, which two would you choose?

Chapter Review

1. Peptic ulcer disease (PUD) usually affects the stomach by causing excessive acid production.

2. Causes of PUD include *H. pylori,* NSAID use, and acid hypersecretion.

3. Various medications are geared toward relieving pain and promoting ulcer healing in patients with PUD.

4. The retrograde movement of stomach contents into the esophagus is called GERD.

5. The most common complaint associated with GERD is heartburn.

6. Wearing loose fitting clothes, eating appropriate foods, and using antacids or prokinetics can alleviate and control GERD.

7. Diarrhea is commonly caused by bacteria or contaminated foods.

8. The primary treatment for diarrhea includes replacing fluids and determining etiology so that proper medication therapy can be started.

9. Constipation can be avoided through proper diet, exercise, and fluid intake.

10. Intestinal gas is a naturally occurring event that may be limited with diet.

11. Most GI disorders can be treated with OTC medications.

12. Abuse of any OTC medication for GI disorders can cause unwanted or severe adverse effects.

References

1. Archer, DL, and Young, FE: Contemporary issues: Diseases with a food vector. Clin Microbiol Rev 1:377–398, 1988.
2. Ateshkadi, A, et al.: *Helicobacter pylori* and peptic ulcer disease. Clin Pharm 12:34–48, 1993.
3. Barradell, LB, et al.: Lansoprazole: A review of its pharmacodynamic and pharmacokinetic properties and its therapeutic efficacy in acid related disorders. Drugs 44:225–250, 1992.
4. Berardi, RR, and Dunn-Kucharski, VA: Omeprazole: Defining its role in gastroesophageal reflux disease. Hosp Formul 30:216–225, 1995.
5. Bertomeu, A, et al.: Chronic diarrhea with normal stool and colonic examinations: organic or functional? J Clin Gastroenterol 13(5):531–536, 1991.
6. Cavanaugh, J: Assessment of the effect of sucralfate on the bioavailability of lansoprazole and omeprazole. Am J Gastroenterol 90:1577, 1995.
7. Dodds, WJ, et al.: Pathogenesis of reflux esophagitis. Gastroenterology 81:376–394, 1981.
8. Donowitz, M, et al.: Evaluation of patients with chronic diarrhea. N Engl J Med 332:725–729, 1995.
9. Drumm, B, Perez-Perez, GI, et al.: Intrafamilial clustering of *Helicobacter pylori* infection. N Engl J Med 322:359–363,1990.
10. Ganiats, TG, Norcross, WA, et al.: Does Beano prevent gas? A double-blind crossover study of oral alpha-galactosidase to treat dietary oligosaccharide intolerance. J Fam Pract 39:441–445, 1994.
11. Garnett, WR: Efficacy, safety, and cost issues in managing patients with gastroesophageal reflux disease. Am J Hosp Pharm 50(Suppl 1):S11–S18, 1993.
12. Gattuso, JM, and Kamm, MA: Adverse effects of drugs used in the management of constipation and diarrhea. Drug Safety. 10(1):47–65, 1994.
13. Gelfand, MD: Gastroesophageal reflux disease. Med Clin North Am 75:923–940, 1991.
14. Graham, DY: Treatment of peptic ulcers caused by *Helicobacter pylori*. N Engl J Med 328:349–350, 1993.
15. Greenhalf, JO, and Leonard, HS: Laxatives in the treatment of constipation of pregnant and breast-feeding infants. Practitioner 210:259–263, 1973.
16. Hatlebakk, JG, and Berstad, A: Pharmacokinetic optimization in the treatment of gastro-oesophageal reflux disease. Clin Pharmacokinet 31:386–406, 1996.
17. Hetzel, DJ, et al.: Healing and relapse of severe peptic esophagitis after treatment with omeprazole. Gastroenterology 95:903–912, 1988.
18. Hogan, WJ, and Dodds, WJ: Gastroesophageal reflux disease (reflux esophagitis). In Sleisenger, M, and Fordtran, JS (eds): Gastrointestinal Disease: Pathophysiology, Diagnosis, Management, ed. 4. Philadelphia, WB Saunders, 1989, pp 594–619.
19. Isenberg, JI, et al.: Acid-peptic disorders. In Yamada, T, et al., (eds): Textbook of Gastroenterology, ed. 2. Philadelphia, JB Lippincott, 1995, 1347–1430.
20. Johnson, NJ, et al.: Acute treatment of reflux oesophagitis: A multicenter trial to compare 150 mg ranitidine BD with 300 mg ranitidine QDS. Aliment Pharmacol Ther 3:259–266, 1989.
21. Kahrilas, PJ, and Gupta, RR: Mechanisms of acid reflux associated with cigarette smoking. Gut. 31:4–10 1990.
22. Kitchin, LI, and Castell, DO: Rationale and efficacy of conservative therapy for gastroesophageal reflux disease. Arch Intern Med 151:448–454, 1991.
23. Kozarek, RA: Complications of reflux esophagitis and their medical management. Gastroenterol Clin North Am 19:713–731, 1990.
24. Levitt, MD, et al.: H_2 excretion after ingestion of complex carbohydrates. Gastroenterology 92(2):383–389, 1987.
25. Longe, RL: Antidiarrheal products. In American Pharmaceutical Association: Handbook of Nonprescription Drugs, ed. 11. Washington, D.C., American Pharmaceutical Association, 1996, p 258.
26. Maddock, WG, Bell, JL et al.: Gastrointestinal gas: Observations on belching during anesthesia, operations and pyleography and rapid passage of gas. Ann Surg 130:512–537, 1949.
27. Maton, PN: Drug therapy: Omeprazole. N Engl J Med 324: 965–975, 1991.
28. McNulty, CM: Bismuth subsalicylate in the treatment of gastritis due to *Campylobacter pylori*. Rev Infect Dis 12(Suppl. 1):S94–S98, 1990.
29. Mofenson, HC, and Caraccio, TR: Magnesium intoxication in a neonate from oral magnesium hydroxide laxatives. J Toxicol Clin Toxicol 29(2):215–222, 1991.
30. Navab, F, and Texter, EC: Gastroesophageal reflux: Pathophysiologic concepts. Arch Intern Med 145:329–333, 1985.
31. Olin, B, ed: Drug Facts and Comparisons. Facts and Comparison, St. Louis, Mo., 2001.
32. Orenstein, SR: Gastroesophageal reflux disease. Sem Gastrointestinal Dis 5(1):2–14, 1994.
33. Quik, RFP, et al.: A comparison of two doses of nizatidine versus placebo in the treatment of reflux oesophagitis. Aliment Pharmacol Ther 4:201–211, 1990.
34. Read, NW, et al.: Chronic diarrhea of unknown origin. Gastroenterology 78:264–271, 1980.
35. Silverstin, FE, et al.: Misoprostol reduces serious gastrointestinal complications in patients with rheumatoid arthritis receiving nonsteroidal anti-inflammatory drugs. Ann Intern Med 123:241–249, 1995.
36. Sontag, SJ: The medical management of reflux esophagitis. Gastroenterol Clin North Am 19:683–712, 1990.
37. Spencer, CM, and Faulds, D: Lansoprazole: A reappraisal of its pharmacodynamic and pharmacokinetic properties, and its therapeutic efficacy in acid related disorders. Drugs 48:404–430, 1994.
38. Steggerda, FR: Gastrointestinal gas following food consumption. Ann N Y Acad Sci 150:57–66, 1968.
39. Traube, M: The spectrum of the symptoms and presentations of gastroesophageal reflux disease. Gastroenterol Clin North Am 19:609–617, 1990.
40. Valle, J, Seppala, K, et al.: Disappearance of gastritis after eradication of Helicobacter pylori. A morphometric study. Scand J Gastroenterol 26:1057–1065, 1991.

Chapter Questions

1. A chronic inflammatory disorder of the mucosa of the stomach is called:
   A. PUD
   B. GERD
   C. Irritable bowel syndrome
   D. Kuder-Richardson syndrome

2. Which of the following is NOT a pathophysiological mechanism of GERD?
   A. Relaxation of the lower esophageal sphincter
   B. A low resting lower esophageal sphincter pressure
   C. Odynophagia
   D. Obesity

3. Which of the following compounds is NOT an antacid?
   A. Calcium citrate
   B. Calcium carbonate
   C. Magnesium salts
   D. Aluminum salts

4. Which of the following drugs is classified as a proton pump inhibitor?
   A. Pepcid
   B. Axid
   C. Aciphex
   D. Milk of magnesia

5. Acute diarrhea can be caused by which of the following?
   A. Shigella
   B. *H. pylori*
   C. Psychogenic origin, *S. aureus*
   D. Flatulence

6. Select the appropriate drug used to treat constipation:
   A. Loperamide
   B. Docusate
   C. Lansoprazole
   D. Pantoprazole

7. This type of laxative draws water from the wall of the small intestine into the stool and stimulates intestinal motility:
   A. Bisacodyl
   B. Mineral oil
   C. Magnesium sulfate
   D. Senna

8. Which of the following examples of drugs are causes of PUD in individuals who are not infected with *H. pylori*?
   A. Lansoprazole
   B. Erythromycin
   C. Bismuth subsalicylate
   D. Ibuprofen

9. This drug is often used to treat traveler's diarrhea:
   A. Pepcid
   B. Imodium
   C. Colace
   D. Senna

10. Which of the following is an alpha-galactoside used to treat intestinal gas?
    A. Beano
    B. Bisacodyl
    C. Simethicone
    D. Ex-Lax

9

Drugs for Bacterial, Viral, and Fungal Infections

Chapter Objectives

After reading this chapter, the student should understand the following concepts:

1 The difference among the following types of microorganisms: bacterial, viral, and fungal.
2 The role of the physician in prescribing medications to alleviate infections.
3 The different categories of antibiotic drugs and how each works.
4 The problems associated with antibiotic resistance.
5 The types of antiviral medications available and how they are used.
6 The treatment options for topical fungal infections.
7 The use of the Internet as a source of information about microorganisms.

Chapter Outline

*A*t certain times, we become susceptible to different types of infections caused by bacteria, viruses, or fungi. Typically, the immune system in the body is strong enough to repel or destroy the invading microorganism. Situations do occur, however, when the body's immune system is not able to combat and control an invasion by one or more of these microorganisms. When microbes overload the natural immune system, the body requires assistance to control the invasion. During these instances, chemotherapeutics (chemical agents that fight organisms such as bacteria, viruses, and fungi) are prescribed to control or eliminate the infection. In this chapter, we will study three categories of chemotherapeutic agents—antibiotics and antiviral and antifungal agents—and discuss their mechanisms of action in fighting invading microorganisms.

*A*ntibiotics

Bacteria

Bacteria are classified according to their general structure and makeup. They are small unicellular microorganisms (about the size of mitochondria) contained within a cell wall. Their genetic material is not contained in a true nuclear membrane. Bacteria cells lack the processes of mitosis and meiosis, and their genetic organization is simpler than that of cells in multicellular plants and animals.[16] Bacteria are able to maintain cellular metabolism. However, they require nutrients and prefer to steal from their host the necessary amino acids, sugars, and other products they need to sustain life. By understanding the needs of bacteria, we can begin to appreciate how they compete with their human host for these nutrients.

Some bacteria are beneficial to humans. For example, the bacteria in the gastrointestinal (GI) system assist in the digestion of food and help to limit the growth of other microorganisms and excess production of some stomach acids. These helpful bacteria, the normal flora of the GI system, should not be destroyed on a regular basis. However, they are sometimes casualties of antibacterial treatment. It is sometimes necessary to restore these normal GI flora after an antibiotic regimen.

■ Types of Antibiotics

Bacterial infections must be diagnosed and treated by a physician. Treatment of a bacterial invasion is typically accomplished by a regimen of antibiotic therapy. There are several ways to classify antibiotics. For this book we will use the categories of spectrum of activity and method of bacterial control. Antibiotics can be described by their spectrum of activity: either narrow or broad. Narrow-spectrum antibiotics are active only against very specific microorganisms. Conversely, broad-spectrum antibiotics are active against many different categories of bacterial microorganisms. For example, when treating someone with an ear infection, you may want to fight only the bacteria causing the infection. You would use a narrow-spectrum antibiotic so that your treatment regimen does not destroy other bacteria found in the body. A broad-spectrum antibiotic is used when the exact invading bacteria have not been identified. For example, if a person is admitted to the hospital with pneumonia, broad-spectrum antibiotics are started immediately until cultures have been taken and the exact microorganism causing the infection is known.

Antibiotics can also be classified as bactericidal or bacteriostatic. Bactericidal antibiotics can completely destroy the bacteria. Bacteriostatic antibiotics suppress bacterial growth but cannot destroy the bacteria by their own mechanisms. They must rely on support from the immune system of the host.

Once the exact invading bacterial microorganism is known, it is important to choose the appropriate antibiotic. This choice depends on three criteria: (1) identification of the organism, (2) drug sensitivity of the invading organism, and (3) host factors.[8]

To effectively identify the invading organisms, Gram stain tests are ordered. Gram staining is the process of using crystal violet solution and iodine to identify the type of cell wall structure as either gram positive or gram negative. Gram-positive bacteria cell walls retain the violet stain, whereas gram-negative bacteria cell walls stain red. Through this quick method, the type of organism can be identified and appropriate treatment can be started. Samples used for gram staining can be obtained from various sources, but usually are from pus, sputum, urine, blood, or other bodily fluids. Taking direct samples from the site of infection is usually warranted.

Defining drug sensitivity to the invading organism is a common practice because of the emergence of drug-resistant organisms. There are two common methods to assess drug sensitivity: a disk-diffusion (Kirby-Bauer) test or a broth dilution procedure. Although a discussion of how they work is beyond the scope of this text, both procedures are effective in identifying the types of antibiotics to which certain bacteria may be resistant, thereby identifying the appropriate antibiotic treatment. The disk and broth diffusion procedures also help to determine the immunity of the microorganisms to a particular antibiotic. Later in this chapter we discuss in detail some of the emerging causes and problems associated with bacterial resistance.

The last step in choosing the appropriate antibiotic is determining host factors. One of the primary host factors is the natural defense mechanism (immune system). Someone with an impaired immune system will need different antibiotics from someone with a normally functioning immune system. The site of infection and the concentration of the antibiotic at the site of infection also play an important role in effective treatment. The blood-brain barrier, vascularity, or other impediments can alter the function and concentration of antibiotic therapy. Other factors, such as age, pregnancy, and genetic disposition, can also alter drug therapy. All these factors must be taken into consideration when a health-care professional chooses an antibiotic.

An athletic trainer's knowledge regarding antibiotic therapy does not have to be as complete as the attending physician's. However, it is important for the athletic trainer to be able to understand and explain to the athlete the general process by which an antibiotic works in the body. Therefore, in this section of the chapter, we will discuss antibiotics according to their mechanisms of action: (1) inhibition of bacterial cell-wall synthesis, (2) inhibition of bacterial protein synthesis, (3) inhibition of bacterial DNA synthesis, and (4) inhibition of folic acid synthesis. As we describe the mechanism of action for each drug, we will also refer to the class of the drug so that the reader will have a second way to remember each of these antibiotic drugs.

Antibiotics That Inhibit Cell Wall Synthesis

Penicillin

Penicillin was discovered in 1928 in Alexander Fleming's laboratory when mold was mistakenly introduced into bacteria being grown in a Petri dish. Initially, the scientist was going to discard the contaminated Petri dish, but then he noticed that the bacteria in the dish were dying around this contaminated area. Fleming looked closely at the contaminant and determined that it was mold. After it was determined that the penicillin produced by the mold would kill bacteria, he proceeded to experiment with the amount needed to destroy the microorganisms. Fleming went on to determine whether or not this new substance was toxic to life forms by injecting a rabbit that had an infection with what he termed "mold broth," and the rabbit appeared to get better. Over the next 15 years, as the result of still more research and development and the discovery of how to produce it in mass quantities, penicillin became available to the general population.[19] It was the weapon needed to fight infections that previously been life threatening. Penicillin is able to effectively inhibit bacterial cell wall synthesis by passing through the small pores on a bacterium's cell membrane and binding to penicillin-binding proteins (PBPs). By attaching to PBPs, penicillin is able to inhibit specific enzymes that allow construction of the bacterium's cell wall. The bacterium cannot maintain its structure because of the decreased stability of the cell wall. The wall then collapses and the contents of the bacterium are forced out. Because mammalian cells lack a cell wall, penicillin has virtually no effect on the cells of the host.[9] Most bacterial cell walls contain PBPs that are not found in animal cells. Therefore penicillin can be effective in selectively destroying some bacteria without affecting the animal or human host cells.[12]

Penicillins all have the same basic chemical structure, called a beta-lactam ring (Fig 9–1). This ring is essential for the antibacterial activity of penicillin. Unfortunately, the beta-lactam ring of the penicillin is a very weak structure. Some bacteria are able to produce an enzyme called beta-lactamase that cleaves the ring structure and inactivates the antibiotic. This is one example of a method by which bacteria are starting to develop resistance to antibiotics.

Penicillins are available in oral and injectable formulations and are used to treat infections, particularly those caused by gram-positive bacteria. These include ear infections, pneumonia, and skin infections. Other penicillin classes are able to treat gram-negative bacteria, which cause problems such as urinary tract infections, gynecological infections, and pneumonia.

The most common adverse effect of penicillin is hypersensitivity reaction, otherwise known as allergic reaction. The patient may develop a rash, itching, swelling, or a more serious anaphylactic reaction involving bronchospasm, vasomotor collapse, and laryngeal edema.[6] Rashes and fevers usu-

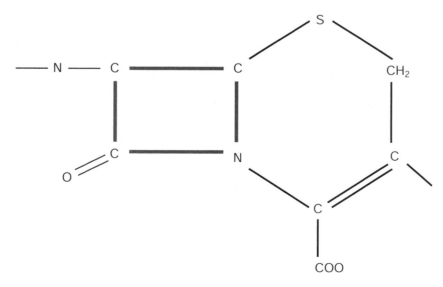

Figure 9–1. Beta-lactam ring structure in bold lines.

ally do not appear until after several days of therapy, but anaphylaxis may occur within 10 minutes. Other adverse effects are usually related to disrupted GI function. Patients may experience nausea, vomiting, or diarrhea. Hypersensitivity and gastrointestinal reactions can occur with any antibiotic class; therefore, maintenance of allergy information for each patient is vital to ensure correct antibiotic selection.

Patients receiving any antibiotic treatment should be asked if they have an allergy to the medication and, if so, the type of reaction that occurred. If the patient reports a minor reaction, such as itching, he or she may be able to continue that specific drug therapy. In more severe reactions, the patient should change therapy to another drug class. In either case, the physician must be made aware of any abnormal reaction to a medication.

Implications for Activity

Athletes experiencing bacterial infections must be aware that whenever they have a fever, the physician is going to be reticent to allow them to participate in sports. Taking penicillin or an antibiotic will not reduce the fever, and just because the athlete is taking antibiotics, it does not mean that he or she is immediately cleared to participate. Antibiotics will not improve athletic performance, nor will they control viral infections. If an athlete with a bacterial infection wants to accompany the team to an event, he or she should be particularly careful not to communicate the infection to teammates.

Cephalosporins

The first cephalosporin was isolated in 1948 from the sea near the Sardinian coast. Today cephalosporins are among the most commonly prescribed classes of antibiotic agents by physicians in outpatient and inpatient settings. Cephalosporins have a mechanism of action and structure (beta-lactam ring) similar to those of the penicillins. Because of this ring, cephalosporins are also susceptible to beta lactamase destruction.

Unlike the penicillins, the cephalosporin agents have developed into a hierarchical classification by chemical structure generation. Cephalosporins are currently divided into four generations, each based on general features of its antimicrobial activity. First-generation cephalosporins are most effective at fighting gram-positive bacteria. Second-through fourth-generation cephalosporins have increasing effectiveness against gram-negative bacteria while at the same time fighting gram-positive bacteria.

Because of this wide range of effectiveness, cephalospo-

rins are used to treat many different types of bacterial infections. They are effective in treating skin and soft tissue infections, respiratory tract infections, and even meningitis. Cephalosporins are available in oral and injectable formulations. Most are effectively absorbed by the body and excreted via the kidneys.

Cephalosporin hypersensitivity reactions, similar to those of the penicillins, are the most common adverse effect noted. Because of the drugs' similar beta-lactam structures, patients who are allergic to penicillins may develop a cross-reactivity to cephalosporins.[14] However, many patients who have mild allergic reactions to penicillins are able to take cephalosporins. If a patient develops severe hypersensitivity reactions to penicillins, cephalosporins can be prescribed, but with great caution.

Internet Resource Box

More information about penicillin can be found on a number of Websites set up to provide the consumer with general information:

http://www.fda.gov/cder/drug/infopage/penG_doxy/default.htm
http://www.informed.org/100drugs/penitoc.html

Antibiotics That Inhibit Protein Synthesis

Another mechanism of action of antimicrobial agents is the inhibition of bacterial protein synthesis. These antibiotics are able to bind to bacterial ribosomes and block the production of new amino acids needed for protein synthesis.

Common classes of agents that inhibit bacterial protein synthesis include tetracyclines, macrolides, and clindamycin. These antibiotics are also bacteriostatic and suppress bacterial growth. Another class of antibiotics that inhibit bacterial protein synthesis is the aminoglycosides. They are a little different because, in addition to inhibiting bacterial protein synthesis, they exert bactericidal activity. There are other agents that inhibit protein synthesis, but they will not be included in this discussion because they are used specifically in the treatment of hospitalized patients.

Tetracyclines

Tetracyclines are a broad-spectrum class of antibiotics. These agents are effective against a variety of gram-positive and -negative organisms. Importantly, they are also effective in treating infections caused by rickettsias, such as Rocky

Mountain spotted fever; and spirochetes, such as Lyme disease and syphilis. Commonly used agents include tetracycline, doxycycline, and minocycline.

Tetracyclines are readily absorbed from the stomach and small intestine. This absorption is impaired by concurrent administration of any products containing calcium, magnesium, aluminum, iron, or zinc. Therefore tetracyclines should not be taken with dairy products, iron, antacids containing aluminum, calcium or magnesium, or supplements containing zinc. If an athlete needs any of these supplements, tetracyclines may be administered 1 hour before or 2 hours after ingestion of the calcium, vitamin, or other mineral product.

The most common adverse effect of the tetracycline class is GI upset. To decrease the incidence of this upset, these agents can be taken with food as long as it does not contain the previously mentioned products. Photosensitivity reactions have also occurred with tetracyclines. When photosensitivity reactions occur, the skin becomes more sensitive to ultraviolet light. This is commonly recognized as an exaggerated sunburn. Patients should be advised to avoid prolonged exposure to the sunlight, wear protective clothing, and apply sunscreen to exposed skin. Tetracyclines also bind to calcium in the developing teeth of children and can result in a yellow or brown discoloration of the teeth. This discoloration is permanent and is related to dose, not duration of therapy.

Macrolides

Macrolides are another class of agents that have the ability to inhibit bacterial protein synthesis and are bacteriostatic in nature. These agents have a spectrum of activity similar to that of penicillins and are effective for persons who have an allergy to the penicillin class. Common agents in this class include erythromycin, azithromycin, and clarithromycin.

These agents are all available in oral formulations; some also have intravenous forms. It is important to note that some of these agents may be taken with or without food. This will affect the absorption rate, and therefore the athletic trainer should ensure that the athlete reads the instructions for taking the medication.

The most reported adverse effect of macrolides is GI disturbances. These effects are most severe with erythromycin. Macrolides have also been reported to have drug interactions with other agents. Because of the drug interactions, it is important to have all prescription medications dispensed from the same pharmacy. This will ensure that all potential drug interactions are reviewed by a pharmacist.

Clindamycin

Unique unto itself, clindamycin is the only agent in its class. Clindamycin has antibacterial activity that is similar to that of erythromycin but is effective against anaerobes, bacteria that can flourish without oxygen. Clindamycin absorption is not affected by food. Diarrhea is the most common adverse effect. It occurs in 2 to 20 percent of people taking this drug.[2]

Aminoglycosides

Aminoglycosides are agents that inhibit bacterial protein synthesis, are bactericidal in nature, and most commonly provide coverage against gram-negative bacteria. Aminoglycosides are formed by two or more amino sugars connected by a glycoside linkage, hence their name. Drugs in this class include gentamicin, tobramycin, amikacin, and neomycin. Neomycin, is commonly found in topical preparations for treatment of infections of the eye, ear, and skin.

Aminoglycosides are effective antibiotics but are reserved for hospitalized patients because most of them can be given only via intravenous infusion. Aminoglycosides are rapidly distributed throughout the body after IV administration and collect in the urine. They can also be used topically for some wound care. Because of their exclusive elimination by the kidney, the pharmacist or physician must continually monitor these drugs to determine if dose adjustments are necessary based on the individual's renal function. These agents can also cause ototoxicity and thus may result in impaired hearing or balance.

Antibiotics That Inhibit DNA Synthesis

Fluoroquinolones

Fluoroquinolones are popular agents used to treat broad-spectrum bacterial infections.[13] These agents exert their antibacterial activity by inhibiting the coiling process of the bacterial DNA. Some agents included in this class are ciprofloxacin, levofloxacin, gatifloxacin, and moxifloxacin. Most are available in oral and intravenous formulations.

Adverse effects that sometimes occur with fluoroquinolones include central nervous system (CNS) effects such as headache and dizziness, GI upset, and arthropathy. This class of agents is not commonly used in children.

Recently, animal studies have reported an incidence of

tendon rupture in fluoroquinolone use. The Achilles tendon is most commonly involved.[7,20] Fluoroquinolones disrupt the extracellular matrix of the cartilage and therefore should be discontinued if tendon pain or inflammation occurs. They have a food-drug interaction similar to that with tetracyclines, and therefore fluoroquinolones should not be administered concurrently with aluminum, magnesium, calcium, iron, or zinc products because of the decreased absorption of fluoroquinolones by the body.

Antibiotics That Inhibit Folic Acid Synthesis

Sulfonamides

Sulfonamides ("sulfa drugs") were used even before penicillin to treat bacterial infections Initially, these drugs were used because they significantly decreased morbidity and mortality from invading bacterial infections. However, they are not the most effective antibacterial agents for fighting many different types of bacteria. After the introduction of penicillin, this class of agents slowly lost favor. Sulfonamides are still used today; however, they are mainly used in the treatment of urinary tract infections. They are able to eradicate bacteria by inhibiting folic acid synthesis, thereby producing a bacteriostatic effect. Common agents include sulfadiazine and sulfamethoxazole (a component of Bactrim). Common adverse effects are usually of the hypersensitivity type.

■ Adverse Effects of Antibiotics

In our discussion of the different types of antibiotics we have mentioned some of the adverse effects, however it is important for the athletic trainer to have an awareness of the general adverse effects associated with antibiotics. Hypersensitivity to antibiotics is not a common reaction in most people, but it can occur even after the athlete has been taking the medication for a few days or longer. Adverse effects that an athlete might experience when taking antibiotics include diarrhea, gastrointestinal upset, nausea, vomiting, itching, swelling, skin rashes, and difficulty breathing. In some individuals this hypersensitivity can result in an anaphylactic reaction, leading to severe bronchoconstriction and cardiovascular collapse.

Additionally, as mentioned, some antibiotics may produce an ultraviolet sensitivity, also known as a photosensitivity reaction. An athlete taking an antibiotic may become more susceptible to sunburn or other ultraviolet insult to the skin. It is always wise to warn athletes of this potential problem because of the outdoor location of many sports. Also, there have been a few anecdotal reports of a reduction in the effectiveness of birth control pills during the course of an antibiotic regimen.[4] It is wise to tell female athletes who take birth control pills that the pills' effectiveness may be diminished during the period of antibiotic therapy.

Because the drugs are antibacterial, the helpful bacteria that normally exist in the gastrointestinal tract may also be contained and destroyed. To more rapidly replenish normal gastrointestinal flora, the athlete can eat yogurt after he or she has finished taking the entire course of antibiotics.

Minor Skin Infections

Athletes participating in almost any sport will at some time experience a minor cut or laceration to the skin. If these minor accidents result in a superficial skin infection, or if the athletic trainer wants to avoid minor complications from this trauma, readily available OTC topical antibiotics can be used. Many OTC antibiotic ointments are triple antibiotic preparations; that is, they typically contain the three main types of antimicrobial agents in smaller concentrations. Generally, these ointments contain small amounts of antibiotics that (1) inhibit cell wall activity, (2) inhibit protein synthesis, or (3) inhibit DNA synthesis of bacteria. Topical application of one of these ointments can destroy the microbes that may exist on or around the infected area.

■ Antibiotic Resistance

A growing health-care problem that appears to be getting worse as time goes on is the reduced efficacy of antibiotics to contain or destroy bacterial organisms.[3,23] Some strains of bacteria are becoming resistant to existing antibacterial drugs, and the greatest resistance patterns are in the United States and Latin America.[15] This resistance has various etiologies. One is the beta-lactamase enzyme, which was discussed previously. This enzyme is becoming more prevalent in society and therefore causes more bacterial resistance. Stuart Levy, a diligent researcher in this area, has written an article about antibiotic resistance that will be informative to those interested in this ongoing problem.[10] In monitoring the effectiveness of tetracyclines over three decades, it has been demonstrated that the growth in resistance in some strains of bacteria over that period has increased from 30 to

Table 9-1

General Antibiotic Summary Chart

Antibiotic Class	Generic Name	Brand Name	Mechanism of Action
Penicillin	Penicillin VK Aminopenicillins Amoxicillin Amoxicillin plus clavulanate	Veetids Ampicillin, Omnipen Amoxil Augmentin	Inhibits bacterial cell wall synthesis (bactericidal)
First-generation cephalosporin	Cephalexin 1st Cefadroxil 1st	Keflex Duricef	Inhibits bacterial cell wall synthesis (bactericidal)
Second-generation cephalosporin	Cefprozil 2nd Cefaclor 2nd	Cefzil Ceclor	
Third-generation cephalosporin	Cefixime 3rd Cefpodoxime 3rd	Suprax Vantin	
Fourth-generation cephalosporin	Cefepime 4th	Maxipime	
Aminoglycoside	Tobramycin Amikacin	Nebcin Amikin	Inhibits bacterial protein synthesis (bactericidal)
Fluoroquinolone	Ciprofloxacin Levofloxacin Gatifloxacin Moxifloxacin	Cipro Levaquin Tequin Avelox	Inhibits bacterial DNA synthesis (bactericidal)
Tetracycline	Minocycline Doxycycline Tetracycline	Minocin Vibramycin Sumycin	Inhibits bacterial protein synthesis (bacteriostatic)
Macrolide	Erythromycin Azithromycin Clarithromycin	E-Mycin Zithromax Biaxin	Inhibits bacterial protein synthesis (bacteriostatic)
Sulfonamide	Sulfamethoxazole/ Trimethoprim	Bactrim	Inhibits bacterial folic acid synthesis (bacteriostatic)

Please note that the brand names listed are only examples and other brand names for the same drugs may exist. Consult a physician or pharmacist if you have questions regarding any medication.

80 percent. This can be considered a major setback for tetracycline effectiveness over time,[21] and other antibiotics are experiencing antibiotic resistance as well.

Other researchers discuss the mutations that occur in bacteria over the years.[17] Many people who take antibiotics take only a portion of the dosage. For example, they may start to feel better and stop taking the antibiotic. However, the entire colony of bacteria may not be contained or destroyed, and the surviving bacteria can mutate and become more resistant to the antibacterial medication being taken. This is a good reason to consistently remind athletes taking an antibiotic to be fully compliant and take the entire course of the prescription, even if they start to feel better before they have completed the total prescription. Even if an athlete has 2 or 3 days of medication left to take and insists that he or she feels "fine," continue to encourage the athlete to finish the entire prescription.

Internet Resource Box

The U.S. Food and Drug Administration presents some interesting information about antibiotic-resistant infections at http://www.fda.gov/fdac/features/795_antibio.html.

Additional information is available at http://www.bact.wisc.edu/Bact330/lecturebactres.

The World Health Organization has a dedicated Website about controlling antimicrobial resistance, global strategies, and antibiotic use in developing countries: http://www.who.int/emc/amr_interventions.htm.

A Washington D.C. organization, Keep Antibiotics Working, that works to preserve the effectiveness of antibiotics maintains a Website at http://www.keepantibioticsworking.com.

Another reason that has been suggested for the increase in bacterial resistance is the overprescribing of antibiotics by physicians. Swain and Kaplan[22] boldly state that antibiotics are overused in the treatment of upper respiratory infections. The prescription of antibiotics is beyond the scope of practice of the athletic trainer. However, we mention this issue so that the athletic trainer can explain to athletes why a physician will not prescribe antibiotics for a sore throat. Most sore throats are a symptom of a viral infection, such as a common cold, on which an antibiotic will not have any effect. Medications for the common cold will be discussed farther on in this chapter under the heading "Antiviral Agents."

Recently there has been a growing discussion regarding the use of antibiotics to prevent infection in farm animals raised for human consumption.[5] Some farmers and ranchers have been using antibiotic supplements in animal feed to maintain health in the animal during its growth period and before it goes to market. It is suggested that residual antibiotics in meat allow bacteria in the body to mutate. Once the bacteria mutate, they become difficult to control by the normal defense mechanisms of the body. This theory is of recent origin, and research in this area is ongoing. There is not a great deal of definitive information at this time. In 1997 the United States, in collaboration with a number of other countries around the world, began collecting data on antimicrobial resistance.[15] The antibiotic resistance scheme used in the United States is called SENTRY Antimicrobial Surveillance and includes 30 sites that report to a main center at the University of Iowa. This system is linked to similar systems for monitoring antibiotic resistance in Europe, Asia, and Central and South America. The objective of SENTRY is to provide a worldwide network of laboratories that will monitor and provide timely information about hospital- and community-acquired infections, among other priorities.[15] In the United States there are state- and county-level groups that are attempting to reduce bacterial resistance by educating the public about the proper use of antibiotics.

In response to the problems of antibiotic resistance numerous scientists and laboratory personnel are working diligently on developing new antimicrobial drugs. One of the most recent advances is a drug called quinupristin-dalfopristin, which was approved by the FDA in 1999 for serious or life-threatening illnesses associated with severe bacterial infections.[11] This is a new class of antibiotic. Its desired action is to impair bacterial protein synthesis. It is currently being successfully implemented in the hospital setting. Additionally, scientists and drug companies are continuing research to discover new types of drugs that will successfully destroy or deter microbial activity in humans and animals.

Antiviral Agents

When a virus invades the human body, it brings with it only the necessary DNA or RNA to replicate. The capsid holding the DNA or RNA invades the body either via an airborne mechanism or through an opening in the skin. When the capsid enters the body, it finds a host cell and releases its replication materials into that cell. The virus, in essence, takes over one of the cells of the human body and uses the cellular mechanism to reproduce more DNA or RNA, which is released and takes over other cells within the same host. The virus causes the host's cells to cease functioning normally and utilizes cellular mechanics to propagate the virus. This continues until the body can produce enough appropriate antibodies to destroy the virus without destroying its own system.

A virus invading a human host is a very small microorganism and can be relatively benign, severe, or fatal, depending on its type. The common cold is a good example of a viral infection that typically has only minor repercussions for the human host if cared for properly. However, the common cold can also be extremely debilitating and can develop into a possibly fatal illness if proper care procedures are not followed. In contrast, almost everyone is aware of the ramifications of the human immunodeficiency virus (HIV), and most people do everything possible to avoid contact with this virus because it is almost always lethal in the long term.

Implications for Activity

There are many viral infections that can impair an athlete's performance. Viral infections typically produce problems in the athlete for weeks, although some may cause a decrease or impairment in performance only for a day or two. Antibiotics do not have any effect on viral infections, and therefore athletes need to be constantly reminded that a common cold virus will not respond to penicillin or any other antibiotic. When an athlete is suffering from a viral infection, he or she may have a fever, chills, nausea, vomiting, diarrhea, or other flulike symptoms. Many times an athlete with an active virus has to wait out the initial infection, and may miss a practice or competition while his or her body is building an immune response to the virus.

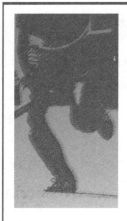

Scenarios from the Field

A 20-year-old collegiate male soccer player returning for twice-daily practices at the beginning of the fall semester presented to the athletic trainer with a rash contained within the trunk area (mostly bilateral along the ribcage). When questioned at the initial presentation, the athlete did not report that he was taking an antibiotic prescribed by his hometown physician before arriving on campus. The next day, the rash began to spread and was starting to progress into all four extremities. On the second day, the athletic trainer again questioned the athlete to see if he was taking any medications. At that point, the athlete admitted taking the antibiotic before arriving on campus. Previously he had not wanted to admit taking the medication. The athletic trainer immediately had the athlete stop taking the medication and see the team physician. A different antibiotic prescription was issued to the athlete and no further adverse effects were reported.

An 18-year-old female athlete reported to her athletic trainer that she had a significant rash that had erupted overnight. When she was asked if she was taking any medications, she replied that she had been taking an antibiotic (Keflex) for 8 days and had 2 days remaining on the prescription, but had experienced no adverse effects until the previous night. The athletic trainer immediately sent her back to her physician, who told the athlete to immediately stop taking the prescription and start taking a different drug. The physician explained to the athlete that she had developed an allergic reaction to the drug well into the prescription. This latent-response phenomenon can and does happen, and therefore the athletic trainer should keep this potential problem in mind.

A 16-year-old male athlete was with his team in a foreign country when the team decided to take a day trip to the beach. The athletic trainer warned the players of the dangers of sun exposure and told them to reapply sunscreen multiple times during the day. Late that night, this young man presented to the athletic trainer with a severe second-degree sunburn on his back and chest. On questioning, the young man revealed that he was taking an acne medication that was determined also to be an antibiotic. He was not able to participate in any games following this sunburn until the skin healed.

As mentioned, a viral infection can manifest as a cold, flu, or other system-wide disturbance. It can also be localized: for example, a cold sore or wart located on one small part of the body. Many, if not all, athletes experience some type of viral infection at some point in their athletic career. Therefore the athletic trainer should be familiar with viruses and their treatment.

▪ Oral Medications

One of the more common antiviral medications is acyclovir, commonly prescribed to contain an outbreak of the herpes simplex virus. It is prescribed for treatment of initial and recurrent episodes of the herpes virus, including cold sores and chickenpox, as well as genital herpes outbreaks. Acyclovir inhibits viral DNA replication in the host cell. When the genetic material cannot be replicated and passed on, the virus eventually succumbs to the host's immune system.

Acyclovir and other prescription antiviral agents are described in Table 9–2.

Internet Resource Box

The CDC provides a weekly flu update, flu shot information, questions and answers, and a number of other informative topics on their Website: *http://www. cdc.gov/ncidod/disease/flu/fluvirus.htm#part3*

New drugs are being developed for viral infections. Some of those are OTC medications for the care of minor viral infections such as cold sores and fever blisters. One of the most recent is docosanol (Abreva). It has a 10 percent active ingredient, can be purchased OTC, and claims to shorten the healing time for cold sores.

Other antiviral medications target the influenza virus. Drugs such as zanamivir (Relenza, see Table 9–2) work with the body's immune system to decrease the duration of flu

Table 9-2

Examples of Prescription Antiviral Medications

Generic Name	Trade Name	Common Indication(s) for Viruses
Acyclovir	Zovirax, Zovirax ointment	Shingles, genital herpes, chickenpox, other herpes simplex infections
Famciclovir	Famvir	Shingles, genital herpes
Valacyclovir	Valtrex	Shingles, genital herpes
Amantadine	Symmetrel	Prevention/treatment of flu
Oseltamivir	Tamiflu	Prevention/treatment of flu
Zanamivir	Relenza	Treatment of flu
Rimantadine	Flumadine	Prevention/treatment of flu

symptoms. If you want an athlete to use antiviral drugs to reduce flu symptoms, it is critical to get the athlete to the physician as soon as the flu symptoms start. The sooner the athlete starts taking the prescription medication, the quicker the symptoms will subside. Relenza and similar antivirals must be taken within 48 hours of the onset of symptoms to be effective.

■ Vaccines

Vaccines are most commonly associated with the influenza virus but are also available for other viral infections. Vaccines are prepared by a method in which either an entire virus or part of a virus is completely or partially inactivated through laboratory procedures so that it does not replicate. This attenuated virus is then injected into the human host. The immune system of the human host, stimulated by an inactive invader that resembles a live virus, proceeds to generate and store antibodies to this virus in the body. If the actual live virus does invade the body, there is a supply of antibodies to immediately attack and stop reproduction of the virus in the human host.

The development of vaccines has been extremely helpful in avoiding many viral infections, some of which can be fatal to their human host (Table 9–3). Vaccines are not yet available for every type of virus. Most notably, no vaccine exists for HIV, which leads to acquired immunodeficiency syndrome (AIDS). Treatment of HIV and AIDS is beyond the scope of the athletic trainer and will not be discussed in detail here.

*A*ntifungal Agents

There are many thousands of fungus species in nature. A very small percentage of these species can cause an infection on or in the human body. A fungus is a plantlike organism that can exist in either air or soil. Many fungal infections in the human are considered opportunistic infections and occur on the epidermis. A cutaneous fungal infection needs three environmental conditions to develop, multiply, and sustain life in a human host: warmth, darkness, and moisture. Proper hygiene and the normal defense mechanisms of the body are the common tactics for reducing the possibility of fungal infections in athletes. However, when these normal modes of control are not available, fungal infections can occur on, or sometimes in, the body.

Many times a cutaneous fungal infestation is referred to as a "tinea" infection. *Tinea* refers to the skin, and most athletic-related fungal infections have the word "tinea" in their names. For example, tinea capitis is ringworm of the scalp; tinea corporis is a fungal infection on the trunk area; tinea cruris, commonly known as "jock itch," occurs in the perineal area, and tinea pedis is athlete's foot. This last infection is very common in athletes playing a variety of sports and can occur in athletes of any gender or age. Nail fungus (onychomycosis) is another common fungal infection experienced by athletes.

Table 9-3

Vaccines

Viral Infections with Vaccines	Viral Infections without Vaccines to Date
Polio	Common cold
Smallpox	HIV/AIDS
Chickenpox/shingles	Mononucleosis
Rabies	Herpes simplex
Measles	Warts
Rubella	Hepatitis C, E, F, G
Hepatitis A, B, D	
Influenza (yearly composition)	

Fungal infections can be spread by direct or indirect contact. Using community showers, having bodily contact with the skin of infected athletes (as in wrestling), lack of good hygiene on the part of the athlete, or any of numerous other contamination procedures can lead to a fungal infection in the athlete. Fungal infections that are allowed to develop over a longer time period usually take longer to resolve.

Internet Resource Box

For more information regarding this and other cutaneous fungal problems, review the information provided by the American Podiatric Association at *http://www.apma.org/topics/fungal.htm*

Some types of fungi find a way to get inside the body and multiply. This produces a much greater threat to human function than the conditions described in the previous few paragraphs. One way in which fungi get into the human body is through inadequate care of a cutaneous fungal infection, allowing it to become so advanced that the skin dries and cracks, opening the inside of the body to the infection. Another inopportune type of infection occurs when fungal spores become airborne and an athlete inhales the airborne fungus, resulting in a respiratory infection. Respiratory fungal growths such as coccidioidomycosis require the use of prescription antifungal medications. Systemic fungal growth is beyond the scope of the athletic trainer's duties and will not be discussed here.

■ Oral and Topical Medications

There are prescription oral and topical medications that the physician can prescribe if a fungal infection is not controlled by an OTC preparation. However, the antifungal medications most commonly seen by athletic trainers are OTC topical medications. Most topical antifungal preparations take from 1 week to 1 or more months (depending on the severity of the infection) to completely control the fungal infection. Athletes need to understand that a fungal infection will not go away overnight, and might not even go away in a week. But, with the correct antifungal (Table 9–4), the athlete should be able to derive some benefit from the medication after the first week and be encouraged that further treatment will completely resolve the fungal problem.

The main control mechanism of topical antifungals is the impairment of cell membrane synthesis. An antifungal

Table 9-4

Topical Antifungal Medications

Generic Name	Mechanism	Formulation	Brand Name(s)*
Tolnaftate	Inhibition of cell membrane function	Cream 1% Gel 1% Powder 1% Solution 1% Spray powder 1% Spray liquid 1%	Tinactin Aftate Quinsana Plus Tinactin Tinactin Jock Itch Spray Powder Absorbine Footcare
Econazole	Broad-spectrum antifungal—many suggested mechanisms	Cream 1%	Spectazole
Terbinafine	Decreases sterol biosynthesis	Cream 1% Solution 1%	Lamisil AT Lamisil
Miconazole	Decreases cell membrane permeability	Cream 2% Powder 2% Spray 2% Spray powder 2%	Monistat-Derm Micatin (foot or jock) Lotrimin AF Zeasorb-AF
Clotrimazole	Alters permeability of cell membrane	Cream 1% Solution 1%	Lotrimin AF Cruex Lotrimin AF
Naftifine	Suspected to decrease sterol biosynthesis	Cream 1% Gel 1%	Naftin
Ketoconazole	Impairs synthesis of cell membrane	Shampoo 2% Cream 2%	Nizoral

Examples of each type provided; other brand names may exist.

typically controls some of the key enzymes that help to build or maintain the cell membrane. Thus, the cell cannot function normally and the fungus dies.

Internet Resource Box

Websites available for more information on fungal infections:

http://www.nlm.nih.gov/medlineplus/fungalinfections.html includes links to a variety of resources for fungal infections and links to related Websites for Spanish-speaking athletes.

http://www.e-antifungal.com provides information about fungi and alternative therapies for fungal infections.

■ Adverse Effects of Antifungal Agents

Topical antifungal agents are generally very safe and have few, if any, adverse effects. There is a possibility that an athlete may be allergic to one of these topical preparations. Oral antifungals can demonstrate a variety of toxicities to the hepatic, cardiovascular, and other systems. Check with the athlete's physician to determine if there are any signs or symptoms of adverse effects that you should watch for. Observe the area being treated and speak with the athlete daily regarding any adverse effects.

What to Tell the Athlete

Athletes are at a higher risk than the general population for all types of infections because of the communication of germs among teammates. The use of antibiotics is very specific, and these drugs should not be overused. It is important for the athlete to understand when the use of antibiotics is indicated. Infections should be monitored closely by the athletic trainer and physician. Here are some tips for the athletic trainer when educating the athlete about these drugs:

■ Antibiotics must be taken as directed to ensure that they are effective in controlling the bacterial infection. Read the instructions carefully with the athlete and answer any questions.

■ Antibiotics can produce allergic responses, even after the athlete has taken them for a number of days.

■ The athlete should be reminded to take the entire prescription of antibiotics.

■ Viral infections do not respond to antibiotics, and the athlete should be counseled not to demand a prescription for antibiotics if the physician does not recommend it for his or her specific illness.

■ Athletes can be vaccinated against some viral infections, such as influenza.

■ Fungal infections need to be controlled before they become systemic.

■ Control of fungal infections is multifaceted; it is better to prevent them than to use an antifungal to destroy fungal growth on the body.

Scenarios from the Field

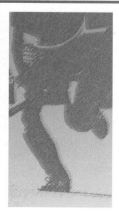

A 17-year-old female basketball player who worked out regularly both at school and a local health club contracted tinea corporis just above her left scapula. It was finally determined that she contracted the fungus while wearing a tank top and doing sit-ups on an unclean mat surface at the local health club. She used a topical antifungal for about 2 weeks and the fungus was eliminated.

Encourage your athletes to be cautious when exercising in public places and not to allow their skin to come in contact with surfaces that may contain infectious agents.

Discussion Topics

- When an antibiotic medication has been prescribed for an athlete, what are the main topics you should discuss with him or her before he or she starts taking the medication?

- Can you explain why a physician does not prescribe an antibiotic for an athlete experiencing symptoms of the common cold (e.g., sore throat and runny nose)?

- What vaccines are available to reduce the possibility of disease?

- What can an athlete do to avoid fungal infections?

Chapter Review

- Bacteria reside in humans by bringing their own cells into the body.

- There are a number of classes of antibiotics used to control bacteria in the body.

- *Bacteriostatic* means a condition in which bacteria are under control and unable to replicate.

- *Bactericidal* refers to an agent that destroys bacteria.

- Disk diffusion and broth diffusion are used to assess the sensitivity of microorganisms to antibiotics.

- Penicillin uses cell wall inhibition to help stop bacterial activity in the body.

- Tetracyclines inhibit bacterial protein synthesis to help stop bacterial activity in the body.

- A virus invading the human body requires a host cell with specific cellular components in order for the virus to survive in the human.

- Vaccines work by injecting an attenuated virus into the body so that an immune response is developed.

- Common tinea infections are a result of fungal growth.

- Fungal growth can be stopped by breaking the warm/dark/moist cycle.

- Severe fungal infections may require an oral antifungal medication.

References

1. Bager, F: DANMAP: Monitoring antimicrobial resistance in Denmark. Int J Antimicrob Agents 14:271, 2000.
2. Chambers, HF: Antimicrobial agents: Protein synthesis inhibitors and miscellaneous antibacterial agents. In Hardman, JG, et al (eds): Goodman and Gilman's The Pharmacological Basis of Therapeutics, ed. 10. McGraw-Hill, N.Y., 2001, p 1258.
3. Gold, HS, and Mollering, RC: Antimicrobial drug resistance. N Engl J Med 335:1445, 1996.
4. Greydanus, DE et al.: Contraception in the adolescent: An update. Pediatrics 107:562, 2001.
5. Heilig, S, et al.: Curtailing antibiotic use in agriculture. West. J Med 176:9, 2002.
6. Hirschmann, JV: Antibiotics for common respiratory tract infections in adults. Arch Intern Med 162:256, 2002.
7. Huston, KA: Achilles tendonitis and tendon rupture due to fluoroquinolone antibiotics. N Engl J Med 331:748, 1994.
8. Lehne, RA: Drugs that weaken the bacterial cell wall I: Penicillins. In Pharmacology for Nursing Care, ed 3. WB Saunders, Philadelphia, 2001, p 909.
9. Ibid., p 919.
10. Levy, SB: The challenge of antibiotic resistance. Sci Am 278: 46, 1998.
11. Manzella, JP: Quinupristin-dalfopristin: A new antibiotic for severe gram-positive infections. Am Fam Phys 64:1863, 2001.
12. Nasrin, D, et al.: Effect of (beta)-lactam antibiotic use in children on pneumococcal resistance to penicillin: Prospective cohort study. Brit Med J 324(7328):28, 2002.
13. Oliphant, CM, and Green, GM: Quinolones: A comprehensive review. Am Fam Phys 65:455, 2002.
14. Petri, Jr., WA: Antimicrobial agents: Penicillins, cephalosporins, and other beta-lactam antibiotics. In Hardman, JG, et al. (eds): Goodman and Gilman's The Pharmacological Basis of Therapeutics, ed. 10. McGraw-Hill, New York, 2001. p 1212.
15. Pfaller, MA, et al.: Survey of blood stream infections attributable to gram-positive cocci: Frequency of occurrence and antimicrobial susceptibility of isolates collected in 1997 in the United States, Canada, and Latin America from the SENTRY antimicrobial surveillance program. Diagn Microbiol Infect Dis 33:283, 1999.
16. Prescott, LM, et al: Microbiology, ed 5. McGraw-Hill, Boston, 2002.
17. Priest, P, et al.: Antibacterial prescribing and antibacterial resistance in English general practice: Cross sectional study/commentary. Brit Med J (international), 323(7320):1037, 2001.
18. Rabenberg, VS, et al.: The bactericidal and cytotoxic effects of

antimicrobial wound cleansers. J Athletic Training 37:51, 2002.

19. Ratcliff, J: Yellow Magic: The Story of Penicillin. Random House, New York, 1945.

20. Ribard, P, et al.: Seven Achilles tendonitis including three complicated by rupture during fluoroquinolone therapy. J Rheumatol 19:1479, 1992.

21. Shoemaker, NB, et al.: Evidence for extensive resistance gene transfer among bacteroides spp. and among bacteroides and other genera in the human colon. Appl Environ Microbol 67:561, 2001.

22. Swain, RA, and Kaplan, B: Upper respiratory infections: Treatment selection for active patients. Phys & Sportsmed 26(2):85, 1998

23. Torpy, JM: New threats and old enemies: Challenges for critical care medicine. JAMA 287:1513, 2002.

Chapter Questions

1. Possible adverse effects of penicillin include which of the following?
   A. Hypersensitivity reaction
   B. GI distress
   C. Nausea/vomiting
   D. All of the above

2. Antibacterial drugs work in a variety of ways. Which one of the following is *not* a way in which these drugs work?
   A. Inhibiting cell wall synthesis
   B. Inhibiting prostaglandin release
   C. Inhibiting protein synthesis
   D. Inhibiting DNA/RNA function

3. Bacterial resistance can occur from all of the following except:
   A. Certain strains of bacteria enzymatically destroying the antibacterial drug.
   B. Noncompliance by the athlete in taking the full course of the drug.
   C. Bacterial evolution.
   D. Combining anti-inflammatories with antibiotics.

4. Which of the following adverse effects is quickly noticed in a reaction to antibiotics?
   A. Fever
   B. Tinnitus
   C. Skin rash
   D. Dizziness

5. The cephalosporins are a class of:
   A. Antibiotics
   B. Synthetic hormones
   C. Anti-inflammatories
   D. Antivirals

6. Bactericidal antibiotics are so classified because their mission is to:
   A. Kill and destroy bacteria
   B. Limit the growth or proliferation of bacteria
   C. Cause death to the host organism
   D. Limit the DNA production of the cell

7. An antiviral drug's mechanism of action is usually:
   A. Cell wall destruction
   B. Inhibition of DNA activity
   C. Stopping of cellular activity
   D. Bactericidal

8. Vaccines inhibit viral infections from becoming active in the human body is through the use of:
   A. A live virus
   B. An inactivated virus
   C. Reconstructed antibiotics
   D. All of the above

9. When an athlete is experiencing a common cold, it is advisable for the athletic trainer to do advise the athlete to do which of the following?
   A. Use aspirin to control the fever
   B. Get antibiotics for the sore throat
   C. Use OTC medications to control the head congestion
   D. All of the above

10. In the human, a plantlike microorganism (fungus) can live:
    A. On the skin
    B. Under the dermal skin layer
    C. In the lungs
    D. All of the above

11. Most athletes will be dealing with which type of medication to control their fungal infections?
    A. Topical
    B. Systemic
    C. Intravenous
    D. Antibacterial

12. If an athlete has an allergic reaction to a prescribed antibiotic drug, you should tell him or her to:
    A. Try a different brand of the drug
    B. Tell the pharmacist and see if there is an alternative drug they could use
    C. Stop taking the drug immediately
    D. Take the medication with food

Analgesics and *10* Local Anesthetics

Chapter Objectives

After reading this chapter, the student should:

1 Have a basic history of analgesics and anesthetics.
2 Understand the rationale for treating pain.
3 Be able to differentiate between analgesics and anesthetics.
4 Understand the rationale for the use of prescription and over-the-counter (OTC) analgesics.
5 Be able to differentiate between opioid and nonopioid analgesics.
6 Understand the physician's role in the prescription and monitoring of analgesics.
7 Be able to determine the warning signs of improper use of analgesics by athletes.
8 Understand how local anesthetics can be delivered to the athlete.
9 Understand the proper use of local anesthetics in athletics.
10 Be cognizant of the adverse effects of analgesics and anesthetics.

Chapter Outline

Analgesics
    Endogenous Opioids
    Opioids' Mechanism of Action
    Exogenous Opioids
    Nonopioid Preparations

Local Anesthetics
    Delivery and Use of Local Anesthetics
    Commonly Used Local Anesthetics
What's Next?
Discussion Topics
Chapter Review

*T*his chapter outlines the use of pain-relief preparations and their appropriate application in sports. The team physician should always be the person responsible for advising athletes regarding pain relief and prescribing these drugs. Sometimes athletes, coaches, and others will self-prescribe or encourage the use of analgesics or local anesthetics to allow players to participate in a contest. When recommending an analgesic or anesthetic to allow an athlete to participate in a practice or competition, the athletic trainer must be aware of the ramifications of this action. It is not our intention to outline the instances when using analgesic or anesthetic methods to allow a player to participate would be justified. We feel that participation by an injured athlete is a decision that must be made by the individual athlete in consultation with the team physician. It is well recognized that analgesics and anesthetics should not be used when further tissue damage is expected or may occur.

When an athlete experiences pain, this is an intrinsic signal from a body part indicating that something is wrong at some level in one or more of the tissues. The team physician should evaluate pain signals lasting more than a few days and refer the athlete to a specialist in pain management when it is deemed necessary. Injured athletes experiencing pain for short periods of time (less than a day) can use an over-the-counter (OTC) analgesic for short-term relief. If an athlete is in continuous pain for more than a day, he or she should seek the advice of a physician. The World Health Organization (WHO) has outlined a three-step approach to the management of pain. Table 10–1 outlines these recommended steps.

Many analgesics can be obtained OTC by the athlete and used without the knowledge of the team physician or athletic trainer. When this occurs, the pain experienced by the athlete can be masked, and participation on sports can lead to further damage to tissues. The athletic trainer and team physician should discourage frequent and independent use of analgesics for the purpose of participation. It is important to understand the normal system of pain control in the body. In the human body there is a pain control process initiated by the release of endogenous opioids to assist in diminishing pain perception when various problems occur. As mentioned previously, further pain control using prescription medications must be done under the direction of a physician.

Over the years the term "narcotic" has been associated with the opioid drug class. But, by definition, the term narcotic means "producing sleep or stupor,"[13] which is an adverse effect, and not really the objective of, an opioid compound. Therefore, the more common description for this class of drugs is "opioids," a general term for morphine-type medications. Opioids are defined as "any drug containing or derived from opium." When physicians explain the use of opioids to the lay public, they also refer to similar synthetic drugs as opioids. There are many pain-control options, as outlined in Table 10–2, including both opioids and nonopioids as well as nondrug methods.

*A*nalgesics

Analgesics in many different forms are available for pain relief. An analgesic is a drug or preparation that reduces or eliminates pain. Analgesics can be broken down into two basic categories: opioids and nonopioids. Opioid drugs were originally discovered as naturally occurring substances extracted from the opium poppy. The natural form is derived from the dried seeds of the poppy, which are processed to derive multiple active compounds. The opioids are well known for their ability to relieve moderate and severe pain symptoms. Drug manufacturers have developed semisynthetic and synthetic opioid derivatives that have effects similar to those of the naturally occurring form. Two of the best known compounds are *morphine* and *codeine*. Both morphine and codeine have similar chemical structures (Fig. 10–1)and both produce an analgesic effect in the body. With continued processing of the opium seeds, the drug *heroin* can be extracted. Thus it becomes apparent that this class of drugs is one in which physical dependence is a significant adverse effect.

Physical dependence signs and symptoms are typically demonstrated when a user stops taking the drug. An athlete who is physically dependent on an opioid will demonstrate withdrawal signs and symptoms such as irritability, sweating, insomnia, and tachycardia. An athlete who is psychologically dependent will exhibit behaviors that indicate he or she is craving or seeking the purchase of drugs. If the ath-

Table 10-1

World Health Organization Pain Management Hierarchy

Severity of Pain	Drug Use
Mild to moderate	NSAIDs or acetaminophen
Moderate to severe	Opioid for mild to moderate pain, plus a nonopioid adjuvant drug*
Severe	Opioid at higher dose for moderate to severe pain plus nonopioid adjuvant drug

*The use of an adjuvant medication is recommended in each case to enhance the effectiveness of the analgesic. An adjuvant medication is a drug added to the prescription medication that will hasten or increase the action of the principal ingredient.

Table 10-2

Pain Control Options for Noncancer Pain in Athletes

OTC preparations	Ibuprofen, acetaminophen, aspirin, naproxen, etc.
Therapeutic interventions	Cold, heat, joint mobilization
Prescription preparations	Opioids, nonopioids, local anesthetics
Nontraditional techniques	Hypnotism, acupuncture, acupressure

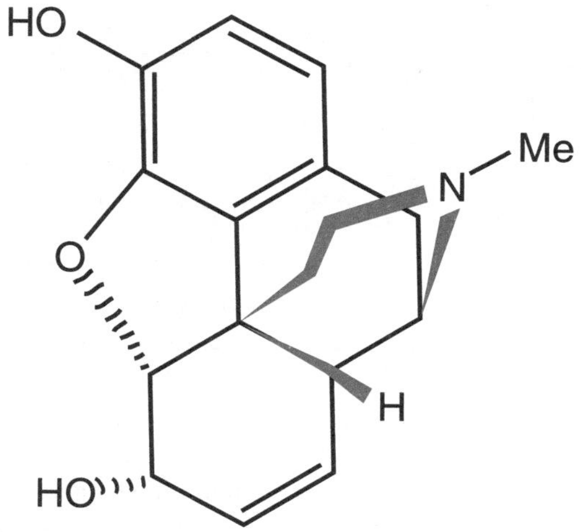

Figure 10–1. Chemical structures of morphine and codeine.

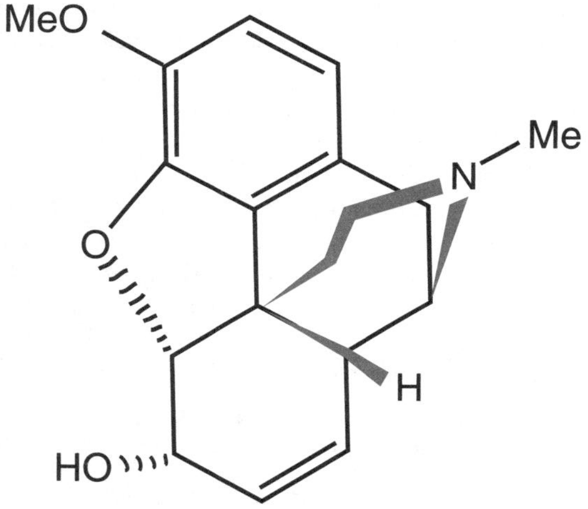

lete is truly experiencing pain, the effect of addiction is diminished.

Implications for Activity

Athletes using analgesics have to be aware that, when they are using these drugs, they have a reduced perception of pain. If an athlete using analgesics gets injured, he or she may not be able to perceive the injury or convey the appropriate pain responses to the athletic trainer evaluating him or her. Athletes should not use analgesics to mask pain in order to continue participating.

■ Endogenous Opioids

Endogenous opioids such as endorphins and enkephalins circulate throughout the body on an "as-needed" basis. The endorphins are naturally occurring morphinelike substances and are thought to bind to receptor sites on the pain-mediating pathways. The enkephalins have a similar function to that of the endorphins; they bind to different receptor sites but provide the same type of pain mediation. These endogenous opioids are considered more potent than morphine. Endogenous opioids are available to the central nervous system (CNS) for analgesic purposes. However, these endogenous substances do not exist in the same concentrations as exogenous opioids.

Opioid receptors have been identified in the peripheral nerves. Circulating endogenous opioids can bind to these sites and decrease the excitability of the peripheral sensory neurons, thereby providing an analgesic effect.[11] The endogenous opioids are thought to be more active in the peripheral tissues when one is dealing with an inflammatory process and analgesia is needed.[10]

Internet Resource Box

To learn more about pain in general, go to the American Association of Pain Management's Website, which contains a great deal of information and links:

http://www.painmed.org

The World Health Organization (WHO) has produced a treatment progression for physicians and others treating pain. The WHO outlined a three-step procedure (see Table 10–1) that health professionals can follow when addressing the problems associated with pain management. The WHO panel described pain in three categories: mild, moderate, and severe.

If the athlete is experiencing pain in the mild category, nonopioid medications such as acetaminophen, NSAIDs, or COX-2 inhibitors are recommended (see Chapter 3 for more details on these drugs). In the moderate pain category, if necessary, the physician may prescribe morphine or the related opioids such as hydrocodone and oxycodone. If the athlete is experiencing severe pain, the physician may choose methadone or a related opioid for pain control. The steps outlined in the WHO ladder (Fig. 10–2) give the medical provider good direction when helping an athlete to overcome pain for any situation. In some athletes there may be individual intolerances or contradictions to the use of NSAIDs or other drugs, which would indicate the use of an opioid for pain relief. Additionally, the athlete may need greater relief from pain, which may require an opioid drug. The physician should be the person who judges the severity of the pain that

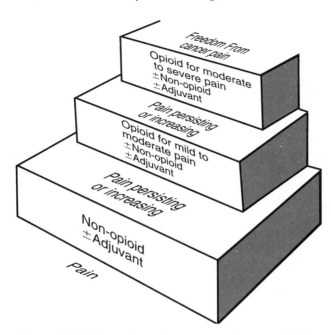

Figure 10–2. Three-step pain management process (World Health Organization, Guidelines for Analgesic Drug Therapy, 2003, p. 25, with permission).

the athlete is experiencing and prescribes the proper analgesic for the level of pain. The specific drugs mentioned here will be discussed in more detail further on in this chapter.

■ Opioids' Mechanism of Action

Opioid receptors were among the first receptors in the brain to be characterized for a specific activity. In addition to receptors in the CNS, there are opioid receptors in peripheral tissues. The opioid receptors are classified into three categories: mu (μ), kappa (κ), and delta (Δ). Theoretically, any of the opioids can attach to any of the receptors and act as an agonist or antagonist. Typically, there are specific drugs that bind to one or two of the three receptors and cause a change based on the drug-receptor combination. When the physician prescribes an opioid, he or she is usually prescribing a mu receptor agonist, which results in pain relief. Sometimes drug-related euphoria is an adverse effect experienced from the use of this type of drug.

Some drugs have an agonist effect on the mu receptor and an antagonist effect on the kappa receptor. Additionally, it should be noted here that the mu, kappa, and delta receptors have other functions in the body. Alteration of their functions can result in an adverse effect of the drug. For example, a mu receptor agonist can also be associated

Table 10-3

Opioid Receptors and Physiological Responses

Opioid Receptor	Related Response
Mu (μ)	Analgesia, euphoria, respiratory depression
Kappa (κ)	Spinal analgesia, general sedation
Delta (Δ)	Euphoria, general sedation

with respiratory depression, pupillary constriction, changes in self-image, and increased energy. These and other adverse effects will be discussed further on in this chapter.

Opioid drugs act on the body by producing a decrease in neurotransmitter activity at both the presynaptic and post-synaptic sites, which alters the nociceptive transmissions to the brain. The excitability of the neuron is altered as the opioid attaches to the potassium, calcium, or cyclic adenosine monophosphate (cAMP) activity at the synaptic site, resulting in a decrease in potassium or calcium conductance or cAMP second-messenger synthesis. These changes in activity at the synapse will result in changes at other sites along the neural pathway. In the case of the spinal cord, the opioid activity will result in an inhibition of the release of substance P (neurotransmitter) at the substantia gelatinosa. This decrease in substance P release produces an analgesic effect.[6]

■ Exogenous Opioids

Physician Prescription

Opioid use must be prescribed and monitored by the physician. This class of drugs is tightly controlled in the United States, mainly because of the potential for addiction. When used properly, these drugs are generally safe and effective. Children and adolescents react to opioids in much the same way as adults. These drugs can be prescribed for both acute and long-term pain syndromes. A common use of opioids is to treat chronic pain in cancer patients. Their use for treatment of chronic noncancer pain was not common in the United States before the early 1980s. In athletics, the physician generally prescribes these drugs for acute pain, such as pain resulting from surgery or severe trauma.

Physicians use a set treatment plan when prescribing an opioid analgesic. This plan will most likely have the athlete taking normal dosages of the prescription drug initially, followed by small increases in the dose until the athlete begins to experience relief from the pain. The dosage will then be leveled off and the athlete will be slowly withdrawn from the drug. In most cases this takes less than a week. By then, the athlete should have suitable pain relief and can begin a rehabilitation program.

Specific Agents

According to Scott-Levin, a pharmacology consulting firm in Newtown, Pennsylvania, the single most prescribed drug in the year 2000 was hydrocodone with acetaminophen (APAP). Scott-Levin estimates that in more than 2.04 billion prescriptions for this drug alone were written in the year 2000. Table 10–4 outlines some of the more commonly prescribed oral opioid analgesics with which athletic trainers should be familiar in order to talk to athletes about their time of onset and duration of action. Hydrocodone (Vicodin, Lortab) is a semisynthetic narcotic analgesic that is combined with acetaminophen in some preparations. It also has an antitussive action and is used in several cough-suppressant formulations. However, this drug is more commonly prescribed for pain.

Oxycodone (prescribed under brand names including Oxy-Contin, Percocet, Percodan, Oxycodone, Roxicodone, Endocet, Roxicet, Roxilox, Tylox, Endodan, and Roxiprin) can be prepared in combination with acetaminophen or other similar analgesics. It is an opioid analgesic and, like other controlled drugs, must be prescribed by a physician. There is a high risk that an athlete will develop a tolerance if he or she uses this drug over a long period of time. These drugs can be abused by athletes and others, and the use of such drugs must be monitored by the athletic trainer. As with other opioids, this drug is contraindicated in conjunction with other CNS depressants such as alcohol.

Codeine is another mild to moderate agonist that can be prescribed by a physician or dentist to alleviate pain. It is also used as an antitussive for those experiencing severe coughing from the common cold or other upper respiratory tract infections. Codeine can also be habit forming, and the athletic trainer should be aware of any athlete who takes codeine for long periods of time. The most common complaint with the use of codeine is constipation.

Adverse Effects of Exogenous Opioids

As mentioned, this class of drugs can be addictive, which is an important concept for the athletic trainer to keep in mind. It is suggested that persons who have other addictive behaviors should be closely monitored when using these drugs. The ability of these drugs to become addictive suggests that the athletic trainer should monitor the athlete during the use of these drugs and discuss their use with the physician.

The opioids in general can cause sedation, nausea, vomiting, and constipation. The use of opioids with alcohol or

Table 10-4

Oral Opioid Analgesics

Drug	Time to Onset (Oral)*	Duration*
Codeine	10–30 minutes	4–6 hours
Hydrocodone Hydrocodone is always combined with other products. (Hycodan—a combination product that also contains homatropine)	10–30 minutes	4–6 hours
Meperidine (Demerol)	10–45 minutes	2–4 hours
Morphine	15–60 minutes	3–7 hours
Oxycodone (Oxy IR)	15–30 minutes	4–6 hours
Pentazocine (Talwin)	15–30 minutes	3–4 hours

* All times are approximate and based on normal hepatic function.

other CNS depressants has an additive effect. Taking hydrocodone or other opioid drugs in combination with alcohol or other CNS depressants can be lethal. This is an important point to stress to the high school or college athlete who may be experimenting with or using alcohol regularly. Respiratory depression when taking opioids, and other drug interactions with alcohol or CNS depressants, all of which may cause other health problems or even death, must be explained to the athlete.

As mentioned previously, the physician will prescribe only a limited amount of an opioid drug after surgery to help reduce the associated pain. In most situations, an athlete will be using the drug for less than 10 days, so the opportunity for developing tolerance or dependence is decreased. If the athletic trainer notices that an athlete is taking an opioid for longer periods of time, it may be that the athlete is obtaining extra medication from multiple sources. Suspicion of inappropriate use should be reported to the physician immediately. In a published article by Jonasson et al.,[5] 22 percent of the orthopedic and chronic pain population they interviewed was considered to have an analgesic use disorder. An even higher percentage, 33 percent, met the criteria for having a substance use disorder.

It is recommended that physicians be aware of whether a patient has addictive behaviors before they prescribe an opioid for analgesia. Coambs et al[3] (1996) developed the Screening Instrument for Substance Abuse Potential (SISAP) (Table 10–5). The athletic trainer can implement it and convey the information derived from it to the team physician.

It should also be remembered that many prescription opioid pain relievers are combined with acetaminophen or aspirin. The maximum amount of acetaminophen that an athlete with a healthy liver can safely take is 4000 mg per day. If the athlete uses alcohol or has impaired liver function, the maximum daily amount is 2000 mg. People with liver failure should not take acetaminophen. Acetaminophen and aspirin are included in many OTC products also. The athlete should carefully read the label of each OTC drug he or she is considering using to determine all of the ingredients it contains. The athletic trainer should check with the physician or pharmacist to determine if any extra acetaminophen or aspirin can be taken along with the prescription medication.

As mentioned previously, the opioids are known to induce a tolerance effect in some individuals. Tolerance in this situation means that an increasing amount of the drug is required to maintain the same level of analgesia. Tolerance development can be affected by dose, frequency of administration, and regularity of dosing. In the case of the opioids, an increase in tolerance alone does not indicate that a person is addicted to the drug, but an increased tolerance can be a part of the addiction process. It has been shown that 10 to 20 times the initial dose may be needed to control pain in some drug-tolerant individuals. Even though a tolerance effect can start in the first days of taking an opioid, it is not common, and the typical athlete's regimen of taking the drug for less than a week seldom initiates a tolerance response. Tolerance is an important concept for the athletic trainer to understand because tolerance development is normal and expected when opioids are used for long periods of time. The physician can increase the opioid dosage over time. Athletes (and all patients) need to be reassured that this increased dosage does not mean that they are becoming addicted to the medication. When opi-

Table 10-5

Screening Questions for Potential Opioid Abuse

Question	Use Caution When:
How many alcoholic drinks do you have on a typical day? In a typical week?	Men have > 4 drinks/day or 16 drinks/week Women have > 3 drinks/day or 12/week
Have you used marijuana or hashish in the past year?	Use extreme caution in prescribing opioid therapy to a patient who uses cannabis. Use for recreational purposes is of concern in this case.
Have you ever smoked cigarettes?	This indicates addictive behavior.
What is your age?	A person under the age of 40 who smokes should be approached with concern.

Adapted with permission from: Coambs et al.: The SISAP: A new screening instrument for identifying potential opioid abusers in the management of chronic nonmalignant pain in general medical practice. Pain Res Manage 1:155–162, 1996.

oids are prescribed for a pain-related condition, addiction does not commonly occur.

Occasionally, opioid drugs can cause respiratory depression and orthostatic hypotension, even at normal doses. The key physiological signs to look for in an athlete possibly overusing these drugs are reduction of respiratory rate and depth, somnolence, euphoria, sedation, slurred speech, and judgment difficulties. If these adverse effects are noted, the dose may be too high or the patient may be overdosing himself or herself. These drugs have an additive effect when combined with other CNS depressants. Ingesting opioids in combination with alcohol or other CNS depressants can result in severe side effects. Opioids taken in conjunction with other CNS depressants have been identified as causes of accidental and self-inflicted fatalities.

As mentioned previously, opioids can create sedation, drowsiness, and an overall mental slowdown. It is wise to schedule rehabilitation or other activities that require mental acuity at times when the drug is at a period of reduced activity. Another possible adverse effect of the opioids is a perception of euphoria, mood changes, or relief from anxiety, which varies from athlete to athlete. This is an adverse effect that needs close monitoring by the physician with help from the athletic trainer.

Because the opioids have an antiperistaltic action, constipation can be an unwanted adversee effect. The physician needs to be aware of any constipation that the athlete may be experiencing. Treatment regimens are available for opioid-associated constipation and should be followed when the athlete is experiencing this adverse effect. Nausea or vomiting can be a problem at lower doses, although at higher doses the vomiting response can be depressed.[9] Taking the medication with food often helps with opioid-associated nausea.

■ Nonopioid Preparations

Nonsteroidal anti-inflammatory drugs (NSAIDs) are used widely for management of pain as well as inflammation. Because of the many types and wide uses of these drugs, we have dedicated a chapter to the anti-inflammatory drugs. Please see Chapter 3 for more information regarding NSAIDs.

One of the most popular nonopioid prescription medications is propoxyphene (Darvon, Darvocet, Darvon-N,), which is a mild to moderate agonist. Propoxyphene has a high propensity for addiction among users and has a significant toxic effect when used with other CNS depressants. The toxic effect is mainly depression of the CNS, which

results in respiratory difficulty and/or failure. This drug is now prescribed for pain control only on an occasional basis. Propoxyphene ranks second to barbiturates in causing prescription drug fatalities.

Another OTC preparation that is being used more and more is capsaicin, also marketed by the trade name Zostrix. Capsaicin is derived from the seeds of hot chili (capsicum) peppers such as habañero, Jamaican hot, cayenne, and jalapeño. Researchers now have determined that capsaicin limits the activity of substance P in transmitting pain messages from the extremities to the brain.[2] Capsaicin is generally marketed for arthritic individuals or persons with some type of atypical pain such as shingles or other neuropathic pain. However, athletes are discovering the use of this product, which is topically applied as a cream. The OTC preparations have a smaller percentage (0.025–0.075%) of the active ingredient, but there are products being tested that have 5 to 10 percent capsaicin. The higher concentrations appear to provide some analgesia and pain relief.[8]

The athletic trainer should be fully aware of whether the athlete is using any OTC preparation before participation in activity. An athlete should not use an analgesic to mask any pain. When an athlete is not physically ready for practice or competition, he or she should not use an analgesic in an attempt to overcome any warning signals the body may be sending to avoid tissue damage.

Athletes' Understanding of Analgesic Drugs

It is interesting to review the comments of collegiate athletes questioned about "painkilling drugs" and the use of those drugs. In a study reported by Tricker,[12] over 2/3 of 563 athletes surveyed responded that they were aware that painkilling drugs were potentially addictive. When asked for a self-report on the use of such drugs, more than half of the athletes indicated that they used painkilling drugs when injured, sick, or sore after workouts, regularly throughout the season. The athletes in this study generally considered themselves to be overusers of painkilling drugs. Additionally, they reported that they did not obtain the painkilling drugs from physicians, but rather from sources such as teammates, friends, and parents. The actual types of painkilling drugs used were not reported in this study, but it gives a sense of how many athletes are using drugs that produce analgesia.

The physician and athletic trainer should monitor any OTC medications taken by the athlete that produce analgesia because a reduction in pain may allow further tissue damage if an athlete participates without regard for the internal warning signals his or her body produces. Additionally, the athlete should report any use of herbal preparations because of the possibility of adverse interactions between many analgesics and herbal medications. Some herbal medications (such as echinacea and kava-kava), when used in conjunction with OTC or prescription analgesics (such as acetaminophen and opioids, respectively), can lead to hepatotoxicity and nephrotoxicity, among other problems. The effectiveness of some analgesics can be inhibited by herbal supplements. A good review of the potential for adverse interactions between herbal medications and analgesic drugs is available in the recent article by Abebe.[1]

The athletic trainer should observe athletes whom they suspect of overusing analgesics for indications of euphoria, judgment difficulties, and excessive sedation or sleepiness. The athlete might also suffer from respiratory rate reduction. It is not uncommon for an abuser of analgesics to attempt to obtain additional prescriptions for the medication from multiple providers. This allows the abuser to take more of the drug, which keeps him or her in an altered state more often.

*L*ocal Anesthetics

The term *local anesthetic* denotes a drug or preparation used to produce partial or complete loss of sensation in a specific area. Typically, this is done by injection, but a decrease in sensation can also be accomplished by using an ice pack. In this chapter section we discuss drugs that are injected to accomplish this sensation reduction.

Local anesthetics are commonly used in a physician's clinical practice. The origin of local anesthetics goes back to the 1500s, when the Incas used the coca leaf as a local anesthetic. Late in the 1800s, cocaine was derived from the coca leaf and a liquid solution of cocaine was used by physicians for local anesthetic purposes. You will note as you study this chapter that many of the local anesthetics have a "caine" suffix. This derives from the original use of cocaine as an anesthetic. The main advantage of using a local anesthetic in the late 1800s and early 1900s was that it avoided the need to use general anesthesia, which then had a very high associated risk of mortality.

Clinically, there are times when the use of an anesthetic to impair sensation is desirable. Examples of these situations are the repair of a laceration with sutures by a physician or when the dentist is performing a simple procedure and needs to eliminate the pain signal being transmitted to the CNS. In addition to decreasing the pain sensation, local anesthetics have the ability to depress other excitable tissues. Other areas that can be affected by a local anesthetic are the brain, heart, and muscles. Compared to general anesthetics, local anesthetics allow more rapid recovery and have few, if any, residual effects such as lethargy or confusion.

Anesthetics targeted for local activity are administered peripherally because systemic usage does not allow the drug to be effective because of dilution, absorption, or metabolism as it is transported to the site.

Epinephrine is often added to local anesthetics to pro-

What to Tell the Athlete

Opioid analgesics can be addictive, and athletes, as well as athletic trainers, should be mindful of how long these drugs are taken.[5] Here are some tips to help the athletic trainer educate the athlete about these drugs:

■ OTC analgesics can be helpful when relief from acute pain is desired.

■ Any time you "recommend" or suggest that an athlete take any type of medication, especially an analgesic, it can be misunderstood by the athlete as a prescription for medication.

■ When consulted by adult athletes, it is best to provide them with choices of different types of OTC analgesics.

■ Analgesics should be taken according to the recommended dosage and at the recommended intervals to reduce adverse effects.

■ Excessive use of analgesics will not produce additional pain relief or any type of ergogenic effect in the athlete.

Athletes should not be using analgesics on a regular basis to reduce or mask pain sensations. If the athlete is continually using an analgesic for pain, you should refer the athlete to a physician, who can determine the source of the pain. This is a much better course of action than trying to mask the pain for long periods of time. It is also possible that more tissue damage may be occurring while the athlete is masking the pain and continuing to participate at a high level of activity.

vide a longer duration of action. The rationale for adding epinephrine is to cause vasoconstriction in the targeted area, which diminishes blood flow and reduces absorption of the anesthetic from the site of activity. Injection of the drug to the desired site allows for almost complete bioavailability of the drug to the area. On injection, the drug rapidly moves away from the injection site. Figure 10–3 illustrates the absorption of anesthetics into different tissues of the body. If the concentration of the anesthetic is appropriate, it will diffuse across the membrane barriers, where it will begin to affect the outer fibers of the nearest peripheral nerve, followed by the inner part of the nerve. After the drug starts to be metabolized by the body, the anesthetic effect begins to diminish. The outer fibers recover first, followed by the more central sections of the nerve. Depending on the type of anesthetic used, this entire process can take from minutes to hours.

A local anesthetic drug affects the nerve fiber by diminishing the ability of the nerve fiber to conduct action potentials and by inhibiting the number of nerve endings that can transmit impulses to the CNS. The local anesthetic does this by inhibiting the Ca^+ and Na^+ activity and the propagation of impulses along the nerve pathways. Thus, the ability of the CNS to receive pain stimuli is decreased and the person does not feel the stimulus being applied to a specific section of the body. After the anesthetic has remained in the area for a period of time, the patient begins to lose motor control

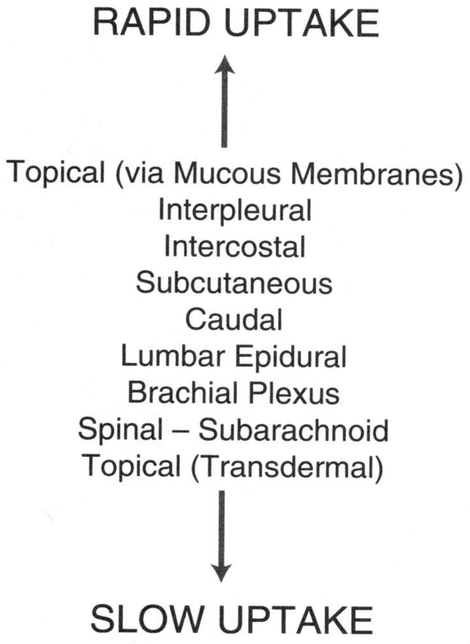

and other muscular activities (including proprioception) at the site of the injection.

Local anesthesia can also be used to provide local analgesia for conditions such as musculotendinous or joint pain. The same basic principle of blocking afferent nerve transmission is applicable in these situations. However, the use of local anesthetics to allow an athlete to participate is much more controversial when the athlete is experiencing musculotendinous or joint pain. For example, an athlete with a mild ligament sprain may be experiencing pain from the initial injury. There might be situations in which the use of a local anesthetic would be appropriate to allow the athlete to participate. The decision to allow an athlete to continue participating after the injection of a local anesthetic must be made by a competent licensed medical practitioner.

■ Delivery and Use of Local Anesthetics

The physician has a number of choices for the application of local anesthetics. Delivery of local anesthetics can be simple, such as applying an ice pack or a topical preparation such as ethyl chloride spray, or sophisticated, such as using an injectable preparation. Topical anesthetics are not as effective as those used within the body. Topical application is also called *transdermal delivery* because the drug has to pass through the skin. Topical application is used for various minor skin irritations. General absorption rates for local anesthetics are presented in Figure 10–3. Parenteral administration (injection) is most often used for suturing or dental work. *Peripheral nerve blocks* involve the injection of an anesthetic close to a nerve trunk to block afferent transmission in minor surgical procedures and tooth extraction and in relieving chronic pain conditions. Anesthetics can also be used as a *central nerve block* or as a *sympathetic nerve block*, usually in connection with more serious conditions not typically associated with athletic participation. The physician should determine the amount, duration, and delivery method of a local anesthetic.

Ice can be a semi-effective anesthetic for reduction of local pain from a sprain or strain, or to decrease temperature and touch sensation in a limited area. The athletic trainer who uses an ice treatment must be careful to watch for allergic reactions such as urticaria. It is also important to make sure the athlete does not have reduced sensation to an area that could receive further tissue injury if improper stresses were applied.

Other topical anesthetics are used for relief of symptoms or for minor procedures. Topical anesthetics may be composed of one or a combination of drugs, and may be applied to the

RAPID UPTAKE

↑

Topical (via Mucous Membranes)
Interpleural
Intercostal
Subcutaneous
Caudal
Lumbar Epidural
Brachial Plexus
Spinal – Subarachnoid
Topical (Transdermal)

↓

SLOW UPTAKE

Figure 10–3. Absorption rates for local anesthetics.

skin, mucous membranes, cornea, or other areas. The physician, rather than the athletic trainer, should be the primary person monitoring an athlete's use of topical anesthetics.

Commonly Used Local Anesthetics

Many years ago, procaine (Novocain) became the first widely used injectable anesthetic. In the mid-20thcentury, other local anesthetics were produced that had better anesthetic properties. However, the term "Novocain" is still sometimes used by the lay public as a generic term for a local anesthetic. Other common local anesthetics and their effects are outlined in Table 10–6. These local anesthetics have similar mechanisms of action and are chosen by the physician based on relevant individual differences among them, such as their duration of action, onset of action, and safety profile.

Cocaine

The origins of cocaine go back to South America and it is a derivative of cocoa plant leaves. Practitioners used cocaine for hundreds of years before it became a drug of abuse by a small portion of the population. Today cocaine can be used in surgical situations when the physician deems it appropriate for use as an anesthetic. Cocaine is still used in some nasal surgeries in a controlled surgical setting as a local anesthetic with vasoconstricting properties. The athlete and general public should understand that cocaine can be toxic and lead to multiple health problems.

Unfortunately, too many people, including some athletes, have determined that cocaine can provide a stimulatory and psychological effect when used for personal pleasure. Cocaine is a highly addictive drug and has extremely serious adverse effects, up to and including death. Athletic trainers should use their role to discourage athletes and

other people from using cocaine recreationally any time the opportunity arises.

Physician Use Considerations

There are three main considerations when a physician uses a local anesthetic. First, time to effect. How long does the drug take to cause enough reduction in pain sensation to begin the surgical procedure? Second, length of time the anesthetic will remain in effect. How long will the drug continue to decrease the pain sensations so that the procedure can be completed? Third, what are the adverse effects? Are there adverse effects that must be considered with respect to the person receiving the local anesthetic? Does the person have heart problems that could be exacerbated by a specific type of local anesthetic? What are the dosage and toxicity limits for this person? The physician should be very familiar with the adverse effects and correct dosages of local anesthetics. If local anesthetics are used illegally or improperly by someone not trained in correct dosages, there can be very serious adverse effects to the athlete.

Adverse Effects of Local Anesthetics

Local anesthetics can have serious and toxic effects if used in excessive dosages. There is a possibility of overdose. An overdose of a local anesthetic can result in multiple problems. There can be altered CNS activity, including both excitation and depression. Signs of CNS excitation can include confusion, agitation, generalized excitation, and seizures. CNS depression can be exhibited as decreased respiration and somnolence. Other possible adversee effects of anesthetics include allergic reactions and cardiac arrest, sometimes leading to death.[7] This class of drugs should not be used by untrained people. There are times when an ath-

Table 10-6		
Parameters of Common Local Anesthetics		
Names **Generic/Trade**	**Onset of Effectiveness***	**Duration of Effectiveness***
Bupivacaine/Marcaine	Up to 30 minutes	3–10 hours
Lidocaine/Xylocaine	Less than 10 minutes	1–3 hours
Procaine/novocain	10–30 minutes	30–60 minutes
*Times of effectiveness are relative depending on dosage, individual metabolism, and other uncontrolled factors such as blood flow.		

What to Tell the Athlete

The use of local anesthetics is uncommon in assisting the athlete to participate in sports. The use of local anesthetics should always be under the direction of a qualified physician. Here are some tips for the athletic trainer when educating the athlete about these drugs:

■ Athletes should not request an anesthetic or analgesic solely for the purpose of participating in a practice or competition.

■ The use of an anesthetic should not be implemented when participation in a practice or competition could result in further tissue damage.

■ If the physician decides to use an anesthetic or analgesic, the decision should be based on the tissues involved, with the understanding that no further tissue damage should occur.

■ The decision to use an anesthetic or analgesic should be made by the physician without pressure from the athlete, parent, or coaching staff.

■ If an athlete receives an analgesic or anesthetic, he or she should be made aware that he or she will not experience the same warning signal (pain) that an injury or other tissue damage would normally produce.

lete may want to use a local anesthetic to reduce the feeling in an area so that he or she can compete. Always make sure that the physician controls the use of local anesthetics in athletes.

■ What's Next?

Curatolo and Bogudk[4] provide an overview of current pain treatments and a brief introduction to new analgesics and anesthetics that are being developed. Techniques are currently being investigated that will utilize biodegradable polymers to encapsulate local anesthetics to provide a longer duration of action. Additionally, researchers are working on developing new types of local anesthetics that will block only the nociceptive impulses and reduce or eliminate the blocking of motor impulses and reduce sensory losses in the local area. They are also working on other types of analgesics that could change the way in which pain is controlled. Some of these new substances include N-methyl-D-aspartate (NMDA) receptor antagonists and cannabinoids. NMDA receptor antagonists appear to affect hyperalgesia and hypersensitivity centrally. Cannabinoids are a derivative of the cannabis plant, which has been used for many years to treat a variety of illnesses. In animal research studies, the cannabinoids appear to reduce pain in a number of experimentally produced pain situations without causing nausea.

Discussion Topics

• Why would you give acetaminophen rather than aspirin to an athlete with a headache before a soccer match?

• If a physician prescribes an analgesic for an athlete, what is the maximum length of time the athlete should take the medication before seeing the physician again?

• What are the most commonly abused analgesics, and how are they being abused?

• What are some of the greatest dangers of analgesic drug abuse?

Chapter Review

• Analgesics can be readily obtained over the counter.

• Physical dependence is a significant side effect of prescription analgesics.

• The WHO has outlined a three-step procedure for dealing with pain management.

• Nonsteroidal anti-inflammatory drugs (NSAIDs) are used for management of pain as well as inflammation.

• Opioid drugs decrease neurotransmitter activity at both the presynaptic and postsynaptic sites, reducing nociceptive transmission to the CNS.

- In athletics the use of opioids is generally limited to acute pain, such as that which occurs after surgery.

- Adverse effects of opioids include sedation, drowsiness, a generalized mental "slowdown," respiratory depression, constipation, somnolence, euphoria, sedation, slurred speech, judgment difficulties, and other problems.

- Local anesthetics can be as simple as an ice pack and as sophisticated as injected preparations.

- Local anesthesia allows a more rapid recovery by the athlete without adverse effects such as lethargy or confusion.

- If local anesthetics are administered at excessive dosages, the athlete can experience serious adverse effects.

References

1. Abebe, W. Herbal medication: Potential for adverse interactions with analgesic drugs. J Clin Pharm Ther 27:391, 2002.
2. Caterina, MJ, et al.: The capsaicin receptor: A heat-activated ion channel in the pain pathway. Nature 389:816, 1997.
3. Coambs, RB, et al.: The SISAP: A new screening instrument for identifying potential opioid abusers in the management of chronic nonmalignant pain in general medical practice. Pain Res Manage 1:155, 1996.
4. Curatolo, M, and Bogduk, N: Pharmacologic pain treatment of musculoskeletal disorders: Current perspectives and future prospects. Clin J Pain 17:25, 2001.
5. Jonasson, U, et al.: Analgesic use disorders among orthopedic and chronic pain patients at a rehabilitation clinic. Substance Use and Misuse 33:1375, 1998.
6. Luty, J, and Harrison, P: Basic and Clinical Pharmacology Made Memorable. Churchill Livingstone, New York, 1997, p 58.
7. Mather, LE, and Chang, DH: Cardiotoxicity with modern local anaesthetics: Is there a safer choice? Drugs 61:333, 2001.
8. Robbins, WR, et al.: Treatment of intractable pain with topical large-dose capsaicin: Preliminary reports. Anesthesia and Analgesia 86:579, 1998.
9. Smith, CM, and Reynard, AM: Essentials of Pharmacology. WB Saunders, Philadelphia, 1995, p 128.
10. Stein, C: Peripheral mechanisms of opioid analgesia. Anesth Analg 76:182, 1993.
11. Stein, C, et al.: Peripheral opioid receptors. Ann Med 27:219, 1995.
12. Tricker, R: Painkilling drugs in collegiate athletics: Knowledge, attitudes, and use of student athletes. J Drug Education 30:313, 2000.
13. Venes, D (ed): Taber's Cyclopedic Medical Dictionary, ed 19. FA Davis, Philadelphia, 2001.

Chapter Questions

1. Which of the following opioid receptors are not located in the brain?
   A. Kappa
   B. Sigma
   C. Delta
   D. Mu

2. Opioid drugs work by which of the following mechanisms?
   A. Decreasing neurotransmitter activity
   B. Increasing neurotransmitter activity
   C. Increasing peripheral vascular activity
   D. Decreasing peripheral vascular activity

3. Endogenous opioids are:
   A. Available for athletes OTC
   B. Taken by the athlete on an "as needed" basis
   C. Produced by the body on an "as-needed" basis
   D. Found in high concentrations when pain occurs in the body

4. True analgesic medications:
   A. Decrease inflammation
   B. Decrease fever
   C. Decrease pain
   D. Decrease blood flow

5. Opioids should not be combined with:
   A. Tobacco
   B. Food
   C. Carbonated drinks
   D. Alcohol

6. What substance was one of the first local anesthetics and is still used medically today, but is illegal for use by the general public?
   A. Procaine
   B. Cocaine
   C. Aspirin
   D. Lidocaine

7. Opioids can induce a tolerance effect during the first week of use.

   True   False

8. An overdose of a local anesthetic can result in the death of the athlete.

   True   False

9. Other than pain, opioids can be prescribed to control:
   A. Weight gain
   B. Cardiac arrhythmias
   C. Eating disorders
   D. Coughs

10. A local anesthetic will eliminate total pain from the entire extremity that it comes in contact with.

    True   False

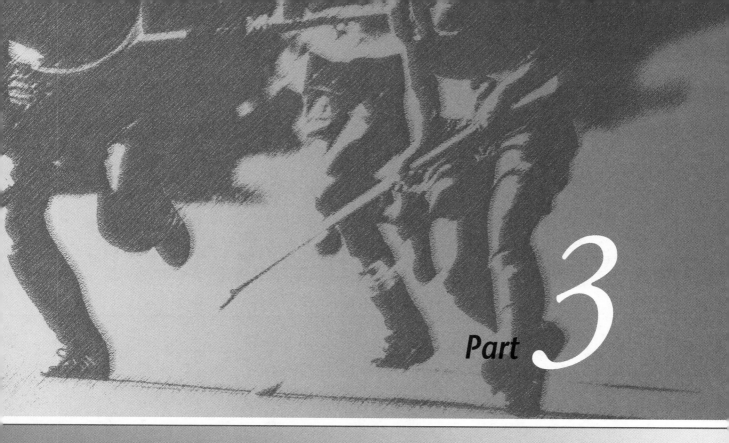

Commonly Abused Drugs in Sports

11

Muscle-Building Agents Used in Sports

Chapter Objectives

After reading this chapter, the student will:

1 Have a brief history of steroid and sports supplement use.
2 Have additional resources to locate information on steroid or sports supplements.
3 Understand the pathophysiology of steroid use on the body.
4 Recognize the signs, symptoms, adverse effects, and complications of steroid abuse.
5 Understand the pathophysiology of human growth hormone, dehydroepiandrosterone and beta-hydroxy-beta-methylbutyrate, and creatine.
6 Recognize the signs, symptoms, and adverse effects of the use of human growth hormone, dehydroepiandrosterone and beta-hydroxy-beta-methylbutyrate, and creatine.
7 Have information with which to counsel athletes using miscellaneous sports supplements.
8 Understand the mechanisms of action of miscellaneous sports supplements.
9 Recognize the signs and symptoms, adverse effects, and/or possible complications of miscellaneous sports supplements.

Chapter Outline

Steroids
   History
   Methods of Use
   Physiological Effects of Steroids
   Adverse Effects of Steroids
What to Tell the Athlete
Scenario from the Field
Human Growth Hormone
   History
   Mechanism of Action
   Effects on the Body
   Adverse Effects of Human Growth Hormone
Dehydroepiandrosterone and Beta-hydroxy-beta-methylbutyrate
   Dehydroepiandrosterone

Beta-hydroxy-beta-methylbutyrate
Creatine
   History
   Mechanism of Action
   Effects on the Body
   Who Uses It
   Adverse Effects of Creatine
   Scenario from the Field
Miscellaneous Agents
   Androstenedione
   19-norandrostendione
   Chromium Picolinate
What to Tell the Athlete
Discussion Topics
Chapter Review

*A*s athletic trainers, we work with many athletes who are enticed to use muscle-building agents in order to become more competitive in their sport. Being more competitive can mean better scholarship opportunities to better schools where the athlete might have a chance to make it to professional sports and possibly make millions of dollars. Typically, in sports such as football and baseball, athletes are more willing to use muscle-building agents to become bigger, stronger, and faster. However, athletes competing in other sports, such as tennis, volleyball, or track and field, are becoming more willing to use drugs for ergogenic purposes. An ergogenic aid is something an athlete might take to increase work output or, more specifically, increase the potential for work output during the athlete's sport or activity.

The disqualification of many Olympic and non-Olympic athletes for the use of steroids has been headline news since the 1960s, when medical personnel from the Soviet-bloc countries were promoting steroid use to all types of athletes.[56] The June 3, 2002 issue of *Sports Illustrated* contained a number of articles discussing the use of steroids in major-league baseball by what is estimated to be over 50 percent of the players. Interestingly, *USA Today* (April 25, 2002) reported that a table-tennis player had been suspended for using steroids. The use of muscle-building agents by both male and female athletes, from baseball players to table-tennis players, continues to grow as the rewards of fame generated by sports performance continue to soar.

Muscle-building agents are abused not only by college and professional athletes; high-school athletes have also been using anabolic steroids for years. In 1988, Buckley et al.[9] published what was then an eye-opening article indicating that approximately 6.6 percent of high-school seniors nationwide had used anabolic steroids starting at an average age of 16. In the years following, other authors have confirmed that high-school athletes continue to use anabolic steroids. Specifically, Whitehead reported that 5.3 percent of the athletes in a rural state were using steroids,[63] and Johnson reported that 11.1 percent of high-school seniors in Arkansas were using steroids.[27] Stigler reported steroid use among Indiana high-school students at an estimated 6.3 percent; he further reported that an estimated 4.6 percent of the student-athletes in Ohio were using steroids.[66] In the southwestern states, the estimate was approximately 3 percent.[65] Nebraska high school students were the lowest, with 2.5 percent reported to be using steroids.[49] Use among the secondary school population is an issue not only in the United States. One report found that 2.7 percent of high–school-age students in Sweden are using anabolic steroids for a variety of reasons other than as muscle-building agents.[31] Thus, the problem of anabolic-

androgenic steroid abuse is growing in many different countries.

In this chapter we discuss the various types of muscle-building agents and miscellaneous sports supplements commonly used today by high school, collegiate, and professional athletes. Some of these ergogenic aids are considered nutritional supplements and are sold in a variety of different stores frequented by athletes. Others are sold via the Internet. Nutritional supplements are not regulated or subjected to Food and Drug Administration (FDA) rules and regulations because they are marketed as food products, unlike prescription medications. (For more information on supplement use, please see Chapter 13). We begin this chapter by discussing one of the most popular ergogenic aids for muscle building in athletes: steroids.

Steroids

Many different hormones are naturally synthesized in the human body. Males produces testosterone in the testes and females produce estrogen and progestin in the ovaries. These hormones are used by the body for the development of secondary sexual characteristics. Females also produce a small amount of testosterone via the adrenal gland and ovaries. These hormones have both *androgenic* and *anabolic* properties. The androgenic part of the compound promotes the male sex characteristics, such as body hair growth, deepening of the voice, and increased muscle mass. The anabolic compounds enhance tissue metabolism. Many times these drugs are referred to as anabolic/androgenic steroids (AAS) by the athlete or public when they are being discussed for their ergogenic properties.

Internet Resource Box

For position statements on anabolic steroids, see:

American College of Sports Medicine:
   http://www.aesm-msse.org
National Strength and Conditioning Association
   (NSCA): http://www.nsca-lift.org

In males, as previously discussed, testosterone is produced in the testes. In females, endogenous testosterone begins in the form of androstenedione and is converted to testosterone as needed. Testosterone is carried in the blood by one of three methods: via sex hormone-binding globulin (SHBG); bound to albumin; or if not bound, in what is called a "free-form" or unbound state. When carried by SHBG, testosterone is tightly bound and is not readily available for use by the tissues in the body. About 30 percent of male-available and 58 percent of female-available testosterone is carried by SHBG. A second method of testosterone movement in the body is via a loose bond to albumin. In males 67 percent of testosterone is carried in this manner, and in females 40 percent of testosterone is loosely bound to albumin. The remaining 3 percent for males and 2 percent for females is free and available to the system. The loosely bound and free testosterones are the most readily available forms for utilization by the body. As can be observed through outward secondary sex characteristics, males have much more testosterone readily available for utilization.

Both sexes naturally produce androgenic and anabolic compounds. Male and female hormones can also be synthetically produced and used for many different types of medical disorders, which will be discussed later. There has yet to be a synthetic steroid that does not produce both androgenic and anabolic properties in the person abusing them. Therefore both genders can experience the development of secondary sex characteristics of the opposite gender if these hormones are "out of sync" in the body or the person is abusing these drugs. Steroid abuse will be discussed in more detail further on in this chapter.

■ History

Throughout recent history, AAS have been used by some to gain an advantage over their competitors or enemies. The illicit use of AAS has been documented in war and athletic competition by numerous authors. It is reported that steroids were used to increase the size and aggressiveness of the German soldiers in World War II.[42] As mentioned, the use of steroids for performance enhancement in athletes can be documented back to the 1970s in East Germany. In the 1960s and 1970s, the sports medicine teams for some Eastern-Bloc countries (East Germany, Poland, and others) were providing steroids to young athletes to increase size and improve performance in all types of sports. Ungerleider[56] reported that steroids were given to these Eastern-Bloc athletes unknowingly. They were told that the pills and shots they were receiving were vitamins that would help their athletic performance. When these athletes found out that they were receiving large doses of steroids, it was usually too late. Many of the female athletes had experienced the masculinizing effects of the steroids. Athletes were also experiencing the physical and mental problems associated with steroid abuse that will be discussed in the adverse effects section.

Because excessive use of steroids is illegal, it is virtually impossible to do scientific testing on athletes using steroids that accurately accounts for the true amounts they use on a daily, weekly, or monthly basis. Most of the information athletes receive about using steroids to generate muscle size and strength comes from people trying to sell steroids, such as teammates or friends who are also using steroids illegally. It is not reasonable to expect persons who are using drugs illegally to maintain accurate and reliable records over many years and then share that information with persons who may oppose the illegal use of these drugs. Essentially, we are aware that AAS will generate muscle mass, but we do not know how much a person needs to take in order to achieve significant gains. To prescribe steroids in the amounts typically used by athletes to build strength and increase body mass would be unethical and illegal in a legitimate scientific research project.

Therefore, in this chapter, we will discuss the prescription of steroids for medicinal purposes and the amounts reportedly abused by some athletes who were willing to divulge information regarding their steroid use. The major difficulty in analyzing self-reported data from illegal drug users is that there is no way to determine if the self reported amounts are correct. This makes it difficult to get objective information for the athletic trainer. The authors of this chapter find it very difficult to believe that information gathered from athletes using drugs is accurate and without bias. We do know that athletes who abuse steroids are taking more than the prescribed therapeutic dosages recommended for the treatment of diagnosed disease processes or other problems that can be treated by medicinal steroid use. The most common types of AAS are outlined in Table 11–1.

■ Methods of Use

Individuals who use excessive dosages of steroids as part of their weight-training activities follow what is called a *stacking protocol* or *cycling*. A stacking protocol consists of simultaneously using multiple types of steroid drugs in high doses. The cycling of drugs means that the athlete follows a timed cycle that begins with small doses and increases to very high doses, then tapers off to a drug-free period. Examples are given in Tables 11–2 and 11–3. The concepts of stacking and cycling drugs have been around for many years. These practices are believed to enhance the effectiveness of the total combination of steroids taken during the cycle. Some users believe that the stacking protocol can reduce some of the adverse effects produced by one or more of the more potent steroids being taken. Again, the recommended length of cycle, combination of steroids used, and daily dosing procedures vary depending on whom you talk to and what they have experienced or learned secondhand about these techniques. According to "experts," cycles range

Table 11-1

Common Types of Anabolic Steroids Used by Athletes

Generic Name	Common or Brand Name	Medicinal Purpose	Recommended Dosage	Reported Dosages by Athletes*	Reference
Oral Preparations					
Fluoxymesterone	Halotestin/Android-F	Hypogonadism	5–20 mg/day		
Mesterolone		Hypogonadism	50–100 mg/day		
Methandrostenolone	Dianabol	Postmenopausal osteoporosis	5–20 mg/day	40 mg/day	bb
Oxandrolone	Anavar/Oxandrin	Anorexia in surgical candidates	5–10 mg/day	25 mg/day	aa
Oxymetholone	Anadrol-50	Severe anemia	50–150 mg/day	1 mg/kg/day	aa
Methylandrostendiole					
Stanozolol	Winstrol	Prophylactic use against hereditary angioedema	2–6 mg/day	150 mg/week	bb
Ethylestrenol	Maxibolin				
Injectable Preparations					
Nandrolone deconate	Decadurabolin	Severe anemia Control of metastatic breast cancer	50–200 mg/week	600 mg/week	aa
Stanozolol	Winstrol	Veterinary use only		100–300mg/week	aa
Trenbolone	Parabolan Finaplex	Veterinary		304 mg/week	aa
Boldenone	Equipose	Veterinary		250 mg/week	aa
Testosterone	Depo-Testosterone	Androgen replacement therapy	50–400 mg/week	1000 mg/week	aa
	Delatestryl	Inoperable breast cancer Male hypogonadism			
Sustanon 250	Testosterone Blend	Available only via underground sources	500 mg/week, some reports of 1000 mg/week	bb	

Contains 4 different types of testosterone:
1. Propionate
2. Phenylpropionate
3. Isocaproate
4. Deconate

*These dosages should not be viewed as recommended for any reason. The figures indicating the dosage per day are sometimes exceeded by a factor of 100 or more by the athlete using steroids to generate muscle strength and body mass.
Source: aa = reference from http://www.geocities.com/hotsprings/7110/
bb = reference from *http://anabolicreview.com/cycles.htm*

from 8 weeks to a year in length. Users may not take steroids every day, but instead may have weeks "on" and weeks "off" that correspond to the type of steroids being taken and the perceived reason for taking each drug.

The propagation of steroid abuse via Internet resources is astonishing. One has only to look for a matter of minutes on the Internet to find dozens of Websites promoting steroid use for a variety of objectives. Many Websites have steroids for sale and contain stacking regimens and question-and-answer pages. The use of commercial Websites as a source of information for athletes using steroids is unconscionable. These Websites can be very convincing, and a

Table 11-2

Steroid Cycling Example

Week	Winstrol mg/week	Primobolan mg/week	Clenbuterol tablets/day
1	100	100	1 tid
2	200	100	1 tid
3	200	200	
4	300	200	
5	300	300	1 tid
6	200	200	1 tid
7	200	200	
8	100	100	
9			1 tid
10			1 tid

Source: http://www.steroids101.com. (Website selling steroids and providing dosages and other information regarding steroid use)

novice athlete could be easily persuaded to use steroids to gain muscle strength and body mass.

Physiological Effects of Steroids

It is difficult to document all of the physiological effects of steroids through scientific research, but many athletes can provide testimonials regarding the increase in body mass associated with steroid abuse. Usually, individuals use AAS to increase muscle strength by increasing muscle protein synthesis, inhibiting the catabolic effects of glucocorticoids, and increasing the aggressive behavior tendencies of the individual, thereby inclining him or her to train harder. Kadi et. al.[30] reported that taking steroids and participating in strength training increases the size of the muscle (*hypertrophy*) and the number of muscle fibers (*hyperplasia*). One must recognize that this study was conducted using subjects (weightlifters) who claimed that they had abused steroids for an average of almost 10 years. The investigators did not

Table 11-3

"Super Cutting Cycle" Example

Week	Mon	Tues	Wed	Thurs	Fri	Sat	Sun
1	100 mg P						
2	100 mg P		150 mg D				
3	150 mg P		200 mg D 50 mg W				
4	150 mg P 50 mg W		200 mg D 50 mg W		50 mg W		
5	200 mg P 50 mg W		200 mg D 50 mg W		50 mg W		
6	200 mg P 50 mg W	50 mg W	200 mg D 50 mg W		50 mg W		
7	150 mg D 50 mg W		150 mg D 50 mg W		50 mg W		
8	150 mg D 50 mg W		150 mg D 50 mg W		50 mg W		
9	150 mg D 50 mg W		150 mg D 50 mg W		50 mg W		
10	100 mg D 50 mg W		50 W 50 D				
11	5000 IU HCG						
12	5000 IU HCG						

Legend (per Website):
P = Primobolan Depot (100 mg/mL)
D = Deca (100 mg/mL)
W = Winstrol (50 mg/mL)
HCG = 5000 IU/injection
Source: http://www.steroids101.com.

make any comparisons of the genetic makeup of the subjects. Some researchers would like to link steroid users' increase in strength to the increase in resistance training that is often associated with the abuse of AAS. Other researchers believe that the increase in strength correlates directly with the use of excessive doses of AAS. They posit that the steroids increase muscle mass; after an athlete has gained muscle mass, he or she is able to lift more weight.

Published clinical studies demonstrate that an increase in the size of a person occurs after the medicinal use of steroids, such as by a physician for growth delay in an adolescent. It is well documented that a person will get bigger when he or she uses supraphysiologic doses of AAS.[7,30,35] However, it is not well documented that the person will generate more strength. In published research, it has been demonstrated that when a person is abusing AAS, typically he or she is also performing a great deal of resistance training on a very regular schedule. This was demonstrated by Bhasin et al.,[7] who demonstrated that either steroid use alone or resistance training alone will individually increase strength in some athletes. However, when steroids and resistance training were combined, the strength gains were greater than those achieved with either of the individual treatments.

It is also suggested that steroids may provide a decrease in reflex latency. A study conducted by Ariel and Saville[3] indicated that there is a quicker patellar reflex response by the muscle from a stimulus in the athlete using AAS. This would indicate that athletes requiring quick reflex movements might benefit from the use of steroids. Almost any athlete would benefit from being quicker in his or her reflex activity; obvious examples include baseball players, hockey goalies, and volleyball players.

The effect of supraphysiologic doses of AAS on aerobic performance is not clear. Over the years, research studies have indicated that there does not appear to be a positive effect on aerobic performance.[4,17,52] However, athletes will explain that steroids give them a psychological advantage that assists them through the aerobic work and that they feel more vigor, energy, and aggressiveness as they exercise. The psychological aspect of the use of AAS is difficult to measure objectively. The use of AAS by endurance athletes has not been documented to improve their performance because the effects of steroids appear to be more generalized to the strength-training athlete.

■ Adverse Effects of Steroids

General

The adverse effects of steroid abuse can be similar in males and females. However, in some athletes, AAS can produce adverse effects that are very specific to the individual. Many times the adverse effects common to both male and female athletes can have long-term consequences on the internal organs of the body. Other types of adverse effects are specific to the male or the female steroid abuser and have signs and symptoms that are more outwardly observable.

In studies conducted on mice, it was demonstrated that testosterone propionate impairs the capillary function in cardiac tissue, which can lead to blood flow difficulties, especially during physical activity.[54] This decrease in blood flow may be one of the factors contributing to sudden death from cardiac failure in steroid abusers. Additionally, an athlete with a compromised cardiovascular system may be subject to a cerebrovascular accident. In addition to vascular and cardiac problems, the athlete can experience damage or drastic changes to other organs and systems.

Another problem that appears to cause difficulty for both genders is the damage to the liver by steroids from first-pass metabolism. Oral steroids are much more toxic and damaging to the liver than injectable steroids as a result of first-pass metabolism. Oral steroids are broken down in the gastrointestinal tract and delivered to the liver via the vascular network. The liver has the job of cleaning the impurities from the blood before it is circulated throughout the body, providing nutrients and oxygen to the rest of the body. The AAS are recognized as impurities, and the liver tries to metabolize these foreign substances and remove them from the blood. However, the liver cannot take all the impurities out of the blood, so some of the oral steroids get through to the other parts of the body. The steroids that are removed for processing are hard on the liver, and can ultimately cause severe and irreparable damage. Over time, the liver becomes chronically damaged and ceases to function properly. Continuing steroid use may cause such conditions as jaundice, peliosis hepatis (blood-filled cysts), and tumors.

Injected steroids appear to be much more effective in building muscle. Steroids taken via intramuscular injection are not subjected to first-pass metabolism, but directly enter the blood and site of action. Therefore they are available to the muscle tissues in much greater amounts. The liver eventually does process some of the injected steroids that remain in the vascular system as blood is returned to the liver to be cleaned. In *The Underground Steroid Handbook* it is mentioned that injectable steroids are much more effective in making the athlete bigger faster. Of course, information provided by this and other nonscientific resources may contain misunderstandings and half-truths. It is easy to understand how a naïve athlete can be led to believe that the authors of these resources are telling the truth in all respects regarding the illegal use of steroids for performance enhancement.

The kidneys also play a role similar to that of the liver in cleansing impurities from the blood. When excessive levels of steroids are passed through the kidneys, this too can result in chronic dysfunction. Conditions such as hyperinsulinism, decreased high-density lipoprotein concentrations, and increased blood pressure are not uncommon in an individual with an AAS abuse problem.

Many, if not all, of the studies of problems associated with the abuse of AAS have focused on male athletes. However, when a female abuses AAS, the physical changes that can occur are typically irreversible. This does not mean that the physical adverse effects are always reversible in males who abuse AAS. Males must realize that when they abuse steroids, their body will go through changes that may not reverse on discontinuation of steroid abuse. For this reason, it is better to discuss the adverse effects of AAS abuse on males and females in separate subsections.

Implications for Activity

Athletes using hormones or prohormones will most likely become bigger, stronger, and faster in their sport. The use of these drugs appears to be common in all sports, from football to track and field. Athletes need to understand that these drugs have many different adverse effects that can affect their participation, from extreme aggressiveness, which may lead to sportsmanship issues, to tendon rupture during activity. The use of hormones definitely affects the participation of the athlete in both positive and negative ways.

Adverse Effects in Males

One of the most talked-about adverse effects of steroids is their effect on the endocrine system. If exogenous testosterone is being taken into the body, there is no need for the endocrine system to produce testosterone. Therefore, the testicles may cease to produce sperm in the AAS abuser. Alternatively, AAS abuse can cause *oligospermia* (small number of sperm), azoospermia (lack of sperm in the semen), decrease in testicular size, and decreased production of testosterone. It is suggested that these effects will reverse

when the exogenous testosterone is withdrawn, but there are no guarantees. Another well-documented side effect in the male AAS abuser is *gynecomastia,* female-type breast enlargement. Gynecomastia is not reversible, and some AAS abusers have their mammary glands surgically removed so that they do not continue to enlarge. Other steroid users augment their cycle or stacking with the drug Clomid, which is intended to counteract the actions of steroids that result in female-type breast growth.

The AAS abuser should also be prepared for premature balding; severe acne problems on the face, chest, or back; premature closure of growth plates in adolescents; enlargement of the prostate; impotence and decrease in libido; glucose intolerance, insulin resistance; ataxia; and tendon rupture in addition to the previously mentioned hepatotoxicity, increased risk of cardiovascular disease, and gynecomastia.[15,33,38] These are the adverse effects documented in the scientific literature. The undocumented adverse effects are just as significant but have not been reported in reputable scientific journals because of the inherent restrictions on how this type of research would have to be conducted (i.e., excessive amounts of the drug would have to be taken by human subjects to produce reproducible and credible results).

Adverse Effects in Females

Females also experience significant adverse effects from AAS abuse. The most common effect is masculinization. When a female takes large doses of the male hormone testosterone, over time she will begin to exhibit many male characteristics. Women may develop facial hair (*hirsutism*), male-pattern baldness, and a deepened voice tone. They may also develop an enlarged clitoris, along with a decrease in breast size, menstrual cycle changes, and amenorrhea.[33] These changes are typically irreversible. Many of the problems males experience (described in the previous subsection) are also common in female AAS abusers. These can include acne problems, reduction in libido, and mood swings.

Adverse Effects in Adolescents

Adolescent athletes who abuse steroids have a significantly greater problem because AAS abuse can lead to premature closure of epiphyseal growth zones. This is a long-term side effect that can result in smaller adult stature. Obviously, this is the opposite effect that is desired: the athlete will not be bigger; he or she will be shorter.

What to Tell the Athlete

It may be true that the abuse of AAS will increase muscle mass and strength, but the adverse effects of AAS must be described to the athletes under your supervision. The premature deaths of several athletes have been attributed to steroids. The athletic trainer should do everything possible to discourage the illegal use of steroids by athletes in any sport. Some tips for the athletic trainer when educating the athlete about these drugs include:

■ AAS are Schedule III controlled drugs, and distribution of these drugs without the proper license is a felony in the United States.

■ The use of AAS is banned by the National Collegiate Athletic Association (NCAA), the International Olympic Committee (IOC), the National Basketball Association (NBA), and the National Football League (NFL), among other sports governing bodies.

■ Many athletes believe that the adverse effects of AAS will reverse on discontinuation. Reversal of the adverse effects of AAS is not guaranteed when the therapeutic dosage is exceeded.

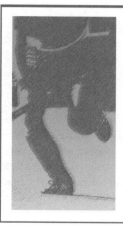

Scenario from the Field

A 14-year-old male was seeing a physical therapist for a shoulder problem. The visits to the physical therapy office went on for a period of months. During the time the boy was visiting the clinic, he was working with an athletic trainer on shoulder exercises. The athletic trainer noticed over the first month how muscular the boy was becoming, and was impressed with his overall conditioning progress. However, the boy continued to get much bigger and then started to get serious acne on his back, chest, and face. The athletic trainer questioned the boy in confidence, and he admitted that he was using steroids to "get bigger." When questioned why he wanted to get bigger, the young man responded that "girls really like muscular guys and I want to be liked by the girls." This indicates that high-school and college athletes are using steroids not only to enhance athletic performance, but for any number of other reasons.

*H*uman Growth Hormone

Human growth hormone (HGH) is produced and released on a regular basis to aid in homeostasis of the body. It is also released as part of the regular hormonal changes that occur during exercise in both competitive and recreational athletes. Exactly how and when HGH is released during or after exercise is being studied on an ongoing basis. It appears that numerous variables influence the increase and decrease of HGH as related to exercise. However, some athletes have promoted the use of exogenous HGH as an ergogenic aid and to give them a competitive edge in their sport.

■ History

Before the mass production of synthetic growth hormone in 1986, HGH was cultivated from the pituitary glands of cadavers, which was costly and could introduce contaminants that could be passed along to the receiver of the drug. Animal GH could not be used because the growth hormone receptors in humans have affinity only for HGH. When HGH was bioengineered, it was developed to assist young people who were short in stature and not producing enough growth hormone to increase their height to normal levels for their age group. Athlete use of HGH has increased dramatically since the introduction of bioengineered or otherwise known as synthetic growth hormone.

In 1996, the Atlanta Olympic games were give the nickname "Growth Hormone Games" because of the impression that fewer athletes were using steroids and more were using HGH. The synthetic version of HGH is now much more affordable for many athletes and is much harder to detect in routine urine samples. Many athletes now use HGH to increase muscle mass, train with increased intensity and frequency, and facilitate quicker training recovery.[48] When these factors are combined with claims of increased size and strength, the unscrupulous athlete has a nearly perfect drug.

▣ Mechanism of Action

HGH is an endogenous substance produced by the pituitary glands in normal people. It facilitates the transport of amino acids across membranes, which increases the RNA in a cell and thereby enhances the protein synthesis of the cell. With enhanced protein synthesis, the cell can function at a higher capacity. HGH also maintains blood glucose levels, facilitates glucose and amino acid uptake into muscle cells, and assists in releasing fatty acids from adipose (fat) cells.

▣ Effects on the Body

HGH has been shown to increase lean body mass and decrease fat tissue in individuals who were deficient in growth hormone.[45] Conversely, when GH-deficient individuals ceased using the supplement, they exhibited a decrease in muscular strength and fiber size and an increase in body fat.[44] When HGH is studied under scientific conditions, the results indicate that neither speed nor strength is enhanced in the athlete who is not deficient in growth hormone.[12,13,16]

Although its ergogenic effects have not been proven, HGH continues to be used by many different types of athletes.

▣ Adverse Effects of HGH

Many athletes are getting their information about the use of HGH on the Internet. These athletes typically do not receive the entire list of adverse effects, many of which are life threatening when using high doses of HGH. Fisher[19] reported that the adverse effects of excessive use of HGH include, but are not limited to, the following: acromegaly, hypertension, cardiomyopathy, respiratory disease, diabetes, abnormal lipid metabolism, osteoarthritis, increased risk of breast and colorectal cancers, development of a "cone-shaped body," and excessive sweating. These are all adverse effects documented in individuals who used HGH for relatively short time periods.

During childhood, excessive secretion of HGH can cause gigantism or, after puberty, acromegaly. Other adverse effects include fluid retention and joint swelling, skeletal deformities, arthritis, and possible visual impairments.[21, 62]

*D*ehydroepiandrosterone and Beta-hydroxy-beta-methylbutyrate

Two other types of supplements have been reported to provide strength and muscle mass for athletes taking these drugs. They are described here.

▣ Dehydroepiandrosterone

History

Dehydroepiandrosterone (DHEA) is a *prohormone* (a precursor to a hormone) that circulates in the blood. It is converted to androstenedione, a precursor to both the male and female sex hormones. DHEA was not commercially available from the mid-1980s until the mid 1990s because the FDA determined that it could cause liver damage if taken in excessive amounts. However, it is currently available commercially under a law that allows it to be marketed as a food supplement. See Chapter 13 for more details on the marketing of this substance.

Mechanism of Action

Blood-borne DHEA, produced in the adrenal gland, is typically converted to androstenedione, then to testosterone. The specific action of DHEA is very complex and depends on several factors, including gender and concentration. Many athletes believe that if they augment their diet with DHEA, they will increase testosterone production. As more testosterone is produced, the body is able to generate more muscle mass and repair damaged tissues. However, the ability of DHEA to increase an athlete's muscular strength, body composition, or other metabolic activities has not been proven.[8,62] DHEA became popular in 1993 as a cure for aging because DHEA levels appear to decrease as we age. However, these claims have been under scrutiny and are not proven. DHEA is used medically for various disorders including cardiovascular disease, obesity, and cancer.[11]

Effects on the Body

In athletes, DHEA may act like a prohormone, increasing levels of androstendiol and eventually testosterone on a short-term basis. DHEA also acts as an antiglucocorticosteroid agent that alleviates the stresses from exercise and training, thus increasing recovery rates. However, evidence-based research in trained human subjects is inconclusive regarding the alleviation of these stresses. Athletes also consume DHEA because of its ability to disguise steroid levels in the body.

Many athletes appear to be spending money on DHEA. However, it has not been scientifically proven to have any effect on their strength or lean tissue mass. The use of DHEA as a supplement may be helpful only to older athletes in reducing cardiovascular problems and lipid levels.[5,18]

In general, DHEA used as a supplement may have more benefit as an anti-aging product.

Adverse Effects of DHEA

DHEA is on the IOC and NCAA lists of banned substances. Long-term adverse effects are unknown, especially in the hormonal and endocrine systems.

▨ Beta-hydroxy-beta-methylbutyrate

Mechanism of Action

Beta-hydroxy-beta-methylbutyrate (HMB) is an amino acid used in the body for cholesterol synthesis. HMB is produced from the amino acid leucine and is believed to have anti-catabolic effects in humans. When HMB is taken into the body, it is broken down and used in cholesterol synthesis. Cholesterol is important to the body in cell building or membrane repair situations. HMB is thought to decrease muscle damage during activity and promote a faster recovery after stressful physical exertion.[20] In addition, HMB may decrease low-density lipoprotein concentrations, increase lean body mass, and increase strength. Thus, it is suggested that the use of exogenous HMB will provide the building mechanism or repair process to continue when the body is running low on the reserves it maintains from normal nutritional consumption habits.

Effects on the Body

HMB has been used for years by athletes wanting to increase strength and lean body mass.[20] Interestingly, there has not

been a great deal of scientific research published on HMB. The scientific evidence published recently indicates that HMB does not appear to have much of an effect on improving strength or muscle mass.[40,51,59]

HMB has also been analyzed for its ability to reduce the damage to muscle during eccentric (muscle-lengthening) exercise. However, HMB did not prove to be any different from other agents in curtailing damage to the muscle tissue.[40,34] It appears that short-term supplementation does not negatively affect the liver functioning, blood lipids, renal function, or immune system.[20] In summary, there is very little evidence that the consumption of high doses of HMB will enhance strength or increase lean body mass in athletes.

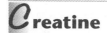reatine

▨ History

Creatine was first discovered in 1832 by the French scientist Michel-Eugène Chevreul. German scientist Karl Lohmann discovered adenosine triphosphate (ATP) in 1927. Only many years later was the connection between creatine and ATP made, and not until the 1980s did athletes start using creatine as an ergogenic aid.[50] Although there are reports of creatine use in the 1920s, not much research was reported between 1928 and the 1980s.

▨ Mechanism of Action

Creatine is a substance that appears to be helpful to the muscle cell in producing energy for muscular activity. It assists in the process of rephosphorylation of adenosine diphosphate (ADP) to ATP and is taken into the system through ordinary dietary intake of meats and fish. Thus, an athlete participating in an exercise that requires short bursts of anaerobic power may benefit from creatine use, if indeed any benefit can be derived from this supplement.

When creatine is taken into the body, it is broken down in the liver and transported to the skeletal muscles, where it is stored mainly as phosphocreatine (PCr). When it is needed, it serves multiple functions. Phosphocreatine is important in energy production because it becomes a phosphate donor to convert ADP into ATP, which can then be used for energy. It is also thought that the PCr works as an energy shuttle to connect sites of energy production with energy utilization sites. The other uses for creatine or PCr are to act as a buffer to maintain normal pH in areas where a great deal of hydrogen is being released from the ATP hydrolysis. Some suggest that creatine is a modulator for glycolysis. When a great deal of energy is being used by a specific muscle or site, the decrease in PCr signals the need for increased glycolysis to that area.

Effects on the Body

In reviewing published research, there is debate as to whether creatine increases both muscle mass and strength in the athlete. Much of the published research indicates that creatine increases total body weight and fat-free mass.[6,41,58] The proponents of creatine postulate a couple of different theories as to why creatine will increase muscle mass and strength in the human body.[14,46,47,58] Dangott et al.[14] reported that, in rats, creatine will increase satellite cell mitotic activity. Satellite cells can donate their nuclei to an enlarging myofibril, which will allow the new tissue to obtain the appropriate DNA to function on its own. Schedel et al[47] explained there is an increase in growth hormone secretion after creatine intake. Growth hormone will provide the environment for tissue growth and development to make the muscle bigger and consequently, stronger. Either of these physiological effects can be linked to an increase in muscle mass and, ultimately, strength.

The opposite argument regarding creatine supplementation is that it does not increase muscle mass or strength in athletes.[1,22,64] Most research indicates that muscle strength is not affected by creatine supplementation. However, the ability of the athlete to recover faster during resistance training episodes leads one to believe that the athlete is able to lift more weight. The maximum isometric contractions of the subjects in most studies has not shown improvement; therefore it would seem that maximal strength is not affected. It should be pointed out that the majority of studies published on creatine supplementation have been completed on males aged 18 to 35 years with little regard to its effects on females or the aging population.

After creatine supplementation, an increase in the athlete's total body weight has been documented and accepted by most researchers. The reason for this body weight increase is a point of contentious debate. Many researchers indicate that the increase in body weight is a result of water retention.[1,26,28,29]

Creatine supplementation techniques are fairly standardized. First, it is generally recommended that creatine powder be mixed with a fruit juice (preferably grape juice) to increase the availability and transportability of the creatine in the body. Many sellers encourage the athlete to begin the creatine cycle with a "loading phase." During the first week, the athlete is told to ingest 20 g daily for 7 days and then take 5 g daily for the remainder of the time they will

be taking the supplement. The idea behind the loading phase is to get as much creatine as possible into the system quickly and then maintain the increased levels with a smaller daily dosage. However, recent information suggests that there is no need to go through the loading phase of 20 g daily for the first week as promoted by most companies.[1,64] With the use of 3 to 5 g of supplemental creatine daily, the body will gain the extra levels over time.

The long-term benefits of creatine loading do not appear to make any difference in the 1 repetition maximum (RM) squat after 10 weeks of supplementation.[64] The total effect of creatine long-term supplementation is questionable when groups of users are compared to nonsupplementing groups in performing resistance exercise. Essentially, there does not appear to be any advantage to a loading phase in a long-term creatine supplementation plan.

An interesting note regarding creatine supplementation are the reports that up to 30 percent of people who use creatine fail to retain adequate storage levels in the body.[50] This indicates that about one-third of all creatine users will not gain any benefit from its use because their bodies are incapable of retaining the supplement. Thus, creatine supplementation cannot produce any type of enhancement effects in these athletes. To date there is no mechanism or technique that can easily and quickly determine who will benefit from creatine and who will not.

■ Who Uses It

Most creatine users would argue that the greatest benefit from its use is in activities that require rapid muscle recovery throughout the exercise period. The population using creatine includes athletes, individuals with muscle diseases, and aging persons. In the athletic population, the largest users of creatine are football players, specifically high-school juniors, seniors, and collegiate-level players.[23,28,36,39] The use of creatine by football players is obviously to make them bigger and stronger. Athletes in other sports use creatine to generate strength.[39] Other reasons why athletes may use creatine are to generate increases in total power, weight, and speed and to decrease body fat content.

When an activity requires the use of two different energy systems (anaerobic and aerobic), the replacement of glucose is critical to the athlete's performance. In a study that presents a new outlook on the types of athletes using creatine, it is argued that creatine could be helpful to athletes participating in sports that alternate between the anaerobic and aerobic systems (soccer, basketball, hockey, etc.) but utilize more aerobic metabolism for the majority of the activity.[43] The idea that creatine supplementation may be helpful to the athlete in a nonsteady-state exercise or when the anaerobic energy supply is diminished and the athlete is performing repeated high-intensity exercise with rest periods in between exercise bouts has some value. Multiple scientific studies replicating these findings in various sports have yet to approve or contradict this latest theory. The advantage of creatine supplementation in assisting with the aerobic power of a muscle is not proven, and there is no evidence of an anabolic effect from creatine supplementation at any dosage.

■ Adverse Effects of Creatine

When athletes were surveyed regarding their perception of the adverse effects of creatine use and the actual documented adverse effects, the athletes demonstrated a good knowledge of the actual reported adverse effects.[39,50] These are kidney damage, fluid retention, muscle cramps, upset stomach, and diarrhea.[1,29,50] Muscle cramping is reported to be more severe during the initial loading phase and is not as problematic during the continuation phase of creatine use.

Although athletes perceive that there are risks to using creatine, they continue to use it as a supplement because they do not believe the risks are long term or cause any physiological changes in their body. Most of the athletes using creatine think their coach is not aware of their creatine use; however, when asked where the most encouragement came from to use creatine, the most common response was "from friends," followed closely by "from coaches."[28,39] The largest source of discouragement for creatine use was parents, followed by friends and then coaches.[39]

Implications for Activity

The use of creatine by athletes who want to become bigger and stronger has increased in the past decade. Research on the effectiveness of creatine in building muscle bulk in the athlete is basically split, but the word of mouth among athletes and coaches seems to overshadow the scientific results. The necessity of the loading phase is very questionable and is thought to be promoted by the manufacturers to increase sales of creatine. The muscle cramping reported in association with the endurance athlete using creatine is confusing because there is no physiological rationale for associated cramping. Some athletes exhibit this cramping problem and will need to stop using creatine in order to reduce or eliminate it.

*M*iscellaneous Agents

■ Androstenedione

Androstenedione, known as andro, is a testosterone or estrogen precursor. It is an androgen produced in the body by either the adrenal gland or the ovaries and is mostly converted into either testosterone in the male or estrogen in the female.

It is suggested that exogenous androstenedione taken by a male has the effect of supplementing the endogenous androstenedione supplies and providing more testosterone. This result is controversial at this time, and different researchers have come to varying conclusions about the ergogenic effect of androstenedione.

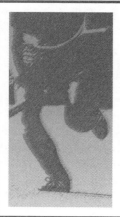

Scenario from the Field

A 17-year-old male soccer player with no history of muscle cramping started to supplement with creatine and follow a very aggressive resistance exercise program. Throughout the 14-week season he experienced some minor cramping in his legs, most commonly in the second half of matches. His team reached the state playoffs and began playing every third day. In the second game of the playoffs, his leg cramps became so severe that he had to remove himself from the game. In the following game, the same cramping occurred, and the player was unable to finish the game. After the high-school season he discontinued the creatine supplementation and during the club league season that followed did not report any cramping episodes. He continued to follow the resistance program and reported continued increases his lean body mass and muscle strength.

The real question is: Does oral androstenedione supplementation provide more of the necessary androgen to build muscle in the athlete? Leder et al[37] concluded that oral ingestion of high doses of androstenedione (300 mg/day) did increase the levels of testosterone in healthy males. Short-term supplementation (1 week) of androstenedione does not increase serum testosterone and does not increase skeletal muscle.[32] Conversely, Earnst[17] concluded that as much as 300 mg/day of oral androstenedione will not produce a positive outcome in young, healthy males. When lower dosages of androstenedione (200 mg/day) were consumed by athletes, plasma testosterone was not elevated.[4] New research following the breakdown of substances in the body via different metabolic pathways suggests that androstenedione may not convert to testosterone in the body. DHEA will convert to androstenedione after ingestion, but after this change still does not increase the serum testosterone levels in the athlete.[17]

Although an athlete may think that supplementing with androstenedione will benefit his or her resistance training, the scientific research does not support that theory. In fact, significant damage can be done by abusing androstenedione, including an increase in estrogen production and an impairment of the body's ability to metabolize lipids in healthy young males.[17] Androstenedione has not been proven to increase muscle size, and has no effect on protein synthesis or muscle mass.

Androstenedione has been marketed as a dietary supplement and can be purchased at many nutritional supplement stores by anyone wanting to take the drug. The International Olympic Committee and the National Football League have banned the use of androstenedione, but other sporting governing bodies continue to allow athletes to use this supplement.

The adverse effects of high doses of androstenedione are similar to those of AAS in both male and female athletes.[37] Damage to the liver and cardiovascular system are in all probability connected with high doses of androstenedione. Long-term masculinizing effects in women are also likely with the abuse of androstenedione.

■ 19-norandrostendione

Some athletes are starting to use 19-norandrostendione, a water-soluble supplement, under the impression that it will convert to nandrolone in the body. Many athletes using 19-norandrostendione have a marked increase in nandrolone in their urine samples. Thus the athlete makes the supposition that 19-norandrostendione is converting to nandrolone in the body and is available for use to generate muscle mass. This supplement has not been studied in detail at this time, but the results currently available from scientifically based research do not indicate that there is any improvement in muscle size or strength with 19-norandrostendione. One adverse effect recognized at this time is that, after just a single dose of 19-norandrostendione, the athlete may test positive for illegal steroid use up to 10 days after the original dose.

■ Chromium Picolinate

Mechanism of Action

In the 1990s there was some suggestion that the use of chromium picolinate supplementation would enhance the strength capabilities of the young athlete, increase muscle size, and decrease the percentage of body fat. In older individuals, chromium may slow down the changes in body

---

What to Tell the Athlete

Supplementation with any type of drug does not take the place of a well-balanced diet. Supplements do not always work in everyone, and there is no way to determine if supplements will benefit any specific individual. Some tips for the athletic trainer when educating the athlete about these drugs include:

■ Many supplements used to enhance athletic performance may be banned or illegal for use in athletics, and some may even be harmful to the athlete.

■ If an athlete consults you, as the athletic trainer, about proposed use of a supplement, make sure that you know the indications and contraindications of the supplement under consideration.

■ Be aware that many athletes will use supplements regardless of the information you provide.

■ Careful monitoring of any adverse effects when a supplement is being used is warranted.

■ Provide printed information to athletes and team regarding commonly used supplements and the problems associated with these drugs.

composition associated with aging. Chromium is a trace element that works in the body with other compounds to assist with the regulation of nutrient metabolism (fat, carbohydrate, and lipid) through insulin activity. The action of chromium on the metabolic pathways may be beneficial for individuals who have blood glucose irregularities (such as diabetes) by improving impaired glucose tolerance and decreasing blood lipid concentrations.[2,25] Exactly how chromium works with insulin in the body is an ongoing debate among many researchers, but it is thought to be connected to the binding of insulin to its specific receptors.

Effect on the Body

Chromium supplementation has been studied and does not appear to have an ergogenic effect on athletes or the aging population in terms of body composition, energy metabolism, or muscular strength or power.[10,24,55,60]

Adverse Effects of Chromium Picolinate

Chromium picolinate supplementation may cause headaches or sleep disturbances, although these adverse effects are based on anecdotal evidence.

Discussion Topics

- What would you do if you knew an athlete was taking anabolic steroids?

- Is it acceptable for athletes to use sports supplements during the off season?

- Is short-term use of sports supplements safer for athletes than long-term use?

- Can athletic injuries be associated with sports supplement use?

- If a sports supplement has little published research regarding its adverse effects, should an athlete take that supplement?

- What are the different adverse effects males and females experience when using excessive amounts of AAS?

- Differentiate among AAS, DHEA, and HMB.

- Explain how endogenous creatine works in the body.

  - Outline the typical use of creatine as a supplement: the amount taken per day and how to get it into the body.
  - Outline the types of athletes that might benefit from creatine use if it provides a physiological benefit to the athlete.

- Differentiate between androstenedione and chromium picolinate.

Chapter Review

- Define the term *ergogenic*.

- Outline the historical development of steroids.

- What countries first used steroids to help their athletes win Olympic medals?

- What is the process of *stacking* or *cycling* steroids?

- Outline the physiological effects of AAS.

- How do excessive doses of AAS effect the anaerobic and aerobic exercise capability of an athlete?

References

1. American College of Sports Medicine: The physiological and health effects of oral creatine supplementation. Med Sci Sports Exerc 32:706, 2000.
2. Anderson, RA, et al.: Chromium supplementation of human subjects: Effects on glucose, insulin, and lipid variables. Metabolism 32:894, 1983.
3. Ariel, G, and Saville W: The effect of anabolic steroids on reflex components. Med Sci Sports 4:120, 1972.
4. Ballantyne, CS, et al.: The acute effects of androstenedione supplementation in healthy young males. Can J Appl Physiol 25:68, 2000.
5. Barrett-Connor, E, and Goodman-Gruen, D: The epidemiology of DHEAS and cardiovascular disease. Ann NY Acad Sci 774:259, 1995.
6. Becque, D, et al.: Effects of oral creatine supplementation on muscular strength and body composition. Med Sci. Sports Exerc. 32:654, 2002.
7. Bhasin, S, et al.: The effects of supraphysiologic doses of testosterone on muscle size and strength in normal men. N Eng J Med 335:1, 1996.

8. Brown, GA et al.: Effect of oral DHEA on serum testosterone and adaptations to resistance training in young men. J App Physiol 87:2274, 1999.
9. Buckley, W, et al.: Estimated prevalence of anabolic steroid use among male high school seniors. JAMA 260:3441, 1988.
10. Campbell, WW, et al.: Effects of resistance training and chromium picolinate on body composition and skeletal muscle in older men. J Appl Physiol 86:29, 1999.
11. Corrigan, B: DHEA and sport. Clin J Sport Med. 12:236, 2002.
12. Cuneo, RC, et al.: Growth hormone treatment in growth hormone-deficient adults, I: effects on muscle mass and strength. J Appl Physiol 70:688, 1991.
13. *Ibid.,* at 695.
14. Dangott, B, et al.: Dietary creatine monohydrate supplementation increases satellite cell mitotic activity during compensatory hypertrophy. Int J Sports Med 21:13, 2000.
15. David, HG, et al.: Simultaneous bilateral quadriceps rupture: a complication of anabolic steroid abuse. J Bone Joint Surg [Br] 77:159, 1995.
16. Deyssig, R, et al.: Effect of growth hormone treatment on hormonal parameters, body composition, and strength in athletes. Acta Endocrinol 128:313, 1993.
17. Earnst, CP: Dietary androgen "supplements". Phys Sportsmed 29(5):63, 2001.
18. Ebeling, P, and Koivisto V: Physiological importance of dehydroepiandrosterone. Lancet 343:1479, 1994.
19. Fisher, PJ: Growth hormone and exercise. Clin Endocrin 50:683, 1999.
20. Gallagher, PM, et al.: ?-hydroxy-?-methylbutyrate ingestion, part I: Effects on strength and fat free mass. Med Sci Sports Exerc 32:2109, 2000.
21. Gill, GN: Endocrine and reproductive diseases. In Wyngaarden, JB et al., eds: Cecil Textbook of Medicine, ed. 19. WB Saunders, Philadelphia, 1992, p 1234.
22. Gilliam, JD, et al.: Effect of oral creatine supplementation on isokinetic torque production. Med Sci Sports and Exer 32:993, 2000.
23. Greenwood, M, et al.: Creatine supplementation patterns and perceived effects in select division I collegiate athletes. J Sports Med 10:191, 2000.
24. Hasten, DL, et al.: Effects of chromium picolinate on beginning weight training students. Int J Sport Nutr 2:343, 1992.
25. Hermann, J, et al.: Effects of chromium supplementation on plasma lipids, apolipoproteins, and glucose in elderly subjects. Nutr Res 14:671, 1994.
26. Hultman, E, et al.: Muscle creating loading in men. J Appl Physiol 81:232, 1996.
27. Johnson, M: Anabolic steroid use in adolescent athletes. Pediatr Clin North Am 37:1111, 1990.
28. Juhn, MS, et al.: Oral creatine supplementation in male collegiate athletes: A survey of dosing habits and side effects. J Am Dietetic Assoc 99:593, 1999.
29. Juhn, MS, and Tarnopolsky, M: Potential side effects of oral creatine supplementation: a critical review. Clin J Sport Med 8:298, 1998.
30. Kadi, F, et al.: Effects of anabolic steroids on the muscle cells of strength-trained athletes. Med Sci Sports Exerc 31:1528, 1999.
31. Kindlundh, AMS, et al.: Factors associated with adolescent use of doping agents: Anabolic-androgenic steroids. Addiction 94:543, 1999.
32. King, DS, et al.: Effect of oral androstenedione on serum testosterone and adaptations to resistance training in young men. JAMA 281:2020, 1999.
33. Koziris, L: Anabolic-androgenic steroid abuse. Phys Sportsmed 28(12):67, 2000.
34. Kreider, RB, et al.: Oral androstenedione administration and serum testosterone concentrations in young men. JAMA 283:779, 2000.
35. Kuipers, H, et al.: Influence of anabolic steroids on body composition, blood pressure, lipid profile and liver functions in body builders. Int J Sports Med 12:413, 1991.
36. LaBotz, M, and Smith, BW: Creatine supplement use in an NCAA division I athletic program. Clin I Sports Med 9:167, 1999.
37. Leder, BZ, et al.: Oral androstenedione administration and serum testosterone concentrations in young men. JAMA 283:779, 2000.
38. Liow, RY, and Tavares, S: Bilateral rupture of the quadriceps tendon associated with anabolic steroids. Br J Sports Med 29:77, 1995.
39. McGuine, TA et al.: Creatine supplementation in high school football players. Clin J Sports Med 11:247, 2001.
40. Paddon-Jones, D et al.: Short term beta-hydroxy-beta-methylbutyrate supplementation does not reduce symptoms of eccentric muscle damage. Int. J Sport Nut and Exerc Metab 11:442, 2001.
41. Pearson, D, et al.: Long-term effects of creatine monohydrate on strength and power. J Strength Cond Res 13:187, 1999.
42. Reents, S: Sport and Exercise Pharmacology. Human Kinetics, Champaign, Ill., 2000, p 162.
43. Rico-Sanz, J, and Mendez Marco, MT: Creatine enhances oxygen uptake and performance during alternating intensity exercise. Med Sci Sports Exerc 32:379, 2000.
44. Rutherford, OM, et al.: Changes in skeletal muscle and body composition after discontinuation of growth hormone treatment in growth hormone deficient young adults. Clin Endocrinol 34:469, 1991.
45. Salomon, F, et al.: The effects of treatment with recombinant human growth hormone on body composition and metabolism in adults with growth hormone deficiency. N Engl J Med 321:1797, 1989.
46. Sasa Mihic, JR, et al.: Acute creatine loading increases fat-free mass, but does not affect blood pressure, plasma creatine, or CK activity in men and women. Med Sci Sports and Exerc 32:291, 2000.
47. Schedel, JM, et al.: Acute creatine loading enhances human growth hormone secretion. J Sports Med and Phys Fitness 40:336, 2000.
48. Schnirring, L: Growth hormone doping: The search for a test. Phys Sportsmed 28:16, 2000.
49. Scott, D, et al.: Anabolic steroid use among adolescents in Nebraska schools. Am J Health Syst Pharm 53:2068, 1996.
50. Silber, ML: Scientific facts behind creatine monohydrate as a sport nutrition supplement. J Sports Med Phys. Fitness. 39: 179, 1999.
51. Slater, G, et al.: Beta-hydroxy-beta-methylbutyrate (HMB) supplementation does not affect changes in strength or body composition during resistance training in trained men. Int J Sport Nutr Exer Metab 11:384, 2001.

52. Smith, DA and Perry, PJ: The efficacy of ergogenic agents in athletic competition. Part I: Androgenic-anabolic steroids. Ann Pharmacother 26:520, 1992.

53. Stigler, VG, and Yesalis, CE: Anabolic-androgenic steroid use among high school football players. J Community Health, 24:131, 1999.

54. Tagarakis, CVM, et al.: Testosterone-propionate impairs the response of the cardiac capillary bed to exercise. Med Sci Sports Exerc 32:946, 2000.

55. Trent, LK, and Thieding-Cancel, D: Effects of chromium picolinate on body composition. J Sports Med Phys Fitness 35:272, 1995.

56. Ungerleider, S: Faust's Gold: Inside the East German Doping Machine. Thomas Dunn Books, New York, 2001, p 35.

57. Volek, JS, et al.: Performance and muscle fiber adaptations to creatine supplementation and heavy resistance training. Med Sci Sports Exerc 31:1147, 1999.

58. Volek, JS, and Kraemer WJ: Creatine supplementation: its effect on human muscular performance and body composition. J Strength and Cond Res 10:200, 1996.

59. Vukovich, MD, and Dreifort, GD: Effect of beta-hydroxy-beta-methylbutyrate on the onset of blood lactate accumulation and vo2 peak in endurance trained cyclists. J Strength and Cond Res 15:491, 2001.

60. Walker, LS, et al.: Chromium picolinate effects on body composition and muscular performance in wrestlers. Med Sci Sports Exerc 30:1730, 1998.

61. Wallace, JC, et al: Responses of markers of bone and collagen turnover to exercise, growth hormone (GH) administration, and GH withdrawal in trained adult males. J Clin Endocrinol Metab 85:124, 2000.

62. Wallace, MB, et al.: Effects of dehydroepiandrosterone vs. androstenedione supplementation in men. Med Sci Sports Exerc 31:1788, 1999.

63. Whitehead, R et al.: Anabolic steroid use among adolescents in a rural state. J Fam Pract 35:401, 1992.

64. Wilder, N, et al.: The effects of low-dose creatine supplementation versus creatine loading in collegiate football players. J Ath Train 36:124, 2001.

65. Windsor, R, and Dumitru, D: Prevalence of anabolic steroid use by male and female adolescents. Med Sci Sports Exerc 21:494, 1993.

66. Yonker, R, et al.: Anabolic-Androgenic steroids: Knowledge about, attitude toward, and the use by high school students. Report No. CG02-3-758, Bowling Green State University (ERIC document reproduction service no. ED338 947).

Chapter Questions

1. An ergogenic substance is something that has:
   A. A genetic beginning
   B. Eggs in the supplement
   C. The ability to increase exercise output
   D. To be injected into the body

2. Steroid use has been traced to which of the following athletic populations?
   A. High school
   B. College
   C. Professional
   D. All of the above

3. Only males produce testosterone.

   True   False

4. The term endogenous means:
   A. Originating within the organism
   B. Contains eggs in the supplement
   C. Will increase work output
   D. Has a genetic ending

5. Irreversible adverse effects of steroids in females include:
   A. Increased foot size
   B. Increased acne
   C. Masculinizing effects
   D. Sterility

6. When an athlete is simultaneously using multiple types of steroids in high doses, the athlete is said to be:
   A. Injecting
   B. Stacking
   C. Maximizing
   D. Producing

7. By using high doses of AAS, an athlete will definitely experience:
   A. Adverse side effects
   B. Faster running speeds
   C. More wins in their sport
   A. Stronger muscles

8. Which of the following AAS are least affected by first-pass metabolism?
   A. Androgenic
   B. Oral
   C. Anabolic
   D. Injected

9. HGH is now mainly available from what source?
   A. Human cadavers
   B. Monkeys
   C. Synthetic production
   D. Pig pituitary glands

10. DHEA is a precursor to:
    A. Androstenedione
    B. Human growth hormone
    C. HMB
    D. Creatine

11. Creatine is reported to result in an increase in weight mainly because of an increase in:
    A. Calories consumed
    B. Strength
    C. Bone size
    D. Water retention

12. The physiological argument for creatine use is that it provides an increase in:
    A. Strength
    B. Energy production
    C. Anaerobic capacity
    D. Aerobic capacity

Stimulants *12*

*A*s our society develops more interest in sports and athletics, we become more fixated on winning matches, races, or games. To win, athletes must be in top physical and mental condition every time they compete. A close analysis of most sports calendars indicates that, despite an increasing number of games, none of the sports-governing bodies want to encroach on another sport's season, so athletes in each sport are required to play more games in a shorter time period. This abbreviated schedule requires athletes to be ready to play almost daily in certain sports like basketball

and baseball. For athletes, competing every day or almost every day can be both physically and mentally fatiguing.

To keep up with ongoing participation requirements, some athletes elect to use a drug, such as a stimulant, to increase their energy level. For the purposes of this book, the term *stimulant* is defined as "any agent temporarily increasing functional activity".[33] These drugs provoke a stimulating action on the central nervous system (CNS) through a number of different actions. Because this book cannot discuss every drug that can provoke a stimulatory effect on the athlete, this chapter focuses on the over-the-counter (OTC) drugs that appear to be most commonly used as stimulants by athletes. Because OTC stimulants are more available to athletes than prescription drugs, the athletes may choose to use these drugs to maintain energy during the playing season. Some also use prescription drugs that stimulate the CNS (such as methylphenidate/Ritalin). These drugs are available legally by prescription only, but can be obtained illegally and abused by an athlete. As with other products, the spectrum of available ways to achieve a stimulatory effect can broaden as new products or alternative uses for current drugs are discovered.

Sympathomimetics are drugs that produce a stimulation of the sympathetic nervous system that is similar to the normal excitation response by the body. They are available in different forms.

In this chapter we begin by discussing products containing the OTC formulation of ephedra, and conclude by summarizing the effects of caffeine on athletic performance. As you will read, many manufacturers are now combining ephedra and caffeine in their products because both are stimulatory in nature. Some of the other drugs that are used as stimulants are discussed in Chapter 14 because they are better classified as social drugs than as actual performance-enhancement drugs for athletes.

*E*phedra (Ma Huang)

In the United States we have a variety of cultures. As our society continues to evolve, we see the impact of these different cultures on our choices of foods and nutritional supplements. An interesting evolution in the American society is the influence of Eastern medical philosophy and practice in our health-care system. One of the most visible signs of the Eastern health-care philosophy is the use of herbal preparations for a variety of reasons. More and more athletes are using herbal preparations, including stimulants, in their quest for enhanced athletic ability, and are suggesting the same to their teammates and friends. Most of the herbal stimulants come from the *ma huang* (pronounced "ma-wong") plant.

The ma huang plant is harvested and processed into two types of stimulants: ephedra and pseudoephedrine. These two drugs are classified as sympathomimetics because of their stimulatory effect on the sympathetic nervous system. This is the system that stimulates the heart, lungs, and blood vessels to promote the "fight or flight" mechanism. Ephedra is removed from the plant and processed into alkaloid form. This form, known as *ephedrine*, is preferred because of its improved water solubility, which makes it easier for the human body to read-ily assimilate and utilize. Ephedrine's basic effects on the human body are threefold. It dilates the bronchial muscles, contracts nasal mucosa, and increases blood pressure. All of these are stimulatory actions on the physiology of the body. Pseudoephedrine, an isomer of ephedra, is more commonly found in OTC oral decongestants. It is helpful in producing a vasoconstriction of the blood vessels in the nasal passages and upper respiratory tract. It is also used for the illegal production of methamphetamine, as explained later in this chapter.

Implications for Activity

The use of stimulants to increase energy levels can have far-reaching effects on the athlete. Athletes are constantly trying to find a technique or supplement that will give them an edge. It is easy for athletes to use a pill or a drink if they think the drug will give them that "little extra edge" they are looking for to be better than the competition. What athletes do not understand is that the combination of exercise with supplements or drugs taken together can become a lethal combination. The use of ephedra has been linked to deaths in a variety of amateur and professional sports. It is important that the athletic trainer educate athletes so that they will understand how these drugs can affect their performance and possibly their lives.

As of early 2004, ephedra was banned for OTC sale in the United States by the FDA. However, it remains available via the Internet, as do many other drugs. Therefore it is important for the athletic trainer to have a good understanding of this drug. To locate the FDA laws that banned ephedra and products that contain ephedra, please visit *http://www.fda.gov*. Ephedra is a compound commonly found in OTC "metabolism boosters"; weight-loss agents; decongestants; and cold, flu, and asthma medications. The potential for serious adverse effects is greater with "natural" or unprocessed ma huang because the amount is not always accurately described on the product label. There are numerous reports of herbal products containing substances (such as lead, diazepam, and codeine) that are not listed on the packaging.[8,22] One such case involved a product labeled "Chinese ginseng" that had the words "no side effects" on the label, when it actually contained 45 mg of ephedrine in combination with 20 mg of caffeine. If the athlete were to use 5 tablets of this preparation, as suggested on the container, he or she would be consuming approximately 10 to 11 times the OTC recommended dosage for ephedrine. Obviously, this would be dangerous, and the athletic trainer must be aware of these issues.

During the late 1990s, the federal government attempted to stop the sale of OTC preparations containing the caffeine-and-ephedra mixture by proposing a law that would stop its sale.[10] Ultimately, however, the government was not able to stop sales of these preparations, even though the FDA continues to receive reports of adverse reactions (over 17,000 reports as of April 2003), including deaths linked to the improper use of these products and similar preparations sold illegally on the street.[11,12] The deaths linked to caffeine and ephedra mixtures should now be reduced with the ban on ephedra sales in the United States.

Pseudoephedrine, an ephedrine isomer, can also be used to produce—legally or illegally—other drugs with stimulatory effects on the body, such as methamphetamine. This alternative use of ephedrine is an unfortunate fact that should be recognized by the general public. In an effort to prevent sales of OTC ephedra-based drugs to people with improper intentions, many states require pharmacies to report individuals purchasing large quantities of OTC cold tablets, diet pills, or similar drugs.

◼ Pharmacokinetics

Ephedra is available via the Internet in both natural and synthetic formulations.[18] The natural form has been reported to reach peak plasma levels in approximately 4 hours, whereas the synthetic form can reach peak plasma levels in 1 hour.[29] After absorption and delivery to the tissues, both natural and synthetic ephedra are excreted in the urine in a basically unchanged form. In the "natural" product formulation, it is difficult to determine how much ephedrine is consumed. The packaging of natural ma huang indicates only how much of the actual herb is present and does not provide a reliable indication of the amount of the ephedrine alkaloid in the product.

As pointed out by Winterstein and Storrs in their overview of herbal supplement use by athletes, the manufacturers of herbal supplements are not regulated like prescription pharmaceutical companies.[40] In Chapter 13 it is pointed out that these supplements are marketed as food and therefore do not have to comply with FDA guidelines. In the past 10 years, numerous organizations have studied the composition of many different herbal preparations for concentration and purity. The results of these investigations indicate that different companies produce a wide variety of concentrations and purities in herbal preparations, even when marketed under the same or similar names.

Therefore, athletes can unknowingly ingest more or less of the active ingredient than they expect when consuming an herbal supplement. Additionally, because of very limited regulation of the production of these supplements, there are numerous reports of product adulteration during manufacturing. When these products are tested in an independent laboratory, chemicals not listed on the packaging are often discovered in the tablets, powder, or liquid. Some of the unknown chemicals are not safe or may interact with other medications a person might be taking, resulting in unwanted side effects.

One of the claims made about ephedrine is that it is an energy booster. It is commonly touted as a drug that will not only decrease fatigue, but will also improve endurance, reaction time, and strength in all types of athletes. Another drug for which these claims are common is caffeine. Many companies believe that combining these two products will generate even greater stimulatory effects for the athlete. Bell et al. reported in 1998 that the combination of ephedrine and caffeine can be synergistic.[2] This means that the combined effects of the drugs are not just additive to one another, but one can potentiate the other. As a result, an athlete can get an extreme reaction from combining these two drugs. Not surprisingly, drug manufacturers promising an "energy boost" regularly combine these two drugs in their OTC preparations. Table 12–1 outlines some of the more common ephedra-containing OTC supplements used by athletes at all levels of competition.

◼ Effect on Performance

Ephedrine has been demonstrated to be an effective CNS stimulant. However, the ergogenic (performance enhancement capability) effect of ephedra on athletic performance has not been proven in well-controlled scientific studies. Most of the research completed to date on ephedrine in university laboratories does not indicate an increase in an athlete's physical capabilities from ephedra or caffeine use. The lack of any results demonstrating an ergogenic effect has not stopped the sale and marketing of these supplements to recreational and competitive athletes alike.

Many companies are now marketing different types of drugs that include a primary compound and a stimulant as a "secondary" acting drug. The secondary action of the stimulant is sometimes intended to overcome the sedative effect of the main drug. It can also be used to enhance a per-

Table 12-1

Examples of Nutritional Supplements That Contain Ma Huang

Supplement	Manufacturer	Ma Huang Content†(mg)	Caffeine Content (mg)
Xenadrine*	Cytodyne Technologies	20	200
BetaLeen	EAS, Inc	20	150
Diet Stack	Metaform	16	66
Metacuts	Metaform	16.5	150
Metadrene	Metaform	18	100
Hydroxycut	Muscletech Research and Development	20	200
Diet Fuel	Twin Laboratories, Inc.	20	200
Metabolift Diet	Twin Laboratories, Inc.	20	200
Ripped Fuel	Twin Laboratories, Inc.	20	200

Source: Reproduced from Powers, ME: Ephedra and its application to sport performance: Another concern for the athletic trainer? J Athletic Training 36:420, 2001, with permission.
*Also contains 105 mg white willow bark extract (equivalent to 15 mg salicin) and 5 mg Synephrine.
†Ephedrine alkaloid equivalent.

son's energy level so that he or she thinks that the primary drug is more beneficial. Athletes might take a product that is designed to relieve symptoms of allergies and unknowingly also consume a stimulant or sympathomimetic agent. An antihistamine, taken to reduce a runny nose, can create a general sedative effect. To counteract this, the manufacturer often puts a stimulant, such as caffeine, in the preparation so that the consumer will not feel sleepy after taking the antihistamine.

Some competitive organizations, including the National Hockey League, allow the use of many OTC stimulants. Other organizing bodies, such as the United States Olympic Committee, place stimulants on the "banned" list even though these drugs are available as OTC preparations.

Between 1993 and 1996, stimulant use was reported on almost 65 percent of the positive drug tests in International Olympic Committee (IOC) drug testing laboratories.[25]

In this chapter the street drugs that are used by some athletes are not discussed in detail. It is worth noting that drugs illegally sold on the street, such as the various cocaine preparations and methamphetamine, are also considered stimulants. They produce a stimulatory effect in much the same physiologic manner as other sympathomimetics. The street drugs are discussed in Chapter 14. For more information on natural or herbal stimulants, see Chapter 13.

Table 12–2 provides an overview of the supplement problems experienced by athletes in the 2002 Winter Olympics in Salt Lake City, Utah. The supplements, which

What to Tell the Athlete

No published research definitively states that ephedrine has an ergogenic effect on performance in competitive athletes. Many psychologists have noted that the mind is a very powerful tool. If an athlete feels more "energy" or is "stimulated," his or her performance may be increased by a psychologic impetus and not a physiologic enhancement. Some tips for the athletic trainer when educating the athlete about these drugs include:

▪ If the mind is convinced that the body has derived some extra energy from a tablet or a drink, it may

be the mind, not the supplement, that enhances the athlete's performance.

▪ The concentration and purity of OTC stimulants are not consistent.

▪ Stimulants are easy to obtain and are not considered harmful by many people who view these drugs as natural products.

▪ An overdose of an herbal preparation can produce toxicity and adverse reactions, including death, in an athlete.

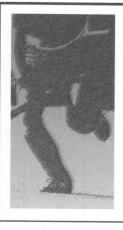

Scenario from the Field

In the 2002 Winter Olympic Games in Salt Lake City, certain athletes were deemed to have a positive drug test either before or after their competition. Many of the athletes who tested positive claimed that the test results were the result of consuming energy supplements from IOC-approved providers. The athletes claimed that they had not used any type of stimulant and that the supplements they were provided with must have contained the illicit substance. It was determined that some of the supplements provided did contain small amounts of ephedra. This is a good example of why the athletic trainer should educate the athlete regarding possible problems associated with energy supplements, no matter how innocent a given supplement may appear.

were available free to the athletes, exceeded the minimum levels for certain banned substances. All testing was completed at the IOC's testing lab in Cologne, Germany.

*C*affeine

Coffee is considered the most popular beverage in the world, and many believe that the caffeine in the drink is what makes it most appealing. The amount of caffeine in coffee varies according to the roasting and brewing technique. Caffeine is only one of many chemicals in coffee; however, it is caffeine that is most recognized by the general public. It can also be found in a variety of other beverages and is frequently an ingredient in food products and medications (cola and other soft drinks, chocolate bars, and medications such as NoDoz and Vivarin). It is well known that coffee and other caffeine-containing beverages and foods have worldwide social acceptance. Additionally, caffeine is a component of many OTC energy-enhancement products.

Table 12-2

2002 Winter Olympics IOC Testing of Nutritional Supplements

Country of Origin	Products Tested	Positive Tests for Banned Substances	Percentage Positive
Austria	22	5	22.7
Belgium	30	2	6.7
France	30	2	6.7
Germany	129	15	11.6
Hungary	2	0	0
Italy	35	5	14.3
Netherlands	31	8	25.8
Norway	30	1	3.3
Spain	29	4	13.8
Sweden	6	0	0
Switzerland	13	0	0
United Kingdom	37	7	18.9
United States	240	45	18.8
TOTALS	634	94	14.8

66 of the samples (10.4%) tested had borderline levels of unlabeled substances.
Source: Adapted from April 4, 2002 International Olympic Committee official press release.

For many years, caffeine has been documented as having an ergogenic benefit for endurance athletes.[4,6,9,13,20,21] The enhancement effect of caffeine on endurance performance is being studied even today, and different theories exist as to why it might be advantageous to the athlete. Spriet outlines the different research lines being followed on the physiology of how caffeine may have an ergogenic effect on the athlete.[30] It is important to keep an open mind and realize that future research on the enhancement effects of caffeine may take us in a totally new direction.

Many suggest that the research that inspired this curiosity about the ergogenic effects of caffeine dates back more than 20 years, when a group of researchers was exploring the effect of caffeine on endurance performance.[6,9,20] Early studies were the basis for the long-held hypothesis that caffeine increases fat metabolism. Caffeine, through one or more metabolic processes, increases the free fatty acid (FFA) concentration in the blood, providing an available energy source in the bloodstream, which spares muscle glycogen during exercise. This glycogen sparing in the muscle was thought to be the reason for the test subject's ability to increase cycling endurance by as much as 20 percent.

After these reports, other researchers began to investigate the reason or reasons why caffeine might be ergogenic in nature, and specifically how it affected fat metabolism in the body. Consequently, many research reports have been published in the last 20 years investigating the mechanism that caffeine uses to produce an increase in athletic performance. However, even the most recent published research does not explain the specific mechanism by which caffeine has an ergogenic effect on athletic performance.[4,7,19,32,36] As mentioned, the ability of an athlete to maintain a high level of performance through the use of caffeine supplements has been verified by numerous authors. Figure 12–1 reveals that endurance performance is improved in cycling and treadmill efforts by athletes working at about 80 to 85 percent of their maximum oxygen consumed during each minute of near-maximal exercise (VO_{2max}).

The following section reviews the various ergogenic mechanisms of caffeine that have been postulated. The reader will have the opportunity to consider the results of the major research published on caffeine as a performance enhancement product. Readers particularly interested in this topic should review articles published by Nehling (184 references),[26] Spriet (56 references),[30] and Hawley (160 ref-

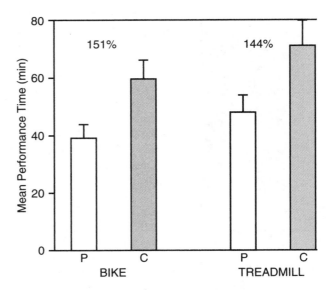

Figure 12–1. Mean performance time for subjects running and cycling to exhaustion (caffeine and placebo). Reprinted with permission from L.L. Spriet, 1995, Caffeine and Performance, International Journal of Sport Nutrition, 5: S88.

erences)[19] for excellent reviews of the literature and discussions of related research.

■ Mechanism of Action

Caffeine belongs to the *xanthine* class of drugs. The xanthines, as one of their actions in the body, act as a CNS stimulant. Caffeine is 99 percent bioavailable, and plasma concentrations peak within 15 to 45 minutes after oral ingestion. Its half-life has been reported to be 3.0 to 7.5 hours in nonexercising adults. The xanthines (e.g., theophylline) are sometimes prescribed by a physician to reduce the incidence of exercise-induced bronchospasm. However, caffeine is not the drug of choice for control of exercise-induced bronchospasm.

There are three different theories that attempt to explain why caffeine has an ergogenic effect on endurance activity in the athlete. All three theories have subtheories, which make it difficult to discern why caffeine exhibits an ergogenic effect on endurance performance.

The *metabolic* theory postulates increases in free fatty acids and catecholamines, which decreases the use of muscle glycogen. One of the effects of caffeine ingestion is an increase in circulating epinephrine levels, which can lead to an increase in free fatty acids (FFAs) in the bloodstream. This could be an argument for enhanced endurance capability in the athlete. However, it is also documented that exercise in general increases circulating epinephrine levels.

The *neurologic* theory suggests that caffeine activity affects the perception of effort at the central nervous system level and reduces the athlete's ability to perceive exhaustion. The *muscular* theory postulates that caffeine has a direct effect on the skeletal muscle via cellular calcium activity during muscle contraction. The general principles of these three theories are presented in the following paragraphs with a brief overview of the history and research supporting each theory.

Metabolic Theory

A common finding in the earlier endurance-related studies found that caffeine enhances fat oxidation during exercise.[5,6,9] In the metabolic theory, the mechanism of action for caffeine to improve endurance performance is by enhancing fat oxidation in the body. This results in an increase in FFAs in the blood. These FFAs are circulating and can be broken down for use as energy by the muscles. When this happens, the enzymes that metabolize carbohydrates are also inhibited.[30]

Because of this increase in FFA mobilization throughout the body, available muscle glycogen stores are spared during exercise. More total energy can be derived from a gram of fat than from a gram of carbohydrate; therefore, during aerobic exercise, the body prefers to gain its energy source from fat stores.[24] It is also known that fat can be stored in the body in much greater quantities than carbohydrates. If more fats are used for energy during aerobic exercise, it is hypothesized that: (1) overall energy production for the body is greatly increased, and (2) muscle glycogen stores are spared so that the system is able to utilize these fuel sources at a later time. When fats are used as an energy source for the body, a greater amount of oxygen is needed to liberate the fat from its storage site. Therefore there is less oxygen for use by the cells, which alters the utilization of the available oxygen in the body during exercise. This is one reason why the metabolic theory is limited in applicability to aerobic exercise (i.e., to times when oxygen is plentiful in the body during exercise).

The metabolic theory has not been as widely accepted recently as it had been in the 1990s as a result of follow-up studies by other researchers who were not able to specifically identify the ergogenic effect of FFAs on the endurance performance of athletes. Specifically, subsequent research projects were not able to positively discern the muscle glycogen-sparing effect of increased FFAs in the bloodstream.[4,14,21,36] The process of muscle glycogen sparing in endurance per-

formance activities has been a basic question for many researchers since the initial metabolic theory information was published. Other researchers have two fundamental questions regarding the effects of caffeine on athletic performance. First, is there an increase in FFAs in the bloodstream with caffeine ingestion? Second, if muscle glycogen is spared in this process, what effect does that have on endurance performance by athletes? The common thought is that aerobic activity is fueled by FFAs and glycogen is not a primary fuel source in endurance activity. If this is true, what does sparing of glycogen do for the system in an endurance activity? Many of the studies published in the late 1990s and after indicate the possibility of a CNS link to the ergogenic effect of caffeine on endurance performance.

Neurologic Theory

Much of the recently published research suggests that caffeine supplementation has an effect on the central nervous system. Specifically, it masks the effects of fatigue.[3,4,21] Different researchers have speculated on how this is done. Bruce et al. suggest that the masking of fatigue occurs in the CNS via alterations in neurotransmitter function or possibly by overruling fatigue signals to the brain during exercise, thus not providing the athlete's brain with the correct information regarding the true level of fatigue.[4] Figure 12–2 demonstrates exercise to exhaustion of well-trained athletes who were given three different dosages of caffeine. The athletes ran at approximately 85 percent of VO_{2max} and there was no significant difference in the time to exhaustion for any of the doses of caffeine administered.

It could also be reasoned that caffeine binds to adenosine receptors in the brain and other parts of the CNS. Normally, when adenosine binds to adenosine receptors, the result is drowsiness and a concomitant dilation of blood vessels (this dilation allows increased oxygen delivery to the brain during sleep). Caffeine looks like adenosine to a nerve cell and will attach to the adenosine receptor, but it has the opposite affect of adenosine in the CNS. Caffeine, in essence, fools the CNS and does not allow the system to become drowsy. Therefore the system remains stimulated and functions at a higher level of activity for a much longer period of time when, in fact, the muscles are tired and ready to slow down.[26] Figure 12–3 shows a typical perceived exertion chart that is used when someone is exercising to exhaustion. Charts like this are a way for exercising athletes to let the examiners know how tired they are getting. Perceived exertion may not match actual time to exhaustion when stimulatory supplements are being used.

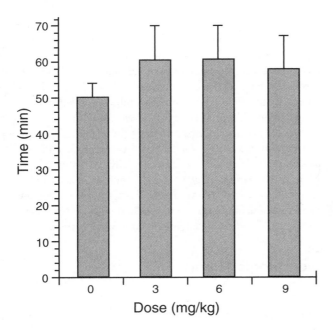

Figure 12–2. Exercise to exhaustion in well-trained athletes with 0 caffeine in their system and 3, 6, or 9 mg/kg of caffeine administered before exercise. The 3, 6, and 9 mg/kg doses are significantly different from the 0 dose, but not significantly different from each other. Reprinted with permission from Graham, TE & Spriet, LL, Metabolic catecholamines and exercise performance responses to various doses of caffeine. J Appl Physiol 78(3):867–874, 1995.

Muscular Theory

During the late 1990s, a number of authors suggested that caffeine has a direct effect at the cell level in producing its ergogenic benefit.[4,21,32] Recently, Tarnopolsky published a study that concluded that there was a direct link between the ergogenic effect of caffeine and the ability of the muscle to perform endurance activity.[33] The subjects in this study were able to increase the contractibility of their muscles with as little as 6 mg/kg of caffeine ingestion. In this study of skeletal muscle force, it was concluded that the endurance effect of the caffeine is via a potentiation of an increase in the calcium release from the sarcoplasmic reticulum. This increase in calcium enhances the ability of the muscle to contract over longer periods of time, thus providing an increase in endurance performance during aerobic activity.

Implications for Activity

Caffeine is a common substance that can easily be obtained by the athlete. Exactly how caffeine works to enhance the athlete's level of performance is not clear at this time. If an athlete is looking to increase his or her exercise endurance, caffeine might be helpful if consumed properly. It is important for athletes to understand that the use of caffeine can hinder their fine motor skills, which may be detrimental to their performance if they need to perform fine motor tasks. Like any drug, caffeine produces adverse effects, and consuming too much caffeine or obtaining it from an unfamiliar source can cause an athlete to feel ill. As a result, the athlete's performance may actually be decreased.

■ Endurance vs. High-Intensity Exercise

Originally, the majority of the research on the ergogenic effect of caffeine was directed at increasing performance

10 9	"I CAN'T GO ANYMORE"
8 7	"REALLY TIRED"
6 5	"TIRED"
4 3	"A LITTLE TIRED"
2 1	"NOT TIRED AT ALL"

Figure 12–3. Example of a perceived exertion chart.

during endurance activities (e.g., activities lasting an hour or more). Trice and Haymes concluded in 1995 that caffeine can have a glycogen-sparing effect during high-intensity moderate-length (30 minutes) stationary cycling.[34] They reported a 29 percent increase in stationary cycling time to exhaustion. The 29 percent increase was attributed to an increase in plasma FFAs, indicating an increase in fat mobilization. In 1996 Jackman et al. published a study that indicated caffeine can be ergogenic in intense activity (lasting approximately 5 minutes).[21] Jackman et al. did not indicate that the caffeine had a glycogen-sparing effect, but they did suggest that there may be a CNS or muscular connection to the increased performance after caffeine ingestion.[21] Similarly, Doherty determined similar findings regarding the effect of caffeine on brief, intense activity. The author suggested that the improvement in short-term, high-intensity treadmill running appeared to be from caffeine either having some type of influence on the CNS or acting directly on the muscle cell.[7] Shortly thereafter, other studies were published that contradicted these results, challenging the general theory that caffeine provides an ergogenic effect during short-duration exercise.[2,17] Essentially, the most recent evidence suggests that caffeine does not provide any ergogenic

assistance to the athlete during brief, high-intensity activities.[28,35] Figure 12–4 demonstrates the results of a study in which anaerobic capacity was measured over three different bouts of exercise on a stationary bicycle with caffeine and creatine ingestion by trained athletes.

■ Habitual Caffeine User vs. Nonuser

The effect of caffeine in the habitual user was questioned early in the search for the most efficient use of caffeine as an ergogenic aide. Tarnopolsky outlined much of the early research and questioned the physiologic responses to exercise of the habitual caffeine-consuming athlete.[33] Earlier results indicted that habitual caffeine users did not experience a metabolic or neuromuscular benefit during exercise following the consumption of caffeine.[33] Nor were any detrimental effects from the caffeine ingestion noticed in the performance of the subjects. However, in his most recent work on the subject, published in 2000, Tarnopolsky concludes that there is an increase in muscle contraction in both habitual users and nonusers of caffeine. It now

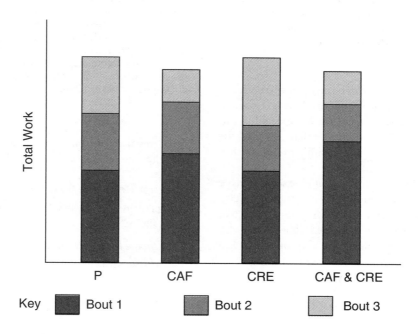

Key — Bout 1, Bout 2, Bout 3

P = Placebo
CAF = Caffeine (dosage: 7 mg x kg-1)
CRE = Creatine (dosage: 3 x 100 mg/kg-1 day-1)
CAF & CRE = Caffeine & Creatine (dosages: CAF = 1 mg x kg-1 & CRE = 3 x 100 mg/kg-1 day-

Figure 12–4. Anaerobic capacity measured for three different bouts of exercise on a stationary bicycle with caffeine and creatine ingestion by trained athletes. Adapted from Vanakoski et. al., 1998, Int J Clin Pharmacol Ther.

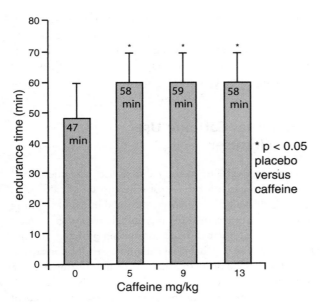

Figure 12–5. Endurance performances. Cyclists' performance to exhaustion with three different dosages of caffeine. The 0 represents no caffeine in the cyclists and the 5, 9, and 13 are doses of caffeine in mg/kg. The caffeine doses are significantly different from the no-caffeine group, but there is no significant difference between the caffeine doses. Adapted with permission from Pasman et al: The effect of different doses of caffeine on endurance performance time. Int J Sports Med 16, 1995.

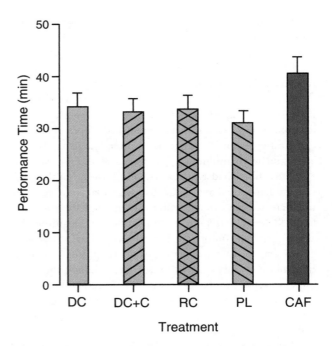

Figure 12–6. Types of caffeine ingestion and time to exhaustion during exercise. Healthy males exercised to exhaustion on a treadmill after ingesting the equivalent of 4.45 mg/kg caffeine in tablet form (CAF), decaffeinated coffee (DC), decaffeinated coffee with caffeine added (DC+C), regular coffee (RC), or a placebo (PL). Caffeine tablet ingestion produced a longer time to exhaustion than the other treatments. Reprinted with permission from Graham, Hibbert, et al.: Coffee, caffeine, and metabolism. J Appl Physiol 85:833, 1998.

appears that caffeine ingestion can be ergogenic to both the regular user and the nonuser of caffeine. This is definitely an area that will be researched in much more detail in the future. Figure 12–5 demonstrates that cyclists in endurance-to-exhaustion tests show a similar result to that in runners.

Athletes using different sources of caffeine seem to have various results in their ability to maintain exercise endurance. Capsules appear to be slightly more effective than beverages in producing this change.[14] The reason why capsules appear to be more effective is also unknown. See Figure 12–6 for a comparison of types of caffeine ingestion and time to exhaustion during exercise.

Athletes need to understand that some of the supplements they can use might contain both caffeine and ephedra.

Internet Resource Box

The following sites will tell you more about coffee and caffeine.

http://home.howstuffworks.com/caffeine.htm
http://faculty.washington.edu/chudler/caff.html

What to Tell the Athlete

The majority of published research in the past 20 years supports the premise that caffeine can have an ergogenic effect on endurance performance in athletes. From a research standpoint, there appears to be a combination of events that may lead to the ergogenic effect of caffeine on the athlete. Some tips for the athletic trainer when educating the athlete about these drugs include:

- High levels of caffeine can be detected in the urine.

- Caffeine is a "restricted" substance according to the NCAA and the USOC.

- The level of caffeine in the system needed to result in disqualification would require an average athlete to consume six regular-size cups of drip or percolated coffee about 1 hour before competition.

- Lower doses of caffeine, such as 5 mg/kg, appear to provide an ergogenic effect to the endurance athlete.[27] To translate this amount into ounces, an athlete weighing 70 kg (154 lb) could consume approximately 20 oz of brewed coffee (135 mg/8 oz) to gain an ergogenic effect.

- It appears that caffeine capsules are more effective than coffee or other highly caffeinated beverages.[14]

- Quite possibly, more is not better in the case of caffeine as a supplement.

Scenario from the Field

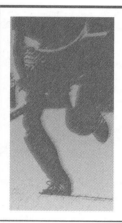

A 21-year-old amateur bicycle racer decided to use caffeine as an ergogenic aid before a 50-km road race. The racer thought that if he drank a large amount of coffee, it would provide a hydration base and the caffeine necessary for an ergogenic effect. He consumed five large cups of coffee starting 1 hour before and finishing the last cup just before the race started. He did not eat very much before the race, anticipating that the caffeine would be more effective on an empty stomach. After the race, he explained that during the race he felt that the caffeine was providing an ergogenic benefit, but he did not feel well enough to capitalize on the advantages the caffeine was supposed to provide. The cyclist suffered from severe stomach pains, and his bladder was extremely active during the race (caffeine has a diuretic effect). This amateur racer had a slower time than in his previous races and was nauseated when he finished.

Discussion Topics

- Does the type of caffeine that an athlete consumes make a difference? (Some familiar types include coffee, soda pop, chocolate bars, No-Doz, Vivarin, and diet pills.)

- By taking ephedra, will an athlete lose weight or get an increase in energy?

- What are the associated factors one must watch carefully when taking ephedra that can lead to a dangerous, possibly fatal outcome?

- What are the newest kinds of stimulants being used by athletes today?

Chapter Review

- Stimulant drugs provoke a stimulating action on the central nervous system (CNS) through a number of different actions.

- Drug manufacturers sometimes combine ephedra and caffeine in OTC products because both are stimulatory in nature.

- The ma huang plant is harvested and processed into two types of stimulants: ephedra and pseudoephedrine.

- Ephedrine is argued to be an effective CNS stimulant, but in scientific studies it does not improve athletic performance.

- The production of herbal supplements does not have to conform to the regulations of the FDA, so the final product may vary in concentration of the included drug.

- Numerous athletes in the 2002 Winter Olympics tested positive for banned drugs after consuming approved energy drinks containing supplements.

- There are three main theories as to why caffeine has an ergogenic effect on athletic performance: metabolic, neurologic, and muscular.

- Caffeine appears to be more ergogenic for the endurance athlete.

- Athletes using caffeine as a performance enhancer do not have to abstain from caffeine at other times for it to be ergogenic.

- Certain urine levels of caffeine in athletes can present a problem because caffeine is categorized as a restricted substance by the National Collegiate Athletic Association and the United States Olympic Committee.

References

1. Anderson, ME, et al.: Improved 2000-meter rowing performance in competitive oarswoman after caffeine ingestion. Int. J Sport Nutrition & Exer Metab 10:464, 2000.
2. Bell, DG, et al.: Effects of caffeine, ephedrine, and their combination on time to exhaustion during high intensity exercise. Eur J Appl Physiol Occup Physiol 77:427, 1998.
3. Bell, DG, et al.: Reducing the dose of combined caffeine and ephedrine preserves the ergogenic effect. Aviat Space Environ Med 71:415, 2000.
4. Bruce, CR, et al.: Enhancement of 2000-m rowing performance after caffeine ingestion. Med Sci Sports Exerc 32:1958, 2000.
5. Chesley, ARA, et al.: Regulation of muscle glycogenolytic flux during intense aerobic exercise after caffeine ingestion. Am J Physiol 275:R596, 1998.
6. Costill, DL, et al.: Effects of caffeine ingestion on metabolism and exercise performance. Med Sci Sports 10:155, 1978.
7. Doherty, M: The effects of caffeine on the maximal accumulated oxygen deficit and short-term running performance. Int J Sport Nutrition 8:95,1998.
8. Ergil, KV, et al.: Chinese herbal medicines. Western Journal of Medicine 176:275, 2002.
9. Essig, D, et al.: Effects of caffeine ingestion on utilization of muscle glycogen and lipid during leg ergometer cycling. Int J Sports Med 1:86, 1980.
10. Federal Register: Dietary supplements containing ephedrine alkaloids: Proposed rule 30677, 1997.
11. Federal Register: Dietary supplements containing ephedrine alkaloids: Docket No. 00N-1200, 2000.
12. Federal Register: Dietary supplements containing ephedrine alkaloids: Reopening of the comment period. Docket No. 95N-0304, 2003.
13. Graham, TE, and Spriet, LL: Performance and metabolic responses to a high caffeine dose during prolonged exercise. J Appl Physiol 71:2292, 1991.
14. Graham, TE, et al.: Metabolic and exercise endurance effects of coffee and caffeine ingestion. J Appl Physiol 85:883, 1998.
15. Graham, TE, and Spriet, LL: Metabolic, catecholamines and exercise performance responses to varying doses of caffeine. J Appl Physiol 78:867, 1995.
16. Graham, TE, and Spriet, LL: Performance and metabolic responses to a high caffeine dose during prolonged exercise. J Appl Physiol 71:2292, 1991.
17. Greer, F, et al.: Caffeine, performance, and metabolism during repeated Wingate exercise tests. J Appl Physiol 85:1502, 1998.
18. Gurley, BJ, et al.: Ephedrine pharmacokinetics after ingestion of nutritional supplements containing ephedra sinica (ma huang). Ther Drug Monit 20:439, 1998.
19. Hawley, JA, et al.: Strategies to enhance fat utilization during exercise. Sports Med 25:241, 1998.
20. Ivy, JL, et al.: Influence of caffeine and carbohydrate feedings on endurance performance. Med Sci Sports 11:6, 1979.
21. Jackman, M, et al.: Metabolic, catecholamines, and endurance responses to caffeine during intense exercise. J Appl Physiol 81:1658, 1996.
22. Ko, R: Adulterants in Asian patent medicines. N Eng J Med 339:847, 1998.
23. Kovacs, EMR, et al.: Effect of caffeinated drinks on substrate metabolism, caffeine excretion, and performance. J Appl Physiol 85:709, 1998.
24. McArdle, WD, et al.: Exercise Physiology; Energy, Nutrition, and Human Performance, ed 3. Lea & Febiger, Philadelphia, 1991, p 118.
25. Mottram, DR: Banned drugs in sports: Does the International Olympic Committee (IOC) list need updating? Sports Med 27:1,1999.
26. Nehling, A, and Debry, G: Caffeine and sports activity: A review. Int J Sports Med 15:215, 1994.
27. Pasman, WJ, et al.: The effect of different dosages of caffeine on endurance performance time. Int J Sports Med 16:225, 1995.
28. Patton, CD, et al.: Little effect of caffeine ingestion on repeated sprints in team-sport athletes. Med Sci Sports Exerc 33:822, 2001.
29. Powers, ME: Ephedra and its application to sport performance: Another concern for the athletic trainer? J Athletic Training 36:420, 2001.
30. Spriet, LL: Caffeine and performance. Int J Sport Nutr 5: S884, 1995.
31. Spriet, LL, et al.: Caffeine ingestion and muscle metabolism

during prolonged exercise in humans. Am J Physiol 26 2:E891, 1992.

32. Tarnopolsky, MA, and Cupido, C: Caffeine potentiates low frequency skeletal muscle force in habitual and nonhabitual caffeine consumers. J App Physiol 89:1719, 2000.

33. Tarnopolsky, MA, et al.: Physiological responses to caffeine during endurance running in habitual caffeine users. Med Sci Sports 21:418, 1989.

34. Trice, I, and Haymes, EM: Effects of caffeine on exercise-induced changes during high intensity, intermittent exercise. Int J Sport Nutrition 5:37, 1995.

35. Vanakoski, J, et al.: Creatine and caffeine in anaerobic and aerobic exercise: effects on physical performance and pharmacokinetic considerations. Int J Clin Pharmacol Ther 36:258, 1998.

36. van Baak, MA, and Saris, WHM: The effect of caffeine on endurance performance after nonselective B-adrenergic blockade. Med Sci Sports 32:499, 2000.

37. Van Nieuwenhoven, MA, et al.: Gastrointestinal function during exercise: Comparison of water, sports drink and sports drink with caffeine. J Appl Physiol 89:1079, 2000.

38. Venes, D, ed.: Taber's Cyclopedic Medical Dictionary, ed 18. FA Davis, Philadelphia, 2001.

39. US Food and Drug Administration: FDA statement on street drugs containing botanical ephedrine.: National Press Office, Rockville, Md., 1996.

40. Winterstein, AP, and Storrs, CM: Herbal supplements: Considerations for the athletic trainer. J Athletic Training 36:425, 2001.

Chapter Questions

1. Ephedra and pseudoephedrine can be found in "natural," OTC, and prescription medications.

   True   False

2. The production and marketing of herbal supplements is regulated by the Food and Drug Agency in the United States.

   True   False

3. Ephedra will NOT enhance the performance of a sprint athlete.

   True   False

4. Wrestlers who are trying to lose weight will lose more weight using ma huang.

   True   False

5. To what group of drugs does caffeine belong?
   A. Amphetamines
   B. Xanthines
   C. Decongestants
   D. Appetite suppressants

6. Caffeine has multiple effects on the physiology of the body.

   True   False

7. Which of the following is NOT a theory of how caffeine works on the body?
   A. Muscular
   B. Neurologic
   C. Metabolic
   D. Stimulatory

8. Which caffeine theory is the original argument for how caffeine works to provide an ergogenic benefit to athletes?
   A. Muscular
   B. Neurologic
   C. Metabolic
   D. Stimulatory

9. What effect does caffeine have on an endurance-type of activity?
   A. Increases reaction times
   B. Increases total exercise time
   C. Decreases reaction times
   D. Decreases total exercise time

10. What effect does caffeine have on a short-term type of activity?
   A. No difference in exercise time
   B. Increases total exercise time
   C. Decreases reaction time
   D. Decreases total exercise time

Natural and *13* Ergogenic Supplements

Objectives

After reading this chapter, the student should understand the:

1 Legal premise of herbal supplements.

2 Legal parameters of medically prescribed ergogenic aids.

3 Risk factors associated with the use of herbal and ergogenic aids.

4 Rationale for consuming sports drinks.

5 Use of amino acids and proteins in an athlete's diet.

6 Types of diet and nutritional changes that athletes might try to enhance their performance.

Chapter Outline

*B*ecause more athletes are now looking for ways to enhance their performance through chemical means, sports-governing organizations are implementing more regulations regarding the acceptability of supplements. Companies such as Twinlab and General Nutrition Center have discovered a potential market in athletes, resulting in more and more "natural" supplements appearing on the natural foods shelf. These new natural supplements are marketed toward athletes, promising that the body will be stronger and faster, and will endure exercise longer, when these supplements are taken regularly. Buchanan and Lemberg estimate that up to 18 percent of Americans regularly use herbal products for medicinal purposes. Americans spend over $3 billion annually on natural supplements, and it is projected that this will increase by approximately 10 percent each year.[7] Reportedly, athletes are more eager to use supplements than their nonathlete peers.[52] Obviously, this is a market niche where natural supplement manufacturers can generate a great deal of income. The United States Congress, realizing the impact of supplements on the consumer market, conducted an investigation of the supplement market in the early 1990s. In this government investigation it was determined that supplements have a potential to be hazardous to health. Since that time, numerous laws have been enacted in an attempt to safeguard the public health.

This chapter is divided into two sections. The first section deals with "natural" supplements, and the second section addresses the ergogenic aids sometimes used by athletes. There will be some crossover in the coverage of the two sections because some ergogenic aids are natural substances and some natural supplements have alleged ergogenic properties. As you read this chapter, try to keep in mind the interrelationship between these two concepts. Additionally, so far in this book we have been discussing prescription and over-the-counter (OTC) medications. In this chapter we introduce the concept *nutraceutical,* a relatively new term that has been circulating since the mid-1980s. A nutraceutical, as the term is used by natural drug manufacturers, is any dietary or nutritional supplement used for general health benefits.[43] This definition may be suspiciously close to the vitamin or the natural supplement concept, but as one looks at the methods by which nutraceuticals are marketed, it is apparent that the manufacturers intend for athletes to use their products in performance enhancement.

The Dietary Supplement Health and Education Act

The United States government passed a law in 1994 that allows a company to promote a natural substance with claims of improved function and health as long as the company does not claim that the supplement will affect a disease process. This law is known as the Dietary Supplement Health and Education Act of 1994 (DSHEA).[2] The crux of the DHSEA is that Americans should have unrestricted access to food supplements. The DHSEA states that, for a dietary supplement to be a food, it must contain one of the following: vitamins, minerals, herbs or botanicals, amino acids, metabolites, constituents, or extracts of any of the above named substances. Manufacturers may claim that their supplement can assist with some aspect of the nutritional needs of humans.

Internet Resource Box

Examples of one Internet distributor's marketing claims include the following:

St John's Wort: "may assist with depression . . ."

Cytosport Muscle Milk "enhances fat metabolism, promotes protein synthesis for workout energy . . ."

Canthaxanthin, the "tanning pill," "acts as an ultraviolet absorber, antioxidant, free radical scavenger protecting DNA from genetic damage . . . may decrease one's chance of getting skin cancer by decreasing exposure time needed to obtain a suntan, thus preventing sun damage."

Source: www.supplementcentral.com (9/16/04)

As is discussed in Chapter 1, the United States Food and Drug Administration (FDA) is the governmental organization responsible for assuring the American public that drugs, food, and cosmetics are safe for use. If a manufacturer wants to introduce a new drug (a product that will affect a disease process), that drug is subject to a long and detailed battery of tests. In order for herbal and natural supplement manufacturers to avoid the FDA's rigorous testing process, they market their natural supplements as food products. Because they are marketed as food, these supplements can be purchased by anyone at any time. Therefore, there are numerous products on the market that purport to be ergogenic in nature but have not been subjected to the same rigorous scientific experimentation as FDA-approved drugs. One of the best examples of the effect of this law is dehydroepiandrosterone (DHEA), a substance initially identified in the 1930s as a testosterone precursor.[6] It is now recognized that if DHEA is taken in excess, it can cause numerous liver problems. The FDA banned the sale of DHEA in the mid 1980s, but in 1994, after the passage of the DHSEA, nutraceutical manufacturers put it back on the market as a health supplement. See Chapter 11 for more information regarding DHEA use by athletes.

Supplement manufacturers can market their products in the same manner as any food. Exactly how many people use natural supplements or, for that matter, how many athletes, whether professional, collegiate, high school, or recreational, are taking a natural supplement to enhance their performance is not known. In one survey of young athletes, 40 to 60 percent of participants self-reported that they have taken some type of nutritional supplement to enhance their performance.[51] There are also plenty of incidental reports of professional athletes claiming they owe their improved performance to a particular supplement or a combination of supplements. None of the reports by professional athletes are based on scientifically collected and published information, yet published testimonials seem to sway the general consumer to believe in and buy something that may or may not be of benefit to them.

Coaches are one of the main conduits of information to athletes. It is important for coaches to understand supplementation and the potential hazards that come when athletes take supplements to enhance their performance. Another way for the athlete to gain information is from their (or their team's) athletic trainer. The athletic trainer needs to be aware of the types of natural supplements athletes might take. The claims made by supplement manufacturers cannot be completely outlined in this chapter because they frequently change. What we hope to provide in this chapter is a basic foundation for understanding what a supplement is and how you, as an athletic trainer, should converse with the athlete about supplements. It is important that the athletic trainer be a resource and educator for the athletes in his or her care. As you read this chapter, please remember that just because a supplement is marketed as "natural," it does not mean that it cannot be harmful. You will learn that there are risks associated with taking certain supplements, and that the combination of natural products with prescription drugs can sometimes cause adverse reactions.

*U*nderstanding "Natural"

The term *natural* is generally accepted as meaning anything that is not artificial, or that is produced by nature. It is a word beloved by companies and manufacturers because it is a term that the public equates with safety. For example, many natural foods—those designated as *organic*—are certified to have been grown without the use of artificial fertilizers or pesticides. Most natural supplements do not qualify as organic, but are marketed as containing only naturally occurring substances.

To many people, the word *natural* means something that comes from the earth and is necessary for human function. Others believe that *natural* means that the body will easily assimilate the product. Most importantly, many people believe that natural products will not harm the body. These beliefs are not based on fact but on advertising and marketing techniques. There are risk factors that are involved in taking natural products, just as there are in taking prescription drugs. Taking almost anything into the body has the potential to create a negative response in the tissues. Even natural foods, such as wheat, can be rejected by the digestive system and cause adverse reactions in certain individuals.

Children maybe at greater risk when they use herbal supplements because differences in physiology, immaturity of the metabolic system, or weight may directly affect the safety and efficacy of a specific supplement.[54]

Many questionable herbal products are still on the market and available for purchase by anyone with an interest in trying an herbal remedy for a current problem.[5] When athletes are using one or multiple supplements, or many athletes on a team are using natural supplements, it is wise to have a number of reliable resources available for study and confirmation regarding the safety of such supplements. One such resource has been compiled by the American Botanical Council, a group that has put a great deal of effort into helping consumers understand the effect of natural and herbal supplements. It has published an exhaustive work on these products entitled *The Complete German Commission E Monographs: Therapeutic Guide to Herbal Medicines.*[5] This document contains only information collected from reliable or scientific resources. It is divided into sections outlining approved and unapproved components.

In 1998 a report by Eisenberg et al.[14] compared the results of two separate national surveys on the use of alternative medicines by the general public. In this report, there was a 47 percent increase in visits to alternative practitioners and use of alternative medicines by the general public between 1990 and 1997. Herbal remedy use in this 7-year period increased 380 percent, and the use of high doses of vitamins increased 130 percent. One of the most alarming factors was the number of people (18 percent) who reported using prescription medications in addition to alternative medical products without informing their physician. As Eisenberg points out, this carries a high possibility of drug interactions.

Implications for Activity

Many athletes believe that taking a "natural" supplement will not harm them if the supplement is a natural product from some earth source. However, even natural supplements can be harmful to the athlete because impurity, inconsistent formulation, toxicity, and interactions with other drugs do occur. When an athlete experiences an adverse reaction from a natural supplement, he or she may fail to report to the treating physician that he or she is taking any drugs or medications. Many athletes do not equate natural supplements with the use of prescription, OTC, or illegal drugs and medications.

If an athlete is having trouble and does not report taking any drugs or medications, the athletic trainer may want to ask specific questions and use specific examples of natural supplements the athlete might be taking.

Risk Factors

A 2001 editorial in *Clinical Pediatrics* pointed out that, because of the many different substances in a natural product, the identification of the active substance or substances in herbal medications is currently not possible. Herbal preparations from various plant materials may contain anywhere from one to hundreds of active chemical substances. The possible presence of contaminants in these supplements from pesticides, heavy metals, bacteria, or other factors makes the outcome of taking these supplements and medications unpredictable in humans.

The risk factors for athletes using natural supplements can be broken down into four basic areas.[40] First, the purity of the supplement may be unknown and should be checked. Second, there can be toxic side effects. Third, as with any combinations of chemicals, there can be interactive effects. Fourth, the production of natural supplements (including growth of plant ingredients as well as manufacturing of the final product) offers multiple opportunities for contamination of the drug. Because the manufacturing process is not regulated by the federal government, there is a greater opportunity for contamination. All of these concepts are important considerations when one is contemplating taking natural supplements.

■ Supplement Purity

The amount of active ingredients stated on a supplement's product label is not always the actual amount found in the tablets or powder in the container.[19] Sometimes supplements contain ingredients that are not included on the label. Some may have higher levels than disclosed of a listed ingredient. Some do not even include the active ingredient. The discrepancies go on and on.

This can create problems for athletes who must submit to random drug testing. Recently a team of physicians and researchers at the University of California at Los Angeles (UCLA) tested the purity of 12 OTC supplements that are commonly used by athletes as muscle-building agents. It was determined that 11 of the 12 products tested did not meet the labeling standards required by law. Some of the products tested contained illegal or improper amounts of a drug. One of the products contained a drug that is legally available only by prescription in the United States. One contained 77 percent more of the active ingredient than was

indicated on the label; the other 11 products contained less of the active ingredient than was listed. Similar results can be seen with other products such as St. John's wort, echinacea,[19] ephedra,[20] ginseng,[10] and other supplements.[23,27] When the amount of a natural substance is not disclosed reliably, numerous different types of problems, including toxicity, may result.

Internet Resource Box

www.consumerlab.com is a Website operated by *ConsumerLab.com LLC,* a private company that provides the "CL Seal of Approval" and evaluates many different natural products for the public.

■ Supplement Toxicity

Although the possibility of toxicity is increased in children as a result of their immature metabolic or physiologic systems, the use of these supplements can be toxic to teenage and adult athletes as well. Admittedly, some of the toxic reactions experienced by adults have been minor in nature. Reactions have varied from simple skin rashes to hepatic toxicity, and some deaths have been reported. Toxicity of an herbal supplement is a function of multiple variables such as dose of the herb taken, other drugs or herbs being taken, duration and frequency of exposure to the herb, and other similar variables.[50] A college wrestler who was taking an herbal product containing, among other substances, ma huang and caffeine reported experiencing syncope and chest pain at practice. He was also attempting extreme weight loss techniques, and it may be that the combination of this practice plus the herbal product created an unmanageable situation.[39] However, this is a good example of how herbal products can build up to a toxic level in the body rather easily.

Internet Resource Box

www.supplementwatch.com is a Website operated by a group of health professionals. It rates supplements and provides a "Recommended Brand" status.

As more reporting is done by attending physicians, larger databases are created that can be used to determine toxic effects of products.

The FDA has pointed out the growing problems with aristolochic acid, a component of several dietary supplements and "traditional" herbal medicines. It has identified over 160 botanical supplements suspected to contain some level of aristolochic acid, which may lead to a variety of kidney problems or, in more severe cases, cancer.[32]

At present, there is speculation regarding the use of ephedra (ma huang) as an herbal supplement. The use of ephedrine is discussed in Chapter 12, but we also mention it here because the literature concerning toxicity of herbal preparations includes a number of published articles regarding ephedra.

Medical literature on the topic of toxicity is loaded with references to energy boosters, weight control preparations, pain control, anti-inflammatory agents, antidepressants, and sleep aids. Other natural supplements have also been suspected of producing toxic reactions. For example, as far back as 1979, it was postulated that ginseng could produce unwanted side effects.[47,48]

■ Supplement Interactions

Many athletes might not believe that a supplement considered natural could interact with other medications, either prescription or OTC. Some prescription medications are affected by certain foods. For example, dairy products are known to reduce the effectiveness of tetracycline. Athletes should be aware that herbal or natural supplements can likewise reduce the effectiveness of a medication they are currently taking as prescribed. Table 13–1 shows common herbal supplements that either decrease the activity of another drug or cause some type of adverse effect when taken in combination with a drug.

■ Supplement Contamination

When an athlete is taking an herbal preparation for ergogenic or other health reasons, he or she should be concerned about the purity of the product. The consistency and purity of herbal preparations is not held to the same standard as that of drugs regulated by the FDA. The DSHEA outlined a provision for the FDA to establish manufacturing practices for companies in the business of producing herbal products. However, the FDA has proposed only a few man-

Table 13–1

Examples of Herbal/Drug Interactions

Common Name	Uses/Properties	Cautions
Chamomile	Internally used for GI spasms and as a mild sedative. Externally used for skin and mucous membrane inflammatory responses.	Allergic reactions are common—pruritus, tongue and throat "thickening," urticaria, and so forth.[36]
Echinacea	Mainly used internally to reduce flu or cold symptoms. External use is for poorly healing wounds and ulcerations.	Three types exist—scientists are investigating "Kansas Snake Root" for effectiveness/complications.[5] Hepatotoxic effects reported with persistent use.[36]
Garlic	Antiseptic, bacteriostatic, antiviral properties, hypocholesterolemic, antihypertensive.	Hypocholesterolemic and antihypertensive properties are not well documented. People also taking an anticoagulant drug should use caution.
Ginkgo biloba	Short term memory deficits, concentration problems, dizziness, tinnitus, headaches, vascular disorders.	People taking anticoagulants should use caution. May result in spontaneous hyphema or subdural hematoma.[7,36]
Ginseng	Increases overall vigor, feeling of well being, physical activity level.	Reduces clotting mechanism.[7,36] Increases nervousness and sleeplessness, should be avoided by persons with manic-depressive disorder.[36]
Kava-kava	Reduces anxiety, stress; promotes muscle relaxation.	Potentates the effectiveness of CNS drugs such as alcohol, barbiturates.[5]
St. John's wort	Alleviates depression, anxiety, sleep disorders.	Increases photosensitivity.[5] May cause breakthrough bleeding when used with oral contraceptives. Decreased theophylline concentrations may occur in persons using a theophylline bronchodilator. Lethargy and mild serotonin syndrome also reported.[15]
Valerian	Alleviates restlessness and sleeping disorders.	Do not use with alcohol or barbiturates.[36]

From Winterstein, AP (2001), with permission.

ufacturing guidelines, and companies are free to adopt these guidelines or not. Even when a manufacturer does adopt the FDA-approved practices, there is little regulation of compliance. A company is investigated only if a formal complaint is lodged.

A variety of factors can affect the purity of a preparation. The species of the plant, soil, fertility, and overall growing environment, along with the part of the plant used and the extraction method, can all lead to contamination of the product. Any or all of these factors can be a potential problem for the athlete taking an herbal preparation. Contamination may also occur at any time during the manufacturing process. Many manufacturers are interested in creating guidelines to implement purity standards for natural products. However, as reported by Nelson Myer et al.,[40] consistency in the production and manufacture of herbal products is difficult to attain because of the many variables in the growing process. The growing process is not amenable to regulation because many of the growers have their own special techniques and are not willing or able to change or standardize them. Differences in the quality of herbal supplements will persist as long as these differences in growing and manufacturing methods exist.

Internet Resource Box

Reliable sources of information regarding herbal products can be obtained from:

American Botanical Council,
  http://www.herbalgram.org
The Herb Research Foundation, United States
  Pharmacopeia, *http://www.usp.org*
  http://www.herbs.org
US Food and Drug Administration Center for Drug
  Evaluation and Research, *http://www.fda.gov/cder*

Supplement Use and Popularity

In China and India, the use of herbal treatments for all sorts of diseases and disorders is a traditional and valued part of the culture. In the United States, the treatment of disease with herbal remedies was once common but was supplanted by treatment with manufactured medications. Today there is a resurgence of interest in herbal medicine in the United States, encompassing both Eastern and Western traditions.

Herbal supplements are popular with consumers across

the United States, and athletes are no exception. Athletes use herbal supplements for a variety of reasons. Some use herbs for relaxation purposes; others take them expecting an energy boost; and still others use them to achieve a complete integration of the body systems. Some supplement salespeople suggest that a combination of herbal preparations will integrate all the systems of the body so that everything in the body is functioning properly, thereby making the athlete more efficient.

Some of those potential problems occur because of the interference with the activity of prescription medications, especially those prescribed for cardiovascular disorders.[18,24,46] Cardiovascular problems are not the only contraindications of which the athlete and athletic trainer need to be aware; there are problems when herbal supplements are combined that may result in depressive disorders and hormonal and other imbalances.[24] Table 13–2 lists some toxic effects of herbal supplements.

Internet Resource Box

The main Website for the FDA is found at
www.fda.gov

Athletes must be aware that people from different backgrounds and with different motivations will suggest that they try various performance-enhancing products. They need to understand which types of products are "natural" supplements and which ones are technically drugs. The use of performance-enhancing drugs is a widespread phenomenon, and is laden with controversy and problems. Take the time to educate athletes on which types of supplements are illegal, which ones might be beneficial, and which ones are marketed with all hype and no fact. Remember, young athletes are willing to do almost anything to get bigger, stronger, and faster in their quest to be the best athlete in their school, town, or state. There will always be a newer and better supplement available to enhance athletic performance. Athletes need to be aware of the constant marketing barrage and the athletic trainer has to be up to date on the latest and greatest supplement claims.

"Natural" Ergogenic Aids

There are many different substances that an athlete might use as an ergogenic or performance enhancement aid. Ergogenic means "having the ability to increase work, especially to increase the potential for work."[59] The substances can be as simple as a type of food, a sports drink, or a natural sub-

Table 13–2

Examples of Potentially Toxic Herbs

Herb	Toxicity
Borage (*Borago officinalis*)	Liver toxicity and cancer of the liver
Cocoa (*Cacao semen*)	Migraine headache
Coltsfoot (*Farfarae folium*)	Liver toxicity and carcinogenic potential
Comfrey (*Symphytum officinale*)	Liver cancer in laboratory animals and veno-occlusive disease in humans
Ephedra (*Ephedra sinica*)	In high doses can lead to asphyxiation and heart failure
Kelp	Hyperthyroidism
Licorice (*Glycyrrhiza glabra*)	Large doses over extended periods can produce liver toxicity
Sassafras (*Sassafras albidum*)	Has caused liver cancer in laboratory animals

Sources: Muirhead, 1999; Blumenthal, 1998, with permission.

stance taken to enhance energy; or as sophisticated as a prescription drug that can cause physiological changes. One thing the athletic trainer should bear in mind is that the use of ergogenic substances will mainly augment the ability of the athlete to continue in an activity longer or respond a little more quickly to a stimulus. In the majority of instances, performance-enhancing substances do not provide the athlete with an increased skill level (e.g., an increased ability to make free throws in a basketball game).

Some ergogenic substances are illegal and have a higher potential for being life threatening. Many other substances are readily available to the athlete and are relatively safe. In this section, we discuss those substances that are either marketed as ergogenic or have been scientifically studied to determine their effectiveness in assisting an athlete to perform at a higher level. Substances considered ergogenic include sports drinks; dietary techniques; vitamin, mineral, and amino acid supplements; and prescription drugs.

■ Sports Drinks

Over the years many companies have aired television commercials, or used print media along with team sponsorships, to promote their specific sports drink as being the most efficient at replacing lost water and electrolytes in the exercising athlete. The amount spent on advertising indicates that this is a very lucrative market for the sports drink companies. If one looks closely at the published literature over the last 10 years, all of the major sports drink companies have, at some time, laid claim to the title of being the best at rehydration and replacing electrolytes lost during exercise.

The first widely available commercial sports drink was Gatorade, developed in a University of Florida exercise physiology laboratory to help the college's football players (nicknamed the Gators) to rehydrate during the hot and humid days of summer and early fall. Whether or not it really helped the Gators with rehydration, they subsequently had a winning season and thus attributed their success to this new drink. More and more teams wanted the drink, and the increasing demand for it initiated thoughts of a commercial enterprise. Gatorade was first marketed as a way to help athletes compete longer at a higher level even in the heat and humidity. We are all familiar with the financial success of Gatorade. Now many other companies have cashed in on the growing market with their own sports drink formulations that they claim work better than the rest.

There have been numerous research projects to determine the rate of absorption of fluid and electrolytes from sports drinks. Most, if not all, of the manufacturers in this area are now using similar carbohydrate types and concentrations in their products because researchers have determined the levels of both that are most efficiently absorbed by the intestinal tract. The slight variations in carbohydrate type and concentration that do exist are used by sports drink manufacturers as marketing tools. For example, Gatorade is formulated with 5 percent carbohydrate and POWERade contains 9 percent.[9]

Possibly the most important variable influencing an athlete's consumption of a sports drink is the taste. If an athlete likes the taste of the drink, he or she will consume more of the drink and therefore rehydrate faster. The actual benefit of a sports drink as a performance enhancement product has been shown to be effective in some studies involving prolonged exercise, but other published research does not provide the same conclusion.[9] However, as long as there is a profitable market for sports drinks, their effectiveness will continue to be argued.

■ Energy Drinks

A new entry into the sports drink market in recent years is the category of drinks marketed as "energy boosters." These drinks are typically made with high levels of caffeine and other stimulating natural substances. The excessive amounts of caffeine in some of these drinks can cause upset stomach, produce diuretic effects, act as a laxative, and produce levels of caffeine in the urine large enough to be detected or questioned in a drug test. Energy drinks with added herbal or natural substances can present the same types of problems regarding purity, toxicity, contamination, and drug interaction as were discussed earlier in this chapter. Table 13–3 lists the ingredients of some popular energy drinks.

Implications for Activity

The consumption of sports drinks and energy drinks has two different objectives for the athlete. A *sports drink* is designed to replace electrolytes lost during exercise and return the athlete's body to a normal state of hydration. Sports drinks are helpful to the athlete during and after exercise and do not produce adverse effects, even when consumed with medications. *Energy drinks* are designed by the manufacturer to provide an energy boost and not to replace lost electrolytes. The use of energy drinks can produce adverse effects in the athlete when they are mixed with other natural supplements or with prescription or OTC medications. Energy drinks can also produce a positive drug test if an athlete drinks significant amounts.

■ Dietary Techniques

Some athletes and researchers have experimented with various styles of dietary supplementation based on the rationale that what and when you eat can provide an ergogenic effect. The most common dietary technique is carbohydrate loading, but other diets are circulated and published every few years.

Carbohydrate loading uses muscular stores of glycogen at the beginning and end of the physical activity. Advo-cates of this technique argue that consuming extra carbohydrate provides increased energy for the endurance athlete. This is the idea behind a pasta dinner the night before a marathon or triathlon. The athlete is putting extra carbohydrates into the body just before the endurance-based competition. The concept of a "depletion phase" (a near-maximal effort that depletes the muscles' glycogen stores about 3 to 4 days before actual competition) before the actual carbohydrate loading begins is now under close scrutiny by many researchers. In the early 1970s, when carbohydrate loading schemes were originally being published in the scientific literature, a depletion phase was said to be critical for the technique to be effective. After what was considered the complete depletion of muscle glycogen, the athlete would eat as many carbohydrates as possible with the idea that the "starving" muscle tissue would grasp and hold on to all the carbohydrates eaten. This, then, would provide more carbohydrate and muscle glycogen availability for the body to access during the competition. For competitions lasting over an hour, carbohydrate loading was viewed as the best technique to improve performance.

A major drawback to this tactic was the adverse effects associated with the nutritional imbalance created by complete depletion of carbohydrate stores. Athletes who strictly followed their high-intensity workouts without any carbohydrates in their diet complained of overwhelming fatigue, generalized irritability, and a reduction in overall performance during the training cycle leading up to the competition. Additionally, the athletes complained of not being able to find foods that they liked to eat, which were composed mainly of fats and proteins. In the 1980s further research indicated that this strict depletion period was not essential to carbohydrate loading, and some athletes then began eating some carbohydrates during the depletion phase. There are still athletes who believe that complete abstinence from carbohydrates is critical for the scheme to work properly.

Today most athletes claim that a closely followed carbohydrate loading scheme will improve their performance in an endurance competition by about 2 to 3 percent. Table 13–4 is an example outline of how an athlete could utilize carbohydrate loading before an important competition.

Other dietary techniques are being promoted by various authors and researchers as ways to improve athletic performance. One of the diets with a vast following is the Zone Diet, which has been given credit for improving performance by a number of United States swimmers who won gold medals in the 1992 Barcelona Olympics and a variety of other athletes who won gold medals in the 1996 Atlanta

Table 13–3

Energy, Carbohydrate, and Additional Ingredients Found in Selected Energy Drinks

Product	Energy (kcal/8 oz)	Carbohydrate (g/8 oz)	Additional Ingredients
Arizona Extreme Energy Shot[b]	124	32	Caffeine, taurine, ribose, ginseng, carnitine, guarana, inositol, vitamins
Arizona Rx Energy[b]	120	31	Caffeine, ginseng, Schizandrae, vitamins
Battery Energy Drink[b]	114	27	Caffeine, guarana
Bawls Guarana[b]	96	27	Caffeine, guarana
Dynamite Energy Drink[b]	95	25	Caffeine, taurine, inositol, vitamins
Effervescent Glutamine Recovery Drink[h]	24	0.8	Glutamine, electrolytes
Gatorade Energy Drink[k]	203	52	Vitamins
G3 Endurance[d]	90	24	Galactose, protein, chromium, green tea, ginseng, vitamins, minerals
G4 Recovery[d]	110	27	Ginseng, galactose, green tea, vitamins, protein
Hansen's Energy[b]	107	31	Taurine, ginseng, caffeine, Ginkgo biloba, guarana, vitamins
Hansen's Slimdown[c]	0	0	Pyruvate, carnitine, chromium, vitamins
Jones Whoop Ass Energy[b]	107	27	Caffeine, royal jelly, guarana, taurine, inositol, vitamins
Mad River Energy Hammer[b]	110	27	Guarana, ginseng, bee pollen
Nexcite[a]	100	21	Guarana, damiana, Schizandrae, mate, ginseng, caffeine
Oxytime+ Sports Drink[h]	80	18	"Stabilized oxygen," carnitine, aloe vera, protein
Prozone Fat-Reducing Energy Drink[g]	184	19	Protein, medium-chain triglycerides, borage oil
Pripps Amino Energy Sports Drink[i]	71	17	Protein, branched-chain amino acids, electrolytes
Pyru Force[f]	2	0.4	Caffeine, pyruvate, guarana, choline, chromium, inositol, carnitine, vitamin C
Red Bull[b]	109	27	Taurine, caffeine, inositol, vitamins
Red Devil Energy Drink[b]	80	21	Caffeine, taurine, guarana, ginseng, Ginkgo biloba, vitamins
Sobe Adrenaline Rush[b]	135	35	Caffeine, taurine, ribose, carnitine, inositol, ginseng, vitamins
Sobe Energy[b]	113	30	Caffeine, guarana, arginine, L-cysteine, yohimbe, vitamin C
Sobe Power[b]	107	28	Caffeine, taurine, creatine, proline, vitamin C
Ultrafit Liquid Endurance[e]	N.A.	N.A.	Glycerol, carnitine, chromium, vitamin B_6
VAAM[j]	56	10	17 amino acids
Venom Energy Drink[b]	127	28	Caffeine, taurine, mate, bee pollen, guarana, ginseng, protein, vitamins
180 Energy Drink[b]	117	32	Guarana, vitamins

[a]**Source:** *www.excitebluebottle.com*
[b]**Source:** *www.bevnet.com*
[c]**Source:** *www.hansens.com*
[d]**Source:** *www.gpush.com*
[e]**Source:** *www.ultrafit-endurance.com*
[f]**Source:** *www.getbig.com*
[g]**Source:** *www.prolithic.com*
[h]**Source:** *www.maxperformance.com*
[i]**Source:** *www.nutrinox.com*
[j]**Source:** *www.vaam-power.com*
[k]**Source:** Package label
From Bonci, L: "Energy" drinks: Help or hype? Gatorade Sport Science Institute 15(1), 2002.

Table 13–4

Carbohydrate Loading Scheme

Breakfast	3 cups low fiber cereal with 1½ cups low-fat milk 1 banana 1 glass orange juice
Midmorning Snack	Muffin (with honey or jam) 18 oz. sports drink
Lunch	2 sandwiches (4 slices bread; low-fat meat, e.g., turkey) 8 oz. yogurt 12-oz. drink of choice
Afternoon Snack	Smoothie with low-fat milk (banana, etc.) Cereal bar
Dinner	2 cups cooked pasta with 1 cup sauce 3 slices bread (garlic, etc.) Drink (18 oz. sports drink, etc.)
Night Snack	Muffin (with honey or jam) 18 oz. sports drink

The Zone Diet requires an athlete to have a fairly extensive understanding of nutrition and physiology. The idea behind this diet is to closely monitor nutritional intake and consume specific percentages of fats, proteins, and carbohydrates. The recommended percentages in the Zone Diet are 40 percent carbohydrate, 30 percent protein, and 30 percent fat. This diet requires a personalized program for each athlete that focuses on the total nutrients consumed. Once an athlete knows the exact amount of nutrients he or she consumes and can determine which group each food source fits into, he or she can consume the correct percentages. This diet requires a great deal of attention to what is being eaten each day. Improving athletic performance through the use of the Zone Diet has not been demonstrated through controlled research studies published in scientific journals.

■ Vitamins and Minerals

Athletes are sometimes taught that adding vitamins, minerals, or amino acids to their diet can increase their athletic performance. In the United States, the general population and most athletes are getting enough vitamins and minerals in their daily diet. The exception may be the economically disadvantaged athlete. If an athlete is not getting a normal diet, as may be the case with a wrestler who must follow a calorie-restricted diet for many months, he or she might benefit from vitamin or mineral supplementation.

It is generally accepted that vitamin supplementation, specifically, vitamin E and C supplementation, has no effect on athletic performance or on postexercise recovery of tissues.[11,49,53] However, there appears to be some potential long-term benefit in vitamin E supplementation for endurance athletes. Many endurance athletes use vitamin E as a prophylactic measure to reduce cholesterol buildup and as an antioxidant. A recent study has shown that an endurance athlete using vitamin E on a regular basis has a reduced potential for atherosclerosis and elevated cholesterol levels.[53] It is suggested that this is a result of the vitamin combining with cholesterol and preventing it from depositing on blood vessel walls. This, in turn, reduces the likelihood of clogging and reduction in blood flow.

The use of zinc has also been suggested to be helpful to the athlete because of its role in cellular metabolism. However, the decrease of zinc in the body is difficult to determine.[35] Therefore it is difficult to ascertain if zinc supplementation is beneficial. If an athlete is experiencing a significant loss of body weight, anorexia, fatigue, and decreased endurance capabilities, he or she may be experiencing reduced zinc levels. The way to obtain zinc through the normal diet is by eating proteins, especially absorbable animal fats, along with other known sources of dietary protein.

■ Amino Acids

In an athlete's diet, the consumption of amino acids is important for many reasons. Maybe the most important is for the rebuilding of tissues that have been damaged as a result of activity. Resistance training is especially hard on the muscle tissues, and amino acids are required for rebuilding. Most athletes in America consume a well-rounded diet, which provides the necessary proteins for athletes to repair and rebuild exercise-related muscle damage. The need of the body to rebuild damaged tissue fluctuates according to the type and exercise level of the athlete. Athletes engaged in resistance training on a daily basis contend that amino acid supplementation is critical for the rebuilding of damaged muscle tissue. The human body does maintain a small store of amino acids that are considered free and available to the system.[34]

The marketing of amino acids to the athlete generally follows one of two different methods. First, supplement makers market amino acid supplementation to athletes as necessary to rebuild muscle tissue from training and participation. Second, they claim that the use of amino acids will enhance athletic performance by sparing carbohydrates or by providing an extra energy source for the muscles. Neither of these claims has been demonstrated in well-conducted scientific studies. Studies published in scientific journals report that there is no ergogenic effect from an increased intake of supplemental amino acids.[55]

As an example of how amino acids are marketed, one Website (www.xsportsnutrition.com) sells various types of amino acids. The consumer is encouraged to pick one or more based on their desired outcome. The primary claim is that amino acids will improve muscle-building potential and promote faster recovery and improved performance from training. One particular type of amino acid product is said to contain three essential branch chain amino acids. The recommended dosage is 2 to 4 tablets on an empty stomach 3 times a day before meals. The cost is $34.99 for 160 tablets, and a 6 week minimum is said to be needed before results are seen.

Some companies market a specific type of amino acid, glucosamine, which is alleged to restore or replace articular cartilage. These companies suggest that their products will have a healing effect as the glucosamine combines with the available cartilage fibers and restores damaged cartilage. This is a controversial area, and a significant amount of scientific inquiry is currently being made into this theory. To date, there is no definitive evidence of the long-term effect of amino acids as an articular cartilage repair mechanism. There is sufficient evidence to establish that amino acids, specifically glucosamine sulfate, will not repair damage done to articular cartilage from athletic injuries.[25]

Athletes need to realize that amino acids are water soluble. The body does not store vast quantities of amino acids, but after they are converted into the necessary protein building blocks and used by the body, extra amino acid intake can be converted into glucose and eventually fat which can be stored. Extra nitrogen left over from the conversion of the amino acid is excreted via the urine. The body only uses the amount of amino acids it requires which is typically gained from the regular diet or in some situations from supplementation, providing the necessary requirements for muscle repair and the tissue building blocks.

■ Whey Protein

Another type of amino acid currently being marketed is *whey,* the protein derived from milk. It is sold as a powder to be mixed with either water or skim milk. Whey contains less fat than regular milk (some products actually contain no fat) and the lactose can also be removed, so whey can be used by individuals with lactose intolerance. Whey proteins are considered to have a higher percentage of branch chain amino acids, which accelerate muscle protein replacement. These proteins are considered to have an increased bioavailability and solubility, making them more effective than other amino acids. Whey is marketed as a product that will increase insulin secretion and enhance the anabolic effects

of insulin. The marketers claim that enhanced insulin production will result in an increase in protein synthesis. This resultant increase in protein synthesis will increase the repair of damaged muscle and even increase the size and overall capability of the muscle.

Whey is sold as a powder and comes in different flavors and container sizes. One manufacturer sells a 2-pound container for $59.99. This manufacturer recommends that users mix 2 scoops in 4 ounces of water or skim milk and use the product 2 to 3 times a day. Again, the manufacturer suggests that the product must be used for a minimum of 6 weeks before the consumer will see any changes.

■ Erythropoietin Alpha

Some prescription drugs, meant for use in legitimate medical conditions, are being used by elite athletes to gain an advantage. One of these prescription drugs is erythropoietin alpha (EPO), a blood product that sends a signal to the body to produce more red blood cells (RBCs). RBCs deliver oxygen to the muscles, organs, and tissues of the body. The more oxygen one can get to a muscle, the longer the muscle can function and the longer one can endure muscle contraction after muscle contraction. In an endurance activity such as a marathon, the muscles continually contract for hours at a time. The ability to deliver more oxygen to the muscles in this situation is a definite advantage for the athlete. Therefore, some athletes inject EPO as part of their overall preparation as they are readying for competition. They believe that their training will be enhanced by the extra oxygen available to the muscles and their competitive effort will increase.

Originally, EPO was extracted from the pituitary gland of a cadaver and was expensive and difficult to obtain. It is now synthesized in the laboratory and can be prescribed by a physician, so it is much less expensive and easy to obtain. Typically, EPO is prescribed for chemotherapy patients to increase their energy level and their ability to perform the activities of daily living while they are going through treatment.

Endurance athletes such as marathon runners, swimmers, and long-distance bicycle riders have discovered the advantages of having more red blood cells to transport oxygen. Yearly reports from the Tour de France and other bicycle races suggest that riders are using EPO to enhance their performance. The use of EPO is not easily detected by random drug testing, and the governing bodies of many different endurance-type sports are looking for laboratories that are able to perform tests to detect the use of EPO in athletes.

Theoretically, proof exists that EPO provides a mechanism to enhance athletic endurance. However, athletes

What to Tell the Athlete

When athletes are determined to use some type of substance to improve their performance, it is often difficult to help them understand the adverse effects that can result. Here are some tips for the athletic trainer when educating the athlete about these drugs:

■ Supplements containing ephedra are easily purchased "online" but can be dangerous to one's general health.

■ Athletes with certain types of cardiac irregularities who use ephedra can experience severe side effects and possibly death.

■ Supplements that claim to produce extra energy may contain high levels of caffeine.

■ The athletic trainer can safely encourage the liberal consumption of sports drinks to maintain hydration and electrolyte balance.

■ Encourage the athlete to use water-soluble vitamins, minerals, and amino acids if he or she is determined to use supplements.

■ The athlete should be discouraged from purchasing stimulants and supplements, especially via the Internet.

should be warned not to attempt to supplement with EPO on their own or to use it on the advice of a fellow athlete. Too much EPO can cause the body to produce excessive amounts of red blood cells. This will require excessive work by the cardiac muscle and may lead to heart failure.

Before EPO was discovered, endurance bicycle riders were using a technique they called "blood doping" to improve their performance. The riders were taking blood from themselves 1 to 2 months before a competition, taking the RBCs out of the plasma, and then having them reinfused just before the race. Unfortunately, there was a great deal of experimentation with this method, and numerous bike racers died by reinfusing too many RBCs. This thickened the blood and made the heart overwork, resulting in heart failure and death. Blood doping is no longer a common practice among endurance athletes because EPO is now available.

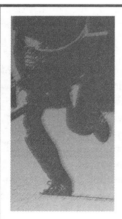

Scenario from the Field

A 20-year-old female soccer player presented to the athletic trainer at her university with the following signs and symptoms. She had experienced bouts of syncope, her skin was pale, and she was experiencing an increase in blood pressure and some tachycardia. Her vital signs were fluctuating and she did not seem stable. She reported that she had been taking an OTC "thermogenic" or diet tablet to lose weight. She was in the athletic training facility at the university when she reported this. The athletic trainer quickly phoned the team physician and learned that he was on his way to campus for a scheduled clinic visit. The athletic training staff decided to wait a few minutes and monitor the athlete until the team physician arrived. When the physician arrived a few minutes later, the athlete was started on IV fluids. She did not respond as well as the physician expected, so she was transported to the local hospital. On arrival at the hospital, the athlete began to respond to the IV fluids and make a slow recovery.

Later it was documented that the athlete was taking an OTC supplement that contained ma huang, caffeine, willow bark, ginger, and some other ingredients. She reported that she was taking twice the amount recommended on the container. It was also determined, after the fact, that she had consumed only a bagel and a couple of diet soft drinks that day.

Athletes should be warned that doubling the dosage of any medication is not wise and that a lack of food intake, combined with exercise and overzealous supplement use, may lead to death. (Example courtesy of A Winterstein, PhD, ATC.)

Class Discussion Topics

- Many athletes try to think of ways to increase their performance without having to work harder. What are some of the pros and cons of the use of the supplements discussed in this chapter?

- An athlete is using herbal supplements, and the team physician prescribes a medication for the athlete, who does not think to tell the physician that she is taking an herbal supplement. As the athletic trainer, should you tell the physician if you know what type of herbal supplement she is taking?

- Are sports drinks more effective than water in rehydrating the athlete during practice? After practice or a game?

Chapter Review

- A natural substance is not intended to improve performance, as is the intent of an ergogenic substance.

- The DHSEA law delineated that food supplements marketed in the United States cannot claim to alter a disease process.

- Supplement manufacturers can legally claim that their products will improve athletic performance.

- Manufacturers marketing supplements do everything they can to make their product enticing for athletes.

- When talking about nutritional supplements, the terms "natural" and "safe" are not the same.

- There are a number of factors that affect the purity of a supplement.

- Sports drink and energy drinks are different in their contents.

- A successful carbohydrate-loading scheme requires a great deal of preplanning by the athlete.

- Amino acids have a significant role in rebuilding damaged tissues but are not a major contributor to the overall general muscle-building process in a mature athlete.

- EPO has been demonstrated to improve an athlete's performance if used correctly.

References

1. Abt, AB, et al.: Chinese herbal medicine induces acute renal failure. Arch Intern Med 155:211, 1995.
2. Are your chronically ill patients turning to herbs? Some cause potentially dangerous interactions. Disease State Management 5:66, 1999.
3. Bahrke, MS, and Morgan, WE: Evaluation of the ergogenic properties of ginseng. Sports Med 18:229, 1994.
4. Berlin, C: Editorial: Herbal medicine. Clin Pediatrics 40:271, 2001.
5. Blumenthal, M, ed: The complete German commission E monographs: Therapeutic guide to herbal medicines. American Botanical Council, Austin, 1998.
6. Brown, GA, et al.: Effect of oral DHEA on serum testosterone and adaptations to resistance training in young men. J App Physiol 87:2274, 1999.
7. Buchanan, K, and Lemberg, L: Herbal or complimentary medicine: Fact or fiction? Am J Critical Care 10:438, 2001.
8. Charatan, F: Fake prescription drugs are flooding the United States. British Medical Journal 322(7300):1443, 2001.
9. Coombes, JS, and Hamilton, KL: The effectiveness of commercially available sports drinks. Sports Med 29:181, 2000.
10. Cui, J, et al.: What do commercial ginsengs contain? Lancet 344:134, 1994.
11. Dawson, B, et al.: Effects of vitamin C and E supplementation on biochemical and ultra structural indices of muscle damage after a 21 km run. Int J Sports Med 23:10, 2002.
12. Dietary Supplement Health and Education Act of 1994. Public Law 103–417. 103rd Congress, 2nd session, S784.
13. Dorn, M, et al.: Placebo-controlled, double-blind study of *Echinaceae pallidaeradix* in upper respiratory tract infections. Complement Ther Med 5:40, 1997.
14. Eisenberg, DM, et al.: Trends in alternative medicine use in the United States, 1990-1997: Results of a follow-up national survey. JAMA 280:1569, 1998.
15. Fugh-Berman, A: Herb-drug interactions. Lancet 355:134, 2000.
16. Gardiner, P, and Kemper, KJ: Herbs in pediatric and adolescent medicine. Pediatr Rev 21:44, 2000.
17. Gatorade Sports Science Institute: *http://www.gssiweb.com/reflib/refs/310/ENERGY_DRINKS_3-12-02cfm?pid=38* (October 8, 2002).
18. Golub, C: Ginseng, cardiac drugs don't mix: Herb interactions you should know. Env Nutr 22:1, 1999.
19. Green, GA, et al.: Analysis of over-the-counter dietary supplements. Clin J Sport Med 11:254, 2001.
20. Gurley, BJ, et al.: Content versus label claims in ephedra-containing dietary supplements. Am J Health Sys Pharm 57:963, 2000.
21. Heiligenstein, E and Guenther G: Over-the-counter psychotropics: A review of melatonin, St. John's wort, valerian, and kava-kava. J Am Coll Health 46:271, 1998.
22. Herbal Rx: the promises and pitfalls. Consumer Reports 64, March 1999.
23. Huang, WF, et al.: Adulteration by synthetic therapeutic substances of traditional Chinese medicines in Taiwan. J Clin Pharmacol 37:344, 1997.
24. Hudson, K, et al.: What you and your patients should know

about herbal medicines. J Am Acad Physician Assistants 14:27, 2001.

25. James, CB, and Uhl, TL: A review of articular cartilage pathology and the use of glucosamine sulfate. J Athletic Training, 36:413, 2001.

26. Jadoul, M, et al.: Adverse effects from traditional Chinese medicine. Lancet 341:892, 1995.

27. Ko, RJ: Adulterants in Asian patent medicines. N Eng J Med 339:847, 1998.

28. Laure, P, et al.: Attitudes of coaches towards doping. J of Sports Med Phys Fitness 41:132, 2001.

29. Lai, RS, et al.: Outbreak of bronchiolitis obliterans associated with consumption of *Sauropus androgynus* in Taiwan. Lancet. 348:83, 1996.

30. Larrey, D, et al.: Hepatitis after germander (Teucrium chamaedrys) administration: Another instance of herbal medicine hepatotoxicity. Ann Intern Med 117:129, 1992.

31. Le Bars, PL, et al.: A placebo controlled, double-blind, randomized trial of an extract of Ginkgo biloba for dementia: North American EGb Study Group. JAMA 278:1327,1997.

32. Lewis, CJ: Letter to industry: FDA concerned about botanical products, including dietary supplements containing aristolochic acid. Rockville, MD, FDA Center for Food Safety and Applied Nutrition, 2000.

33. Melchart, D, et al.: Echinacea root extracts for the prevention of upper respiratory tract infections: A double-blind, placebo-controlled randomized trial. Arch Fam Med 7:541, 1998.

34. Mero, A: Leucine supplementation and intensive training. Sports Med 27:347, 1999.

35. Micheletti, A, et al.: Zinc status in athletes: Relation to diet and exercise. Sports Med 31:577, 2001.

36. Miller, LG: Herbal medicinals: Selected clinical considerations focusing on known potential drug-herb interactions. Arch Intern Med 158:2200, 1998.

37. Mostefa-Kara, N, et al.: Fatal hepatitis after herbal tea. Lancet 340:674, 1992.

38. Muirhead, G, et al.: Herbal medicines you can recommend with confidence. Patient Care 33:76, 1999.

39. Myers, JB, et al.: Syncope and atypical chest pain in an intercollegiate wrestler: A case report. J Athletic Training 34:263, 1999.

40. Nelson Myer, S, et al.: Safety of herbal supplements. Top Clin Nutr 14:42, 1998.

41. O'Neil, CK, et al.: Herbal medicines: getting beyond the hype. Nursing 99:58, 1999.

42. Raloff, J: New support for echinacea's benefits. Science News 155:207, 1999.

43. Reents, S: Sport and Exercise Pharmacology. Human Kinetics, Champaign, Ill., 2000.

44. Scheller, M: Herbal hope or herbal hype? Current Health 2 25:21, 1998.

45. Schulz, V et al.: Rational Phytotherapy, ed.3. Berlin, Springer-Verlag, 1998, p 270.

46. Shaw, D, et al.: Traditional remedies and food supplements. A 5-year toxicological study (1991-1995). Drug Safety 17:342, 1997.

47. Siegel, R: Ginseng and high blood pressure. JAMA 243;32, 1980.

48. Siegel, RK: Ginseng abuse syndrome: Problems with the panacea. JAMA 241:1614, 1979.

49. Singh, A, et al.: Neuroendocrine responses to running in women after zinc and vitamin E supplementation. Med Sci Sports & Ex 31:536, 1999.

50. Smith, CM, and Reynard, AM: Essentials of Pharmacology. WB Saunders, Philadelphia, 1995, p 355.

51. Sobal, J, and Marquart, LF: Vitamin/mineral supplement use among high school athletes. Adolescents 29:835, 1994.

52. Sobal, J, and Marquart, LF: Vitamin/mineral supplement use among athletes: a review of the literature. Int J Sport Nutr 4:320, 1994.

53. Takanami, Y, et al.: Vitamin E supplementation and endurance exercise: Are there benefits? Sports Med 29:73, 2000.

54. Tomassoni, AJ, and Simone, K: Herbal medicines for children: an illusion of safety? Curr Opin Pediatr 13:162, 2001.

55. Trappe, SW, et al.: The effects of L-carnitine supplementation on performance during interval swimming. Int J Sports Med 15:181, 1994.

56. Tyler, VE: What pharmacists should know about herbal remedies. J Am Pharm Assoc (Wash) NS36:29, 1996.

57. Tyler, VE: The honest herbal, ed 3. Pharmaceutical Products Press, New York, 1993.

58. Vanhaelen, M, et al.: Identification of aristolochic acid in Chinese herbs. Lancet 343:174, 1994.

59. Vanherweghem, JL, et al.: Rapidly progressive interstitial renal fibrosis in young women: Association with slimming regimen including Chinese herbs. Lancet 341:387, 1993.

60. Venes, D, ed.: Taber's Cyclopedic Medical Dictionary, ed 19. FA Davis, Philadelphia, 2001.

61. Vogler, BH, et al.: Feverfew as a preventive treatment for migraine: A systematic review. Cephalalgia 18:704, 1998.

62. Winterstein, AP, and Storrs, CM: Herbal supplements: Considerations for the athletic trainer. J Athletic Training 36:425, 2001.

Chapter Questions

1. What is a "nutraceutical"?
   A. A nutrition store
   B. A prescribed medication
   C. Nutritional counseling
   D. A nutritional supplement

2. The DHSEA essentially provides for:
   A. Supplement purity
   B. Supplements for underprivileged children in schools
   C. Unrestricted access to food supplements
   D. Athlete supplementation freedom

3. Supplement manufacturers are not allowed to state which of the following?
   A. That a supplement will prevent cancer
   B. That a supplement will decrease the chance of getting skin cancer
   C. That a supplement will work as a "tanning pill"
   D. That a supplement will cure depression

4. What nutraceutical was taken off the market because it was dangerous to human health and then put back on the market as a result of the passage of the DHSEA law in 1994?
   A. DHEA
   B. St. John's wort
   C. Echinacea
   D. Ginkgo biloba

5. Natural supplements will not cause any harm to the body.

       True   False

6. General drug toxic levels are increased in which population when supplements are used?
   A. Women
   B. Men
   C. Children
   D. Athletes

7. What extra product is included in most "energy" drinks?
   A. Carbohydrate
   B. Caffeine
   C. Sodium
   D. Water

8. Carbohydrate loading is most beneficial to which type of athlete?
   A. Endurance
   B. Sprint
   C. Water sports
   D. Female

9. The athlete can expect to gain, at most, what percent advantage from carbohydrate loading?
   A. 5 to 10 percent
   B. 2 to 3 percent
   C. 15 to 20 percent
   D. 35 to 40 percent

10. Vitamins can be an ergogenic aid for the athlete.

        True   False

11. Whey is a derivative of what product?
    A. Corn
    B. Wheat
    C. Sugar
    D. Milk

14 *Social Drugs*

Objectives

Upon completion of this chapter, the student will have a basic understanding of the following:

1 The types of people that tend to abuse social drugs.
2 Some of the reasons why people use social drugs.
3 The feelings and expectations people have when abusing drugs.
4 Reasons why teenage athletes might choose to abuse social drugs.
5 Reasons why collegiate athletes might choose to abuse social drugs.
6 Social drug abuse patterns in high school and collegiate athletes.
7 Suggestions for the athletic trainer's role in assisting a drug-abusing athlete.

Chapter Outline

"*T*he great majority of people who use drugs never come to the attention of doctors, lawyers, and policemen."[21] The use of social drugs by many in our society is almost a given fact in this new century. People find drug use as a method of gaining social acceptance, an escape from their perceived difficulties, or a habit they obtained inadvertently. In the context of this chapter the term "social drug" is limited to alcohol, tobacco (including smokeless tobacco), marijuana, cocaine, and some examples of the newer club drugs, for example, ecstasy. It would be impossible to discuss all of the social drugs in one chapter. There are entire books written specifically on each of the types of drugs discussed in this chapter. For more details about any of the specific social drugs the reader is encouraged to read one of the available books, articles or other print media available from numerous sources. The United States government has numerous web pages dedicated to curbing drug abuse and have a great deal of up-to-date information that may be found at the following web address: www.cdc.gov. A text by Miller et al (2000) is an excellent source of information to gain a better understanding of the many factors relating to why adolescents begin a drug abuse way of life.

It is argued that most of the socially abused drugs do not have automatic, universal effects on everyone that uses them.[10] That is to say, a person starting to abuse a drug for social reasons may not experience any type of the "claimed" effects until they actually learn and experience the effects that specific drug can have on their individual system. The athlete may have to use the drug on a number of occasions to experience the greatest effects from that drug. Many people who abuse a drug such as alcohol, tobacco, marijuana or similar drugs indicate the first time or first few times they use these drugs they do not experience any euphoric effect. Many relate they have a negative experience when using these drugs initially. It may take a number of drug use experiences for the athlete to begin experiencing any joyful effect, which is an indicator regarding the amount of drug use before he or she admits a problem exists. (Table 14–1)

Many times, the long-term effects of drug abuse are emphasized. However, it is important to remember that there are acute effects of drug use that affect each of us everyday. Examples of acute effects of social drug abuse include the problems associated with alcohol and street drugs. Alcohol is a factor in up to 50 percent of all head injuries.[22] Many times the conflict and disarray in the stands or streets after a game is related to alcohol use by the fans.

The quality control of illegal drugs is nonexistent, thus resulting in overdoses and immediate death to many users. Street drugs may also contain many different substances used as "fillers" or can be adulterated by toxins, pesticides, fungi, bacteria or any one of a number of unknown contaminants as a result of manufacturer, such as in a kitchen, garage, or even the back of a van. These contaminants can cause acute reactions not always related to the drug's intended effect.

There are so many different types of social drugs and many more "street names" for each of these drugs. It is virtually impossible to keep track of all the names of these drugs; therefore, the athletic trainer is encouraged to talk with their athletes regularly to determine the most recent vernacular for street drugs. (Table 14–2)

Additionally, the abuse of drugs is a problem that can start at a young age. Some surveys and published research indicate that drug abuse can begin in the early teen years.[13] Use of alcohol and tobacco can begin in late childhood or adolescents for some children.[13] Increasing emphasis is being put on early education programs in the schools and various youth programs to assist the adolescent and teenager in avoiding drugs all together.

High School Athlete Drug Abuse

High school is a difficult time for teenagers; these young people can be easily influenced in both negative and positive ways. This is a time in their lives when social acceptance is of paramount importance. If a teenager cannot find social acceptance through his or her own experiences he or she may begin to choose other methods of becoming "part of the crowd." Unfortunately, drug use is one way these teenagers may find acceptance and friendship.[23] Out of peer pressure, or the need to "be cool" or for the feel of sophistication, a person may start to use drugs. Other indicators of reasons why adolescents might start drug use are for fun or out of simple curiosity.[23]

The athletic trainer should be aware of the characteristics of a teenager who might become a drug abuser. There appears to be an increase in drug abuse in non-intact families (one parent missing) and homes that have no religious affiliation or activity.[14,24] Interestingly, there does not appear to be large differences in alcohol and drug abuse among ethnic groups in high school seniors.[14] Additionally, there are personality characteristics the athletic trainer can look for in athletes that may be "indicators of a drug user to be." Some of these characteristics are outlined here:

Table 14–1

Summary of Expectations for Alcohol, Marijuana, and Cocaine

Six Alcohol Expectancies	Six Marijuana Expectancies	Five Cocaine Expectancies
Global positive transforming effect	Cognitive and behavioral impairment	Global positive effects
Social/physical	Relaxation and tension reduction	Global negative effects
Sexual enhancement	Social and sexual facilitation	Generalized arousal
Arousal/power/aggression	Perceptual and cognitive enhancement	Anxiety
Increased social assertiveness	Global negative effects	Relaxation and tension reduction
Relaxation/tension reduction	Craving and physical effects	

Jung J: Psychology of Alcohol and Other Drugs: A Research Perspective. Sage Publications, Thousand Oaks, CA, 2001, pg. 169.

Table 14–2

Street Names of Commonly Used Substances

Central Nervous System Depressants

Amobarbital	Blue devils, blue angels, blue heavens, blues, bluebirds
Chlordiazepoxide	Green and whites, libs, roaches
Codeine	Schoolboy, robo, romo, syrup
Heroin	H, horse, junk, noise, pee, scag, shit, skid, smack, boy, doojee, hairy, Harry, TNT
Morphine	M, morph, morphie, morpho, white stuff, cube juice, emsel, hocus, Miss Emma, unkie, white merchandise
Opium	Black stuff, poppy, rat, hop, pin, yen, skee, wen shee, big O
Pentobarbital	Yellow jackets, yellowbirds, nembies, yellows
Phenobarbital	Purple hearts
Secobarbital	Seecy, red birds, red devils, reds
Tuinal	Tooeys, rainbows, double trouble

Central Nervous System Stimulants

Cocaine	Dope, coke, snow, lady, gold dust, rock, crack, Carrie, Cecil, dream, happy dust, heaven dust, joy powder, flake, girl, nose cndy, crystal
Dextroamphetamine	Dexies, oranges, hearts, Christmas trees, wedges, spots
Amphetamine (racemic)	Uppers, bennies
Methamphetamine	Chris, Christine, speed, meth, crystal, whites, ice
Monoethymethylenedroxyamphetamine (MDEA)	Eve
Methylenedioxyamphetamine (MDA)	Love drug
Methylenedioxymethamphetamine (MDMA)	Ecstasy, XTC, Adam
Amphetamine complex	Black beauty, black Cadillacs

Hallucinogens

Cannabis (marijuana)	Acapulco gold, ace, ashes, baby, broccoli, grass, hemp, jive, joint, Mary Jane, pot, THC, weed, Panama red, MJ, loco weed, Texas tea, Sweet Lucy, many others
Dimethyltryptamine (DMT)	Businessman's trip, mind blowing, DMT
Hash, hashish	Black hash (hashish containing opium), black Russian (potent, dark hashish)
Lysergic acid diethylamide (LSD)	Acid, cube, big D, California sunshine, blue dots, barrels, black magic, blue acid, blue heaven, chocolate chips, cupcakes, domes, Hawaiian sunshine, micro dots, peace tablets, squirrels, strawberry field, purple haze, purple ozone, battery acid, Berkeley blood, chief, HCP, sugaar, window pane
Mescaline	Bad seed, big chief, cactus buttons, peyote, pink wedge, white light, mescal, half moon
Phencyclidine (PCP)	Angel dust, dummy dust, PCP, flying saucers, hair hog, mist, peace pill, tranq, whack, Shermans, rocket fuel, sheets
Psilocybin	God's flesh

Anabolic Steroidss

Anabolic steroids	Roids, juice

Gutierrez K: Pharmacotherapeutics: Clinical decision making in nursing. WB Saunders Co., Philadelphia, 1999, pg. 151.

- Alien
- Rebelliousness
- Non-conformity
- Accepts deviant behavior in others
- Lack of ambition
- Lack of commitment to school
- Impulsive
- Preoccupied by pleasure seeking
- Minimal concern for risk
- Poor problem-solving and coping skills

- Low self-esteem
- History of physical and psychological illness[25]

High school student athletes are not of legal age to use alcohol or tobacco and should be discouraged from using these substances if for no other reason than the age requirements. Some local schools, districts, and even states have mandatory penalties for underage use of social drugs.

As an example, the state of Massachusetts Interscholastic Athletic Association (MIAA) has developed and published a "Chemical Health Eligibility Rule" for the high school athletes, coaches and administrators to follow in determining eligibility for an athlete.

> *In part, this Chemical Eligibility Rule reads, "During the season of practice or play, a student shall not, regardless of quantity, use or consume, possess, buy/sell or give away any beverage containing alcohol; and tobacco product; marijuana; steroids or any controlled substance . . ."[18]*

The MIAA then goes on to explain what the penalties are for violating this rule for a first and second time offender. Hopefully, this will provide an impetus for the athlete to start thinking about the harmful effects of social drugs and plan for a healthy lifestyle when he or she is out of high school. Other states and school districts may have similar rules and regulations.

Web Resource Box

The United States Department of Health & Human Services maintains an excellent web site regarding drug use and abuse. On the web site are the results of the National Household Survey on Drug Abuse (NHSDA) which provides excellent and detailed charts and graphs which are updated annually. For information including reports of the users of many different types of illegal drugs go to *www.samhsa.gov/oas/nhsda.htm.*

College Athlete Drug Abuse

The college years are critical years for young adults because this may be the first time the student is out of the parents' home living on their own, making own decisions, and not having to report daily activities to the parents. This is a time when student-athletes are willing to try new activities they were not able do when living at home. Many college students have squandered their first year of higher education by spending far too much time enjoying their newfound freedom. Interestingly, it is noteworthy to remember that after the age of 21, rarely do people try new drugs in an experimental fashion.[13]

To ensure that the college experience is beneficial for the student-athlete, the National Collegiate Athletic Association (NCAA) has been tracking and surveying collegiate athletes for many years in almost every area of their collegiate lives. Other researchers are also interested in determining the substance abuse profiles in collegiate athletes, but as has been pointed out, these studies are reflective of only a small time period.[6] Continued monitoring of national, regional, state

and local drug abuse patterns are imperative to taking control of this ever-increasing problem.

The NCAA has been interested since the mid 1980s in the student-athlete's use of social drugs. Documented now are the types of social drugs athletes might be using and the approximate percentage of athletes participating in social drug use. Even though alcohol use is declining, there still remains a significant percentage of athletes using alcohol on a regular basis. Marijuana use has remained at the same levels since 1989, and smokeless tobacco has seen a minor decline in use. It is also interesting to note that there continues to be a small population of student-athletes using cocaine and psychedelic drugs. (Figure 14–1)

Alcohol

There are records of alcohol availability and use in most every society over the history of the earth. Alcohol use by professional and recreational athletes has been accepted for years. The idea that an athlete goes out to have a beer or two after the game is a common occurrence by athletes in professional sports. By doing this, many fans and other people also drink alcohol after a game or match and this has become a source of concern regarding drunk driving. In vehicle-related deaths, alcohol is the number one killer of teenagers and young adults in North America.[19] The reasons why athletes consume alcohol are as varied as the sports in which they participate. Some athletes actually think the use of alcohol provides them with enhanced ability in their sport. Others consume alcohol for the stress-relieving properties it provides by desensitizing the central nervous system. The American College of Sports Medicine (ACSM) published a "Current Comment" in 2000 to help educate the public about the mixture of alcohol and athletic performance.

In the statement by the ACSM, they point out that a small amount of alcohol in the athlete's system (0.02–0.05 g/dL) can decrease hand tremors, improve balance and throwing accuracy, which might be helpful for an archer or other athletes of that type.[1] However, even this small amount of alcohol can retard reaction time and eye-hand coordination, making it much more difficult to perform at high levels in most other sports. More alcohol in the athlete's system has a negative effect on motor skills. Alcohol will also increase an athlete's speed times in short- and long-distance activity. Chronic alcohol use results in various detrimental effects to the organs of the body, such as liver cirrhosis, heart disease, diabetes, and mental disorders. Alcohol can also create an imbalance in the hormonal status of the body, thus creating a more arduous task for the body in building and rebuilding muscle tissues.

Patterns of Social Drug Use

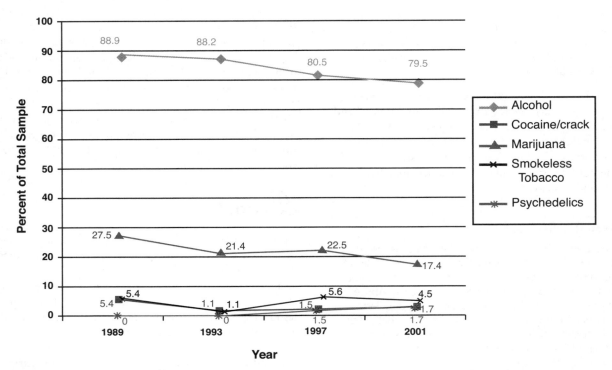

Figure 14–1. Patterns of social drug use by collegiate student-athletes. Adapted from the NCAA Study of Substance Use Habits of College Student-Athletes report presented to the NCAA Committee on Competitive Safeguards and Medical Aspects of Sports, June 2001.

■ Adverse Effects

The detrimental acute effects of alcohol are many times overlooked, as the consumption of alcohol has become a method of reducing stress and increasing joyfulness in many people. Acutely, alcohol is responsible for mental and physical impairment, such as slurred speech, deficits in coordination and reaction time, decreased visual acuity, dehydration and an increase in acidic metabolites. Additionally, it should be stressed to pregnant or possibly pregnant women that alcohol crosses the placenta very easily and can harm the developing fetus.[26] For these reasons, and many others, the athletic trainer should be vigilant in denouncing the use of alcohol by athletes.

obacco

Tobacco was originally promoted for use by people with pain, headaches, labor pains, and a variety of other problems as a medicinal drug to limit the effects of pain. In 1604, King James I tried to limit the use of tobacco as he stated "it

hurt the brain & lungs, was not pretty to look at and smelled bad."[27] As you can see by looking at the percentages of teenagers using tobacco in Table 14–3, there still exists a real problem with young people smoking cigarettes. Tobacco can be a very complex drug that includes many more chemicals than just tobacco but is initially used by many people for social reasons. Some people argue that smoking calms them down in stressful situations and others claim that smoking helps them to reduce their weight. The initiation of cigarette smoking can lead to a physical addiction to the chemicals contained in tobacco.

There are many different chemicals (over 4000) inhaled when a cigarette is smoked, but the most critical is nicotine.[17] When a person smokes a cigarette, nicotine reaches the brain within just a few seconds of being inhaled. Nicotine produces a similar reaction in the brain as the neurotransmitter acetylcholine but also produces other effects. The other effects can include a chemical reaction in the brain producing the enjoyment of smoking, which leads to continued cigarette smoking. Depending on the mental state and mood of the individual at the time of cigarette smoking, nicotine can produce a stimulatory or depressive effect. It has been reported that nicotine will reduce monoamine oxidase B activity, which is involved in dopamine breakdown, thus reducing some motivating behavior.[5]

■ Adverse Effects

In a report by The Centers for Disease Control and Prevention (CDC), more than 430,000 people die annually as a result of cigarette smoking.[2] Outside the central nervous system, the chemicals in cigarette smoke can lead to a great deal of damage to a variety of tissues. Obviously, damage to the lungs is the most commonly reported problem with cigarette smoking. In the lungs the cilia are overworked and damaged, the airway passages are scarred and the tendency for lung cancer is greatly increased. Additionally, cigarette smoke can produce stimulatory effects on the user such as trembling, shaking, agitation, and nausea or vomiting depending on the type of tobacco and the smoking experience of the person. Nicotine can also produce an irregular heart rate, blood flow irregularities, an increased blood clotting mechanism, and increases in the circulating triglycerides leading to myocardial infarction. The possibility of coronary heart disease is much greater in smokers because of the narrowing of the coronary arteries by the excessive fats from the circulating triglycerides. The excess fats also produce an increase in blood pressure and ultimately strokes in these individuals.

Still, there are many adverse effects of cigarette smoking that are less commonly popularized. Problems such as ulcers, tooth and gum diseases, breathing disorders such as asthma or emphysema, skin disorders, complications in pregnancy and the increased possibility of stillbirth, as well as many others are rarely discussed because they are minor in comparison to the more obvious and costly problems (lung cancer) produced by cigarette smoking. Additionally, there is evidence that second-hand smoke is damaging to those who do not smoke. Many of these same problems are associated with people interacting or having regular contact with smokers even though they do not smoke themselves. Children can be greatly affected by passive smoke and can experience many health-related disorders including breathing difficulties and other general health problems.

The good news about smoking is that quitting will be beneficial to everyone. The smoker will enjoy better health and the people around them will also be less prone to breathing and other health problems related to second-hand smoke. Encourage athletes to quit smoking and work with them to find a way to overcome the dependence on tobacco they have acquired. For those who want to stop smoking, there are numerous behavioral programs, chemical products from chewing gums to lozenges to patches and other techniques. A person may find it necessary to use a combination of pharmacological and behavioral interventions to ultimately stop smoking. Physician assistance may be necessary in getting the proper program of smoking cessation prescribed.

The biggest hurdle to smoking cessation is the recidivism of smokers. More than 90% of the people who quit smoking will experience a relapse within 1 year of stopping.[17] Quitting smoking is difficult, and any person in the process of quitting will need a great deal of support to maintain abstinence from this habit.

Table 14–3		
Typical Drug Use Statistics in High School Students (2002)		
(Over 43,000 students in 394 schools nationwide surveyed.)		
Use of an illicit drug (during life time)		
8th grade students	24.5 %	
10th grade students	44.6 %	
12th grade students	53 %	
Cigarette smoker (last 30 days) (Sometime in life)		
8th grade	10.7 %	31.4 %
10th grade	17.7 %	55.1 %
12th grade	26.7 %	57.2 %
Alcohol (last 30 days)		
8th grade	19.6 %	47 %
10th grade	35 %	66.9 %
12th grade	48.6 %	78.4 %

From: Monitoring the Future Study: Trends in prevalence of various drugs for 8th Graders, 10th Graders, and High School Seniors. US government publication accessed at www.drugabuse.gov.

*M*arijuana

The hemp plant commonly used for making rope is the source for marijuana leaves, which are dried and smoked to produce a minor psychedelic reaction for the user. Marijuana is considered a minor psychedelic drug because the user does not have a total and complete break with reality as is the case with major psychedelics like LSD. Marijuana has been written about in many other countries for more than 4,000 years where it has been used as a sedative, to treat constipation, obesity, loss of appetite, and other problems. In the 1960s and 1970s marijuana became a very popular drug among young people who could not legally buy alcohol but wanted a "high" of some type.

The active ingredient in marijuana is tetrahydrocannabinol, but it also contains over 400 other chemicals. It is one of the most debated and talked about illegal substances in the medical and recreational drug user communities. There are numerous groups trying to get marijuana legalized for medicinal purposes in a variety of states. To date, the federal government has not accepted the legalization arguments put forth by any of the medical or other groups attempting to decriminalize or legalize marijuana.

Athletes have been known to smoke marijuana before contests to reduce their stress levels or to relax allowing them, as some argue, to perform better in competition. This relaxation technique however, does not make sense to most athletes. If smoking marijuana produces a lethargic effect why would an athlete want to have less energy and a decreased ability to learn and concentrate during a competitive match? Each individual athlete should find legal and safe methods to reduce pregame stress that allow them to both maintain their ability to concentrate and keep their energy at the greatest levels.

■ Adverse Effects

The use of marijuana has some predictable adverse effects for the user. Some of the acute effects that may accompany the use of marijuana are: anxiety and panic attacks, paranoia, increased mood alterations, increased heart rate, breaks with reality, memory, concentration and learning impairment, decreased ambition and motivation, and other similar side effects. The chronic effects of marijuana smoking also include those problems associated with tobacco smoking, with the inhalation of chemicals leading to lung diseases. Marijuana cigarettes may have more damaging chemicals than regular tobacco cigarettes because of how the drug is processed before being sold to the user. Long-term users can expect many of the same physiological changes as cigarette smokers having sinusitis, chronic cough (smokers hack), shortness of breath and other lung disorders resulting from smoke inhalation. There have been reports of other respiratory diseases, precancerous changes, memory and concentration problems.[4,31]

*C*ocaine

To the surprise of many, there is a medicinal use for cocaine. It can be used as a local anesthetic but is not a common drug selected by most physicians for this purpose. As discussed in Chapter 10 there are many other local anesthetics considered much safer and more effective in their anesthetic properties.

The history of cocaine use goes back thousands of years in South America. Cocoa leaves have been and are still currently used by the natives in South American to provide them with much the same purpose many other people drink coffee; to get a stimulatory effect. Cocoa leaves are the raw materials needed to produce cocaine. Cocoa leaves are processed and made into a paste. The paste is further refined into a powder. Sometimes the paste does not go through further processing and refinement and is utilized by the drug abuser in the paste form. The processing of the cocoa leaves typically takes place in the country of origin. Most of the cocaine produced in the world comes from Bolivia, Columbia, and Peru. The cocaine powder or paste is then shipped out of the country to illegal distributors throughout the world.

Cocaine powder can be "snorted" through the nostrils, which is then taken up into the blood vessels and passed on to the central nervous system, where it stimulates the noradrenaline, serotonin, and dopamine neurotransmitters. The stimulation of these neurotransmitters produces a "high" and is associated with increased pleasure, activity level, and a general feeling of "well being".

For the effects of cocaine to be experienced quicker, the user may elect to use another method of getting it to their central nervous system. The drug user may use the "freebase" method. This method requires the cocaine powder be alkalinized to remove the hydrochloride salt, thus providing a substance that can be heated and smoked. Using the freebase method produces a delivery of the active ingredient to the brain at approximately the same speed as an intravenous injection. If a drug user tries to smoke cocaine powder, the heat required to vaporize cocaine powder destroys the active ingredient. Further processing of the cocaine powder to remove the salt allows the active ingredient to be vaporized at a much lower temperature. Thus, the cocaine can then be smoked. The other form of cocaine that is referred to is "crack," which is a homemade or imitation form of freebase. Crack is usually smoked in a special pipe, piece of aluminum foil or some other crude method by the user to get the rapid desired effect.

Web Resource Box

www.nida.nih.gov/ResearchReports/cocaine/cocaine3. html#how is a government web site that contains comprehensive information regarding cocaine, and its use and abuse.

The use of intravenous injection is possible after the powder is dissolved in water although this is not a common usage technique. Additionally, the user may try to swallow the cocaine to get it into their system. Oral intake of cocaine requires the drug to be absorbed from the intestinal tract, routed via the blood stream to the liver, where it is metabolized. This method results in a much slower and less effective delivery to the brain. Injection is the quickest and most effective way of getting the drug to the brain, and oral intake is the slowest and least effective method of taking cocaine.

■ Adverse Effects

Many cocaine users snort the cocaine through their nostrils which results in a constriction of the blood vessels in the immediate area. With increased use this can lead to necrosis of the tissues in the local area and chronic runny nose and/or collapse of the nasal cartilage, among other related problems. Smoking the drug is very hard on the structures of the lungs and can lead to chest pains and lung disorders such as bronchitis. Possibly the most significant problem is the stimulatory effect it produces on the central nervous system. This stimulation of the nervous system can result in an increase in blood pressure, heart rate, sweating, anxiety, and other central nervous system controlled activities which can sometimes result in death. A single use of cocaine has been reported to cause death. Again, the impurity and contamination of street drugs must be a factor the potential user should be aware of when electing to try this drug. Therefore, the athlete must understand that every person's body will react differently to the use of this and other drugs.

$\mathcal{C}$lub Drugs

■ Ecstasy

Methylenedioxymethamphetamine (MDMA), also better known as ECSTASY, is one of the most popular "club drugs" available today. These drugs are sometimes referred to as entactogens. "Entactogens" is a term that has been coined to describe the class of drugs that increases a person's "warm and friendly feelings" for others. Ecstasy or MDMA is an amphetamine derivative, as can be seen by the amphetamine group at the end of the chemical name. Its chemical structure is related to both amphetamine and mescaline. Over the years, more than 1000 chemical variations of ecstasy have been produced.[28]

According to Robson, the Merck pharmaceutical company takes credit for first synthesizing this drug in about 1912 and obtained the patent rights for it in 1914. At that time it was suggested that it could be used as a weight control drug. However, it was not commercially marketed but did get a restart in the 1950s when the United States Army was testing it for use in psychological warfare. Recreational use started in the late 1960s, and in the 1970s it was used by some psychologists to aid in different types of therapy. In psychotherapy, it was suggested that it allowed people to communicate more effectively.[28]

Ecstasy utilizes the serotonin and dopamine neurotransmitters to create a stimulatory effect in the central nervous system. By stimulating a "flood of serotonin" within the brain, a person feels friendly to everyone he or she comes in contact with during the time period the drug is in effect. When researchers gave ecstasy to animals, it resulted in an increased temperature, heart rate, salivation and actually caused convulsions in high doses. Because it is an illegal drug and cannot be prescribed, it is not used in human research any longer. The use of ecstasy and resulting emergency room visits isncreased dramatically over the period from 1994 to 1999. In 1994 there were about 250 reported emergency room visits compared with an estimated 2850 cases of ecstasy overdose in 1999.[3] In reviewing the most recent United State government drug abuse report,[32] it appears that ecstasy use declined among high school students over the years 2000–2002. High school seniors who reported using ecstasy at some time in their life dropped from 11% in 2000 to 10.5% in 2002. This is not a significant reduction in the number of high school seniors taking ecstasy but a decline in the total number of students trying this drug.

Implications On Activity

Some of the social drugs can have dramatic and even life-threatening consequences on athletes. Because the athlete increases his or her heart rate through exercise, drugs such as cocaine or methamphetamine can cause the heart rate to increase to a point of cardiac overload and result in the untimely death of the athlete. Some of the other social drugs, such as marijuana, are used by athletes on a more frequent basis for performance enhancement through increased relaxation. There are many other ways to increase relaxation in the athlete without use of illegal substances.

Adverse Effects

This drug is an illegal substance with many adverse effects. The main effect that people who take this drug are trying to achieve is the sudden exhilaration that comes anywhere from 20 to 90 minutes after oral consumption of the tablet. The feeling of exhilaration that the person experiences can last from 3 to 5 hours depending on the metabolism rate of the individual. It is also reported that the first experience using ecstasy is the most rewarding for the person, with subsequent experiences being less positive.[29] It should also be remembered that this drug is typically taken in combination with one or multiple other party drugs such as alcohol, tobacco,

What to Tell the Athlete

At the high school and college level, there is a higher incidence of athletes "experimenting" with drug use because social pressure from peers. The athlete needs to be continually reminded of the detrimental effect of social drugs. Some tips for the ATC when educating the athlete about these drugs.

■ Social drugs like alcohol and tobacco are readily available. However, the athlete should be cautioned to not use these substances for acceptance by peers, to prove their independence or for some other superficial reason.

■ Alcohol is an easy drug to abuse, and alcoholism can be initiated at a young age.

■ Marijuana has a high level of social acceptance, but it also has a number of adverse effects the athlete must be aware of when using this drug.

■ Cocaine and club drugs are also easily obtained, and the chance of adverse effects and even death are very high with the use of these drugs.

■ Many times, athletes are the most respected and their behavior is an example to many other non-athlete students.

■ Abstaining from the use of social drugs will show the people around the athlete the real "strength" of the athlete.

marijuana, amphetamines, cocaine, etc. Some of the reported effects of ecstasy include being more friendly with others, and less aggressive and less defensive in interpersonal interactions. People report that they can overcome many of the stresses that are involved in everyday life including obsessive behavior and impulsiveness. It is claimed by many users that speech is enhanced and the perception of time is diminished when using Ecstasy. Adverse effects occurring during the original 3 to 5 hours include nausea and vomiting.

Interestingly, the reported effects of ecstasy use can last up to a week in some individuals. Some report that for 1 week, they have an increased ability to interact with others and experience a decrease in fear, aggression, obsessive behavior, and anxiety. The adverse effects some experience for the week are a decrease in sleep and/or appetite, fatigue, depression, libido, restlessness, and a decreased ability to perform mental and physical tasks.[12]

This drug can have both acute and chronic toxic effects in the athlete.[11] Memory loss and decreased mental functioning is a neurotoxic effect that results from use of even a single dose of ecstasy. Memory loss can include recognition and long-term memory.[15,20] Mental functioning that has

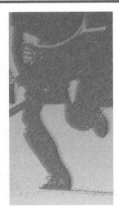

Scenarios from the Field

A very good high school football quarterback was highly recruited to a number of Division I universities. He made his final decision and started fall football the summer after high school graduation at his newly selected university. The university, like all Division I universities, had a random drug testing procedure. This athlete was randomly drug tested his freshman year and tested positive for alcohol and marijuana. The university policy was to put any positive drug tested athletes into counseling and allow them to proceed with their education. The counseling sessions were initiated for this player, but he again tested positive for alcohol and marijuana in his sophomore year. He was removed from the team for 1 year and was again asked to attend drug counseling to determine if he could be helped with his problem. The third year he came back to play football but once again tested positive and was released from the football program as an athlete.

In this scenario the university had a quite liberal testing and counseling policy that allowed the player to continue his relationship with the team during the time he was in drug counseling. There are many universities that do not have a liberal counseling program and when a player tests positive the second time he or she are removed from the athletic department and sometimes the university. Not only do these athletes loose their athletic scholarship but, in some cases, the ability to finish their college education at that university.

been documented to be impaired by Ecstasy use includes both immediate and delayed word recall. Other more obvious acute signs and symptoms include nausea, vomiting, dehydration, fainting, clumsiness, uncoordinated movements, increased body temperature, generalized "hangover" liver damage, and kidney failure,

Athletes could be willing to try ecstasy with their friends on a weekend, during a vacation period, or at some other time for any one of a number of reasons. As the athletic trainer, you should be able to explain the adverse effects the athlete may encounter days or even weeks after taking this drug. Encourage athletes to avoid the use of this drug because it could result in long-term disability or even death.

■ Gammahydroxybutyrate

Gammahydroxybutyrate (GHB) is growing in popularity as a drug that creates a sense of euphoria or a feeling similar to alcohol intoxication in people. Some bodybuilders also use GHB to help them get into the deepest phase of the sleep cycle and remain in that stage for a longer time period.[30] It is suggested that the deepest sleep cycles are associated with increased natural release of human growth hormone which will provide a greater muscle growth potential.[33]

GHB was originally developed as an anesthetic, but the effectiveness to limit or stop pain was never fully developed in this drug. It was determined that it could be of assistance in helping one to sleep. Later it was discovered that it had euphoric properties possibly emanating from its effect on the neurotransmitters in the central nervous system. GHB is rapidly absorbed in the mouth and begins to produce its effects within an hour after ingestion. It can be purchased in tablet or powder form at natural food stores in some states within the United States or on the internet at multiple sites in tablet, powder and solution forms. States such as California, Hawaii, Nevada, Texas, Georgia, Florida, Rhode Island and others have banned the sale of this drug completely. The probability of other states, if not all states, outlawing this drug in the future is great.

■ Adverse Effects

As with any of the social drugs, GHB is usually taken in combination with alcohol or other drugs because occurrence of use is frequently found in nightclubs, bars, and parties. The combined effects of GHB with other drugs can cause nausea, vomiting, muscle weakness, extreme fatigue, respiratory depression, and sometimes coma. The window between a nontoxic and toxic dose is small, and even a little too much GHB can cause an adverse reaction. Athletes should be cautioned from using GHB even to assist them with getting to sleep or other nonthreatening uses. The total effects produced by this drug have not been documented, and there are too many questions still not answered regarding this drug.

Web Resource Box

A lecture on cocaine from the U. of Pennsylvania is located at: www.uphs.upenn.edu/~recovery/pros/cocaine.html

For a good overview of the street drug nomenclature with pictures go to *www.sayno.com/stimulant.html*

Another site with good information for the high school or college athlete is:

www.drugs.indiana.edu/druginfo/stimulants.html

www.pamf.org/teen/index2.cfm (Palo Alto Medical Foundation, excellent source of information for teens about the effects of many different types of drugs)

www.nida.nih.gov/infofax.html (government web site that is updated regularly and provides information regarding the different socially used and street drugs.)

www.cdc.gov/nccdphp/dash/yrbs/index.htm is a web site that you can get reports of youth behavior on health-related risks, not just drug abuse on a bi-annual basis starting with 1990.

www.cdc.gov/tobacco is a web site that provides a regular report of the effects of tobacco on the health of people who use tobacco regularly. Also located on this web site is assistance in smoking cessation programs, sports initiatives, celebrities against smoking, and other educational information. Different pages on this web site give a state by state breakdown of tobacco use by youth, adults, related deaths, etc.

www.quitnet.com is a web site that offers assistance to people trying to quit smoking. This website is interactive and includes counseling and other options to help people quit smoking for good.

www.rwjf.org is a web site offering information and assistance on healthy lifestyles including alcohol and tobacco use. This organization also provides grants and other options for people with ideas about programs to promote a healthy lifestyle.

Class Discussion Topics

- Why do some athletes use marijuana before competition when the central nervous system needs to be highly active?

- What are some techniques (chemical–behavioral) people use for smoking cessation programs today?

- What are some of the reasons teenagers start using alcohol, tobacco, marijuana and other drugs?

- What is the role of the athletic trainer working in a non-traditional setting in assisting the athlete overcome a drug problem?

Chapter Review

- High school is a time when many teens will be more susceptible to experimental drug use.

- Many drug abusers are not aware that there are acute negative adverse effects associated with drug abuse.

- There are signs that indicate current use and personality and behavior indicators that can be interpreted as possible future drug abuse.

- The NCAA has been tracking drug abuse among athletes since the mid 1980's and has implemented programs to reduce drug use among collegiate athletes.

- Alcohol has a depressing effect on the central nervous system, which is the opposite effect the athlete is expecting.

- There are numerous chronic effects of alcohol on the body.

- Tobacco is a complex drug with many chemicals inhaled by the smoker.

- Smoking and the nicotine in the cigarette smoke has been shown to decrease motivation in people.

- There are numerous smoking cessation programs, which include behavioral and pharmacological interventions.

- Some athletes will smoke marijuana with the intent that this will relax them before a competition.

- Cocaine can be used as a local anesthetic by a physician but is also abused by athletes to produce an amphetamine like high.

- Ecstasy is an amphetamine derivative and is abused for the effects of increasing energy and friendliness.

- The effects of ecstasy can begin within 20 minutes of ingestion and last for up to 5 hours.

- Ecstasy use can result in long-term memory loss.

- GHB is used by body-builders to enhance sleep time with the idea that increased growth hormone is released during this sleep period.

- It should be remembered that drug abusers very often combine many different drugs (alcohol, tobacco, marijuana, cocaine, ecstasy, etc.) when they are out with a group or partying.

References

1. American College of Sports Medicine: Current Comment—Alcohol and Athletic Performance, April 2000.
2. Centers for Disease Control and Prevention: Morbidity and Mortality Weekly Report, 46:448, 1997.
3. DAWN Report: Club Drugs: www.health.org/govpubs/phd856/index.pdf. Accessed 10/1/2002.
4. Fried P, et al: Current and former marijuana use: preliminary findings of a longitudinal study of effects on IQ in young adults. CMAJ, 166:887, 2002.
5. Fowler JS et al: Inhibition of monoamine oxidase B in the brains of smokers. Nature, 379(6567):733, 1996.
6. Green GA et al: NCAA study of substance use and abuse habits of college student-athletes. Clin J Sports Med, 11:51, 2001.
7. Gutierrez K: Pharmacotherapeutics: Clinical decision making in nursing. WB Saunders Co., Philadelphia, 1999, pg. 151.
8. Hammersley R et al: Ecstasy and the rise of the chemical generation. Routledge, New York, NY, 2002.
9. Johnson LD et al: National Survey results on drug use from the monitoring the Future Study, 1975–1997. Volume I: Secondary School Students. NIH publication No. 98–4345. 1998.
10. Jung J: Psychology of Alcohol and Other Drugs: A Research Perspective. Sage Publications, Thousand Oaks, CA, 2001, pg. 167.
11. Kalant H: The pharmacology and toxicology of "ecstasy" (MDMA) and related drugs. CMAJ, 165:917, 2001.
12. McDowell DM and Spitz HI: Substance abuse: from principles to practice. Edwards Brothers, Ann Arbor, MI, 1999 pg. 169.
13. Miller MA et al: Adolescent relationships and drug use. Lawrence Erlbaum Associates, Mahwah, NJ, 2000, pg 1.

14. Miller MA et al: Adolescent relationships and drug use. Lawrence Erlbaum Associates, Mahwah, NJ, 2000, pg 7.

15. Morgan MJ: Memory deficits associated with recreational use of "ecstasy" (MDMA). Psychopharmacology, 141:30–36,1999.

16. National Collegiate Athletic Association: NCAA Study of Substance Use Habits of College Student-Athletes. June, 2001, pg 14.

17. National Institute on Drug Abuse: Nicotine Addiction. NIH publication number 01–4342, 2001.

18. Naylor AH, et al: Drug use patterns among high school athletes and nonathletes. Adolescence. 36:627, 2001.

19. O'Brien CP and Lyons F: Alcohol and the athlete. Sports Med. 29:295, 2000.

20. Parrott AC: Human research on MDMA (3,4-methylene-dioxymethamphetamine) neurotoxicity: cognitive and behavioural indices of change. Neuropshychobiology, 42: 17–24, 2000.

21. Robson P: Forbidden drugs. Oxford University, NY, NY, 1999, pg. 22.

22. Robson P: Forbidden drugs. Oxford University, NY, NY, 1999, pg. 19.

23. Robson P: Forbidden drugs. Oxford University, NY, NY, 1999, pg. 9.

24. Robson P: Forbidden drugs. Oxford University, NY, NY, 1999, pg. 14.

25. Robson P: Forbidden drugs. Oxford University, NY, NY, 1999, pg. 11.

26. Robson P: Forbidden drugs. Oxford University, NY, NY, 1999, pg. 48.

27. Robson P: Forbidden drugs. Oxford University, NY, NY, 1999, pg. 55.

28. Robson P: Forbidden drugs. Oxford University, NY, NY, 1999, pg. 139.

29. Robson P: Forbidden drugs. Oxford University, NY, NY, 1999, pg. 144.

30. Scharf MB, et al: Pharmacokinetics of gammahydroxybutyrate (GHB) in narcoleptic patients. Sleep, 21:507, 1998.

31. Schwartz RH: Marijuana: A decade and a half later, still a crude drug with underappreciated toxicity. Pediatrics, 109(2): 284, 2002.

32. United States Government: www.drugabuse.gov, general website accessed 1/10/2003.

33. Van Cauter E, et al: Simultaneous stimulation of slow-wave sleep and growth hormone secretion by gamma-hydroxybutyrate in normal young men. J Clin Invest, 100:745, 1997.

Chapter Questions

1. The initial use of social drugs by many athletes result in effects that are?
   A. immediate
   B. learned over time
   C. delayed
   D. greater than chronic users

2. Acute reactions to drug abuse can be caused by all of the following EXCEPT:
   A. additives to the drug
   B. combining multiple drugs
   C. mood of the drug abuser
   D. environmental temperature

3. According to government and research studies, why do high school students start to use alcohol and tobacco?
   A. legal age in some states
   B. acceptance by peers
   C. parental acceptance
   D. hormonal changes

4. What are the signs or personality characteristics that indicate an athlete could become a drug abuser?
   A. ambitious
   B. committed
   C. deliberate
   D. nonconformist

5. After what age has research shown that experimental drug abuse is reduced?
   A. 18
   B. 21
   C. 25
   D. 30

6. What effect does alcohol have on the gross motor skills of an athlete's performance in basketball?
   A. decreased reaction time
   B. increased reaction time
   C. reduces dehydration
   D. increases hormonal balance

7. Approximately how many chemicals are present in cigarette smoke?
   A. 25
   B. 100
   C. 2000
   D. 4000

8. Which of the following drugs currently has medicinal use accepted by mainstream physicians?
   A. alcohol
   B. tobacco
   C. marijuana
   D. cocaine

9. Most cocaine abusers prefer which method of use to get the most rapid effect from the drug?
   A. snorting
   B. smoking
   C. injecting
   D. oral

10. Ecstasy creates which chemical response in the body resulting in the desired effect to the drug abuser?
    A. increase in serotonin release
    B. decrease in dopamine release
    C. increase in insulin release
    D. increase in beta-endorphine release

11. GHB is used by body-builders to:
    A. increase growth hormone release during sleep
    B. decrease serotonin release during exercise
    C. increase dopamine release during exercise
    D. decrease beta-endorphine release during sleep

Recognition and Rules 15

Chapter Objectives

After reading this chapter, the student should have an understanding of the following:

1 How to recognize the outward signs of drug abuse in athletes.

2 How to respond to an athlete whom they suspect might be abusing drugs.

3 The classes of drugs that are banned by the NCAA and the International Olympic Committee.

4 How the NCAA drug-testing program works.

5 Where to get information regarding starting a drug testing program at an institution.

6 Future implications for high school athletes.

Chapter Outline

Recognition of Drug Abuse

Role of the Athletic Trainer in Drug Abuse Situations

National Collegiate Athletic Association Drug Testing

International Olympic Committee

High-School Drug Testing

Recognition of Drug Abuse

The recognition of drug use is a small part of the athletic trainer's duties, but it can be a major factor in caring for athletes, students, and people in general. Sometimes athletic trainers can inadvertently overlook an athlete's drug or substance abuse problem when they are dealing with other more visible problems that the athlete may be encountering in his or her sports participation. It is much easier for the athletic trainer to care for a sprain, strain, abrasion, or other outward sign of injury than to deal with a problem the athlete is hiding or will not admit exists. The athletic trainer needs to be keenly aware of some of the subtle signs of substance abuse that an athlete might exhibit when he or she is in the athletic training facility or in the company of the athletic training staff members.

Most drug abuse by athletes is for ergogenic purposes. Another athlete or friend may convince an athlete that he or she needs to use some type of a supplement to get bigger, stronger, or faster. Also, some athletes believe that using an ergogenic aid will give them a greater chance at a college scholarship or a professional contract. The NCAA has been surveying collegiate athletes for many years regarding ergogenic drug use.

The 2001 NCAA survey was a continuing effort to determine patterns of drug use among collegiate athletes. A similar survey had been sent to member institutions four times previously since the original results were published in 1989. The survey was sent to a variety of different Division I, II, and III institutions and specified which athletic teams were to be surveyed. For the 2001 survey there were a total of 21,225 surveys completed from 713 member institutions.

As can be seen by reviewing Figure 15–1, the use of anabolic steroids among collegiate athletes has dropped a great deal since 1989, when the athletes were first surveyed. Conversely, the use of amphetamines and ephedrine has greatly increased since the first survey. This indicates that athletes are not as concerned about their size as they are about their energy level. It may be that collegiate athletes are being asked to do too much between their academic requirements and their athletic desires in college.

In Chapter 14 we discussed the student athlete's possible use of social drugs. It is a difficult task for the athletic trainer to watch and wait for an athlete to confide in him or her regarding of an illegal drug or substance. The athletic trainer is not always present to observe the athlete's social behavior or use of illegal drugs. Additionally, there are many college athletes over the age of 21 who can legally purchase alcohol for personal use. This also can lead to problems for the student athlete. In this situation the athlete must take more responsibility for his or her own actions. Athletic trainers can watch the athlete's behavior and, if they see something of concern, approach the athlete privately to see if they can be of assistance. The main clues that the athletic trainer should be watching for are mood swings, depression, anxiety, headaches, and general behavior problems. A fuller list of identifying behaviors is presented in Table 15–1.

There are times when an athlete may not be aware of a drug use problem. This sounds a little odd, but the athlete might be taking one or more herbal and/or dietary supplements purchased over the counter (OTC) that contain any one of a number of illegal substances. Kamber et al.[7] reported that some athletes use 20 or more supplements while training for competition. Sometimes an athlete tests positive for a banned substance when he or she has been consuming only "nutritional supplements." According to test laboratories, it is not uncommon for specific supplements to be mislabeled.[1,3,4,7] Supplements may either contain less than the disclosed amount of the substance named as the main ingredient (a situation unlikely to cause a health problem), or much more of that substance. In one product tested, the concentration of ephedrine was so high that one tablet before competition would result in a drug test that would be positive for doping.[7] The athletic trainer needs to aware that athletes may be taking OTC or herbal supplements as well as illegal ergogenic aids to make them bigger, stronger, and faster.

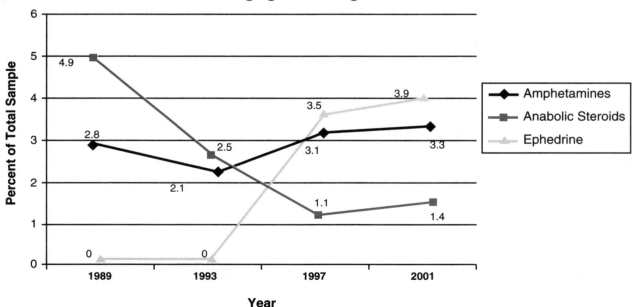

Figure 15–1. Patterns of ergogenic drug use by collegiate student-athletes. Adapted from the NCAA Study of Substance Use Habits of College Student-Athletes. Report presented to the NCAA Committee on Competitive Safeguards and Medical Aspects of Sports, June 2001. (Reprinted with permission of National Collegiate Athletic Association.)

Table 15–1

Characteristics That May Suggest Substance Abuse

Substance	Characteristics	Substance	Characteristics
Alcohol	Arrhythmias, idiopathic cardiomyopathy Behavioral problems in infants Cirrhosis, pancreatitis, splenomegaly Coma Conflicts with legal system (DUI, family violence, MVAs) Depression Eating disorders, malnutrition, gastritis Fetal alcohol syndrome Headaches, neurologic problems House fires Hypersexuality Hypertension Hypothermia Social isolation Unexplained accidents, changes in behavior, suicide attempt	Cocaine	Behavior problems in infants (when consumed by the mother) Epistaxis Headaches Hypersexuality Impotence Masculinization Mood swings Nasal septal defects
		Hallucinogens	Conflicts with legal system (MVAs, violence) Disorientation, fear of surroundings Unexplained accidents, changes in behavior, suicide attempt Psychosis, mood swings, unexplained changes in behavior
Amphetamines	Anxiety, sleep disorders Conflicts with legal system (MVAs, violence) Hypersexuality Malnutrition Membership in high-risk population group Mood swings Multiple skin disorders (infections, ulcerations) Needle marks and bruises on the arms Psychoses, unexplained changes in behavior	Inhalants	Burns around mouth, nose Epistaxis House fires Mood swings Respiratory difficulty, suffocation Social isolation
		Opioids	Malnutrition Multiple skin disorders (infections, ulcerations)
Barbiturates	Coma Depressed responses Endocrine imbalances Hypotension	Steroids	Conflicts with legal system (violence) Depression Hypotension Impotence Masculinization Mood swings Retarded growth in children
Benzodiazepines	Anxiety Coma Suicide attempt		
Caffeine	Arrhythmias Eating disorders Headaches Hyperactivity Hypertension Sleeping disorders		

DUI = driving under the influence; MVAs = motor vehicle accidents
Source: Gutierrez, K: Pharmacotherapeutics: Clinical decision making in nursing. WB Saunders, Philadelphia, 1999, p 157.

Role of the Athletic Trainer in Drug Abuse Situations

One of the major functions of the athletic trainer is to act as a counselor and educator for athletes. Once an athletic trainer has discovered that there is a drug abuse situation with a specific athlete, it is important to determine the options available to both the athlete and the athletic trainer. The athletic trainer must keep in mind that he or she has not been trained specifically in substance abuse counseling and that the athlete may require the assistance of a professional counselor. However, familiarity with basic substance abuse counseling concepts will be helpful to the athletic trainer. There are some general guidelines outlined by Lewis et al. that the athletic trainer can keep in mind:

1. Use a respectful and positive approach to all clients.
2. Adapt treatment to individual client needs, in both goals and methods.
3. Provide a multidimensional treatment that focuses on the social and environmental aspects of long-term recovery.[8]

Understanding that substance abuse treatment is individualized and targeted for long-term recovery should help athletic trainers to be respectful and positive in their daily encounters with these athletes. The athletic trainer should be a good listener and be careful not to provide suggestions of intervention strategies, but he or she should encourage the athlete to follow the course of action outlined by the substance abuse counselor. Be mindful not to suggest an intervention strategy, but provide ideas on how the athlete might avoid getting into a situation that could result in a return to alcohol or drug abuse.

Additionally, the athletic trainer should be actively seeking educational programs that address substance abuse. By putting up antisubstance abuse posters, scheduling guest speakers, and finding time to talk with individuals and groups of athletes about the problems associated with substance abuse, athletic trainers can take a proactive stance in trying to eliminate substance abuse among their athletes.

Internet Resource Box

Resources for substance abuse counseling:

State-by-state listing of alcohol and drug abuse counseling organizations: *http://www.lowefamily.org.*

www.drugabuse.gov U.S. Department of Health & Human Services Website providing links to many different educational programs for alcohol and drug abuse counseling: Website set up to assist people dealing with bereavement and personal loss of various types: *www.griefnet.org*

As mentioned in Chapter 13, it is also important that the athlete understand the implications of OTC supplements and the possibility that those supplements may contain products that are harmful or could result in a positive drug test. One of the OTC products documented to contain unreliable amounts or additional chemicals is androstenedione, used by many athletes in an attempt to generate muscle bulk. In one study, it was documented that two-thirds of the androstenedione samples tested (six out of nine) were contaminated and would produce a positive drug test for steroid use in athletes undergoing standard urine testing.[3]

Additionally, an analysis of nutritional supplements was conducted at the International Olympic Committee accredited doping laboratory in Cologne, Germany. In this study, the researchers gathered 634 nonhormonal nutritional supplements for complete testing. The supplements were gathered from 13 suppliers in 215 different countries. It was determined that more than 21 percent of the prohormone supplements contained anabolic androgenic steroids that were not listed on the product packaging. There were concentrations of anabolic androgenic steroids up to 190 μg/g. The reported contaminated supplements were from one of the following: the United States, the Netherlands, the United Kingdom, Italy, or Germany.[11] Players should be continually reminded that they must be very careful when they select and consume nutritional supplements during their training periods.

*N*ational Collegiate Athletic Association Drug Testing

The National Collegiate Athletic Association (NCAA) has a very strict and detailed random drug-testing program that was first proposed in January 1986 and amended in 1990. The NCAA has a very specific purpose for their drug-testing program. The official NCAA drug-testing manual states, "So that no one participant might have an artificially induced advantage, so that no one participant might be pressured to use chemical substances in order to remain competitive, and to safeguard the health and safety of participants, this NCAA drug-testing program has been created."[10]

Internet Resource Box

http://www.ncaa.org is the official Website of the National Collegiate Athletic Association.

As part of the NCAA membership, each institution agrees to obtain consent for each athlete to be randomly drug tested. Therefore, at the direction of the NCAA, a player must submit to a random drug test. This can be during the season, at a championship tournament, or during the off season for many sports. A few of the highlights of the NCAA drug-testing manual indicate that a student athlete who tests positive for use of an NCAA banned substance (Table 15–2) will be banned from competition for one season. The athlete will be ineligible for any postseason play as well. Additionally, the member institutions must also agree to provide educational programs during each semester of the school year. This educational process includes reinforcing

Table 15–2

NCAA Banned-Drug Classes, 2002–2003

Stimulants

amiphenazole	methamphetamine
amphetamine	methylenedioxymethamphetamine (MDMA) (ecstasy)
bemigride	methylphenidate
benzphetamine	nikethamide
bromantan	pemoline
caffeine[1] (guarana)	pentetrazol
chlorphentermine	phendimetrazine
cocaine	phentermine
cropropamide	phenylpropanolamine (PPA) effective August 2003
crothetamide	picrotoxin
diethylpropion	pipradol
dimethylamphetamine	prolintane
doxapram	strychnine and related compounds
ephedrine (ephedra, ma huang)	
ethamivan	
ethylamphetamine	
fencamfamine	
meclofenoxate	

Anabolic Agents

anabolic steroids	methyltestosterone
androstendiol	nandrolone
androstenedione	norandrostenediol
boldenone	norandrostenedione
clostebol	norethandrolone
dehydrochlormethyl-testosterone	oxandrolone
dehydroepiandrosterone (DHEA)	oxymesterone
dihydrotestosterone (DHT)	oxymetholone
dromostanolone	stanozolol
fluoxymesterone	testosterone[2] and related compounds
mesterolone	other anabolic agents
methandienone	clenbuterol
methenolone	

Substances Banned for Specific Sports: Riflery

alcohol	pindolol
atenolol	propranolol
metoprolol	timolol and related compounds

Diuretics

acetazolamide	hydroflumethiazide
bendroflumethiazide	methyclothiazide
benzthiazide	metolazone
bumetanide	polythiazide
chlorothiazide	quinethazone
chlorthalidone	spironolactone
ethacrynic acid	triamterene
flumethiazide	trichlormethiazide and related compounds
furosemide	
hydrochlorothiazide	

Street Drugs

heroin	THC (tetrahydrocannabinol)[3]
Marijuana[3]	

Peptide Hormones and Analogues

chorionic gonadotropin (HCG—human chorionic gonadotropin)

Corticotropin (ACTH)

Growth hormone (HGH, somatotropin)

All the respective releasing factors of the above-mentioned substances are also banned.

Erythropoietin (EPO) sermorelin

Definitions of positive depend on the following:
[1]For caffeine—if the concentration in urine exceeds 15 micrograms/mL.
[2]For testosterone—if the administration of testosterone or the use of any other manipulation has the result of increasing the ratio of the total concentration of testosterone to that of epitestosterone in the urine to greater than 6:1, unless there is evidence that this ratio is the result of a physiological or pathological condition.
[3]For marijuana and THC—if the concentration in the urine of THC metabolite exceeds 15 nanograms/mL.
Reprinted with permission of the NCAA.

and updating the athletes with the most recent list of banned substances each semester. The educational program should consist of the following points:

1. Review or develop individual team drug and alcohol policies.
2. Review the athletics department's drug and alcohol policy.
3. Review institutional drug and alcohol policy.
4. Review conference drug and alcohol policy.
5. Review institutional or conference drug-testing programs. (if applicable)
6. Review NCAA alcohol, tobacco, and drug policy including tobacco ban, list of banned drug classes, and testing protocol.
7. View the NCAA drug-education and drug-testing videos.
8. Discuss nutritional supplements and their inherent risks.
9. Allow time for questions from student-athletes.

Note: Each athletics department should have a written policy on alcohol, tobacco and other drugs.[10]

The confidentiality of random drug testing is of paramount importance. The athletic trainer must maintain confidentiality in all communications with athletes and with any agencies or professionals providing counseling to the athlete(s). The athletic trainer must also be aware that drug-testing laboratories are capable of reporting a false-positive drug test. For this reason, it is always wise to maintain athlete confidentiality well into the testing and retesting process. If the athletic trainer were to allow some information to inadvertently slip out to the press or other athletes about a positive drug test that had not been rechecked, and it turned out to be a false-positive report, this could be disastrous for the athlete, the athletic trainer, and the institution.

Each member institution of the NCAA is encouraged to have a random drug-testing program in addition to the organization's program. Member institutions are encouraged to involve their legal counsel early in the drug-testing program planning process, have a written plan for the entire program, and follow other recommendations available directly from the NCAA offices.

Implications for Activity

With the advent of random drug testing, athletes are being disqualified from competition for not showing up for a random drug test or because a urine sample tests positive. When this happens, the athlete must suffer the consequences. The urine sample can also be stored and retested at a later date, creating participation problems later in the season or later in an athlete's career.

International Olympic Committee

The International Olympic Committee (IOC) has a long history of antidrug activity and testing Olympic competitors to determine if illegal substances are being used to enhance an athlete's performance. The original impetus for drug testing and control came in 1967, when the Olympic Medical Commission was organized. Since then, the Medical Commission has regularly developed many different methods and strategies to control doping in Olympic athletes. One main function of this commission is to determine which drugs and drug classes will be banned because they are detrimental to the athlete's health, to maintain equality among competitors, or to retain respect for both medical and sports ethics during training and competition. The substances that are banned are broken down into seven specific classes of drugs (Table 15–3).

The IOC is constantly updating the banned substance list. The most recent update to the Anti-Doping Code was promulgated in March 2004. Recently added are new categories on antiestrogenic activity and designer steroidlike

Table 15–3	
Classes of Drug Substances Prohibited by International Olympic Committee	
Class of Drug	**Examples***
Stimulants	amphetamines, caffeine, cocaine, ephedrines
Narcotics	methadone, morphine, heroin
Anabolic agents	19-norandrostenedione, stanozolol, oxandrolone, DHEA, testosterone, clenbuterol, salbutamol
Diuretics	acetazolamide, bumetanide, triamterene
Peptide hormones	corticotrophins, growth hormone, erythropoietin, insulin growth factor, insulin
Mimetics and analogues	aromatase inhibitors
Agents with anti-estrogenic activity	clomiphene, tamoxifen (in males)
Masking agents	diuretics, epitestosterone, plasma expanders

*These are just a few of the drugs named on the IOC list. Some of the named drugs have legal levels (which are small) in injured or female patients or other specifically outlined situations.
Source: www.wada-ama.org

substances. Antiestrogenic drugs are typically used in females to prevent breast cancer (Tamoxifen) or stimulate ovarian function (Clomid). In men, they decrease the development of female sex characteristics, which can result from some types of androgenic steroid abuse. The new designer steroids such as tetrahydrogestrinone (THG) have only recently been documented and are being fully investigated to determine their use by athletes in a variety of sports.

Another addition to the IOC banned substance list is "masking agents." These drugs do not necessarily create an ergogenic effect in the athlete, but they do have a chemical affinity for, and attach to, ergogenic drugs so that, when urine is processed in the laboratory, only the masking agent is detected and the illegal substance is not identified in the testing procedure. Thus the athlete appears to have some benign substance in the urine.

Interestingly, the IOC has added a category to the "prohibited methods" section of the 2003 Anti-Doping Code. Along with to blood doping and identification of oxygen carriers, the IOC has added a "gene doping" category. The concept of using gene therapy has been documented in scientific journals. Ongoing discussion includes how to deliver the materials to the body, what types of improvements could be accomplished, and the dangers involved with this type of therapy.[8] Most of the reported use of gene therapy in sports medicine procedures is to improve tissue healing. It is suggested that gene therapy may be a very good technique to decrease the healing time of muscle tissue or improve the healing capacity of cartilage, meniscus, ligament, and bone.[8] There is a substantial amount of research activity along these lines, and the IOC appears ready to confront the possibility of illegal activity in this new and upcoming area. For more information and current updates regarding the IOC's anti-drug activities and policies, refer to their Website (see below).

Internet Resource Box

The IOC has a separate arm for drug education purposes, the World Anti-Doping Agency (WADA). Their home page is *http://www.wada-ama.org*.

The United States Olympic Committee has set up a similar organization called the US Anti-Doping Agency. Their anti-doping policy statement is found at www. *antidoping.org*

There is also a large confederation of countries that have combined with the IOC to reduce inappropriate drug use in athletes. The Concerted Action in the Fight Against Doping in Sport (CAFDIS) was originally a joint venture between the IOC and the countries of the European Union. Currently, it is funded by the European Union and now has many more members including the International Cycling Union, various non-European national Olympic committees, and some invited organizations as guests. The aim of this consortium is to educate and help athletes avoid the use of drugs for performance enhancement. The organization's Website can be found at *www.cafdis-antidoping.net.*

High-School Drug Testing

The random drug testing of high-school athletes has not become a regular occurrence in most high schools in the United States, but recent legal precedents appear to allow such testing. The drug testing of high-school athletes was originally challenged in the early 1990s in Oregon by a ninth-grade boy who wanted to play football for his public school. His parents refused to sign a form that gave permission to the school to perform random drug testing. Therefore, he was not allowed to participate in football. A court challenge was made questioning the violation of this young man's Fourth-Amendment rights. The Supreme Court of the United States ruled in 1995 that the school district's random drug testing procedure did not violate the Fourth-Amendment rights of the high-school student athlete.[12] Later, in Indiana, another legal challenge went to the United States Supreme Court, which ruled that students involved in extracurricular activities at school can be subjected to random drug testing.[11] This was upheld again by the Court in a 2002 ruling that high school students participating in athletics can be randomly drug tested.[2]

Over the years, Congress has debated legislation that would enact laws requiring random drug testing and counseling for students in schools and public programs.[13,14] There has even been a discussion of the costs associated with such a drug-testing program. The cost of a proposed random drug-testing program in the high schools across the United States was projected to be $1 billion per year, and there was a conceptual 5-year commitment from the federal government to start the program. To date, this concept of random drug testing in public schools is still being debated, and funding the program in each school district is a major issue that needs resolution.

The major obstacle to widespread high-school drug testing appears to be the cost of analyzing the samples. In the future, athletic trainers could be an integral part of random drug testing athletes in high schools if such policies are adopted by the local schools or school districts. The athletic trainer must become extremely proactive in helping the school administration set up policies and procedures for this type of testing if it comes to his or her specific school.

What to Tell the Athlete

Collegiate athletes need to be aware early on that drug testing is going to be a part of the college athletic experience. Each college or university will have its own drug testing rules and regulations. Here are some tips for the athletic trainer when educating the athlete about these rules and regulations:

■ Random drug testing means that athletes can be tested in and out of season.

■ Athletes need to continually document all OTC and prescription drugs they are taking.

■ OTC drugs and herbal preparations can produce a positive drug test.

■ Athletes should be encouraged to confide in someone they trust if they are having a drug problem.

■ Athletes should encourage any friends or teammates who confide in them to seek professional assistance for serious drug problems.

■ The athletic trainer must take the role of counselor and educator seriously when talking to athletes about drug use and abuse.

Discussion Topics

• Your soccer team just won the conference championship. After the game, you overhear some of the players talking about going out that evening to get drunk and "celebrate the win." What should you do? Should you approach the athletes individually? Should you talk with the coaching staff?

• The high school where you work as an athletic trainer does not have a drug-testing program. How do you approach a football player who you suspect is using illegal steroids?

• Some of the athletes you work with ask you, their athletic trainer, about some herb-based energy supplements they are using to increase their energy during twice-daily practice. What should be your explanation to the athletes regarding the use of OTC supplements?

Chapter Review

• The athletic trainer should recognize some of the subtle signs of substance abuse in athletes.

• Abnormal behaviors the athletic trainer might notice in athletes include mood swings, depression, anxiety, headaches, and general behavior problems.

• The athletic trainer should act as a counselor and educator for athletes, and realize when the athlete needs professional assistance.

• The athletic trainer should help the athlete understand the implications of using OTC supplements. He or she should be particularly aware of the possibility that an OTC supplement may contain products that are harmful or could result in a positive drug test.

• The NCAA has a very strict and detailed random drug-testing program for collegiate athletes.

• Each NCAA member institution must agree to provide educational programs each semester of the school year for all athletes at that institution.

• The IOC has a drug-testing program for Olympic competitors to determine if illegal substances are being used to enhance an athlete's performance.

• The IOC has a highly sophisticated drug-testing program that is much more expensive to operate than those at United States educational institutions.

• Drug testing for high school athletes is not a common practice in most school districts throughout the United States because of the costs involved.

References

1. Baylis, A, et al.: Inadvertent doping through supplement use by athletes: Assessment and management of the risk in Australia. Int J Sport Nutr Exerc Metab 11:365, 2001.

2. Board of Education of Independent School District No. 92 of Pottawatomie County v. Earls, 122 S.Ct. 2559 (2002).

3. Catlin, DH, et al.: Trace contamination of over-the-counter androstenedione and positive urine test results for a nandrolone metabolite. JAMA 284(20):2618, 2000.

4. Clarkson, P, et al.: Risky dietary supplements. Gatorade Sports Science Institute 13(2): 1, 2002.

5. Gutierrez, K: Pharmacotherapeutics: Clinical decision making in nursing. W B Saunders Co., Philadelphia, 1999, p. 157.

6. Jung, J: Psychology of Alcohol and Other Drugs: A Research Perspective. Sage Publications, Thousand Oaks, Calif., 2002, p 167.

7. Kamber, M, et al.: Nutritional supplements as a source for positive doping cases? Int J Sport Nutr Exerc Metab 11:258, 2001.

8. Lewis, JA, et al.: Substance Abuse Counseling, ed. 3. Brooks/Cole, Pacific Grove, Calif., 2002, p 4.

9. Martinek, V, et al.: Gene Therapy and tissue engineering in sports medicine. Phys Sportsmed 28(2):34, 2000.

10. National Collegiate Athletic Association. Drug testing program. *http://www2.ncaa.org.* Accessed Dec. 12, 2002.

11. Geyer, H, et al.: Analysis of non-hormonal nutritional supplements for anabolic-androgenic steroids: An international study. Int J Sports Med 25(2):124, 2004.

12. Todd v. Rush County, 525 U.S. 824 (1998).

13. Vernonia School District 47J v. Acton, 515 U.S. 646 (1995).

14. Safe Schools, Safe Streets, and Secure Borders Act of 1999. S. 9, 106th Congress (1999).

15. Bill to Revise and Extend the Safe and Drug-free Schools and Communities Act of 1994. S. 1823, 106th Congress (1999).

Chapter Questions

1. All drugs have an immediate effect on the user.

   True   False

2. An athlete can test positive for drugs when taking only nutritional supplements.

   True   False

3. The NCAA uses drug testing for which of the following purpose?
   A. To stop any one athlete from gaining an unfair advantage in competition
   B. To catch and prosecute anyone using illegal drugs.
   C. To stop illegal drug use on campuses
   D. To eliminate athletes from competition when they use drugs

4. Athletes testing positive on an NCAA drug test will receive which of the following?
   A. A 1-year suspension from competition
   B. A one-game suspension from competition
   C. A referral for counseling and return to competition
   D. A second chance at the next game or tournament

5. Random drug testing for athletes is illegal in the public schools.

   True   False

6. Each NCAA member institution is required to have a random drug-testing process for all the athletes at that institution.

   True   False

Drug Classifications

Generic	Brand	Class	Chapter
Flurbiprofen	Ansaid	Anti-inflammatory	3
Fenoprofen	Nalfon	Anti-inflammatory	3
Ibuprofen	Motrin	Anti-inflammatory	3
Ketoprofen	Orudis	Anti-inflammatory	3
Naproxen	Naprosyn	Anti-inflammatory	3
Naproxen sodium	Aleve	Anti-inflammatory	3
Oxaprozin	Daypro	Anti-inflammatory	3
Diclofenac sodium	Voltaren	Anti-inflammatory	3
Diclofenac sodium/ misoprostol	Arthrotec	Anti-inflammatory	3
Diclofenac potassium	Cataflam	Anti-inflammatory	3
Piroxicam	Feldene	Anti-inflammatory	3
Meloxicam	Mobic	Anti-inflammatory	3
Etodolac	Lodine	Anti-inflammatory	3
Indomethacin	Indocin	Anti-inflammatory	3
Sulindac	Clinoril	Anti-inflammatory	3
Tolmetin	Tolectin	Anti-inflammatory	3
Nabumetone	Relafen	Anti-inflammatory	3
Ketorolac	Toradol	Anti-inflammatory	3
Celecoxib	Celebrex	Anti-inflammatory	3
Rofecoxib	Vioxx	Anti-inflammatory	3
Valdecoxib	Bextra	Anti-inflammatory	3
Methocarbamol	Robaxin	Skeletal Muscle Relaxant	4
Cyclobenzaprine	Flexeril	Skeletal Muscle Relaxant	4
Orphenadrine	Norflex	Skeletal Muscle Relaxant	4
Metaxalone	Skelaxin	Skeletal Muscle Relaxant	4
Carisoprodol	Soma	Skeletal Muscle Relaxant	4
Dantrolene	Dantrium	Skeletal Muscle Relaxant	4
Insulin Lispro	Humalog	Antidiabetic	5
Insulin Aspart	Novolog	Antidiabetic	5
Insulin Regular	Humulin R	Antidiabetic	5
Isophane Insulin	NPH	Antidiabetic	5
Insulin Zinc	Lente	Antidiabetic	5

Generic	Brand	Class	Chapter
Insulin Zinc, extended	Ultralente	Antidiabetic	5
Insulin glargine	Lantus	Antidiabetic	5
Acarbose	Precose	Antidiabetic	5
Miglitol	Glyset	Antidiabetic	5
Metformin	Glucophage	Antidiabetic	5
Repaglinide	Prandin	Antidiabetic	5
Nateglinide	Starlix	Antidiabetic	5
Rosiglitazone	Avandia	Antidiabetic	5
Pioglitazone	Actos	Antidiabetic	5
Acetohexamide	Dymelor	Antidiabetic	5
Chlorpropamide	Diabinese	Antidiabetic	5
Tolazamide	Tolinase	Antidiabetic	5
Tolbutamide	Orinase	Antidiabetic	5
Glimepiride	Amaryl	Antidiabetic	5
Glipizide	Glucotrol	Antidiabetic	5
Glyburide	Diabeta	Antidiabetic	5
Doxazosin	Cardura	Antihypertensive	6
Terazosin	Hytrin	Antihypertensive	6
Furosemide	Lasix	Antihypertensive	6
Hydrochlorothiazide	Hydrodiuril	Antihypertensive	6
Atenolol	Tenormin	Antihypertensive	6
Metoprolol	Lopressor	Antihypertensive	6
Propranolol	Inderal	Antihypertensive	6
Nadolol	Corgard	Antihypertensive	6
Labetalol	Normodyne	Antihypertensive	6
Amlodipine	Norvasc	Antihypertensive	6
Diltiazem	Cardizem	Antihypertensive	6
Felodipine	Plendil	Antihypertensive	6
Nicardipine	Cardene	Antihypertensive	6
Verapamil	Calan	Antihypertensive	6
Captopril	Capoten	Antihypertensive	6
Enalapril	Vasotec	Antihypertensive	6
Fosinopril	Monopril	Antihypertensive	6
Lisinopril	Prinivil	Antihypertensive	6
Losartan	Cozaar	Antihypertensive	6
Quinapril	Accupril	Antihypertensive	6
Ramipril	Altace	Antihypertensive	6

Generic	Brand	Class	Chapter	Generic	Brand	Class	Chapter
Flecainide	Tambocor	Antiarrhythmic	6	Aluminum Hydroxide/ Magnesium Hydroxide/ Simethicone	Mylanta	Antacid	8
Propafenone	Rythmol	Antiarrhythmic	6				
Albuterol	Proventil	Bronchodilator	6				
Levalbuterol	Xopenex	Bronchodilator	7	Magnesium Hydroxide	Phillips' Milk of Magnesia	Antacid	8
Pirbuterol	Maxair	Bronchodilator	7				
Salmeterol	Serevent	Bronchodilator	7	Calcium Carbonate/ Magnesium Hydroxide	Rolaids Extra Strength	Antacid	8
Fluticasone	Flovent	Anti-inflammatory	7				
Triamcinolone	Azmacort	Anti-inflammatory	7				
Prednisone	Deltasone	Anti-inflammatory	7	Calcium Carbonate	Tums	Antacid	8
Cromolyn	Intal	Antasthmatic	7	Methylcellulose	Citrucel	Laxative	8
Montelukast	Singulair	Antasthmatic	7	Polycarbophil	FiberCon	Laxative	8
Zafirlukast	Accolate	Antasthmatic	7	Psyllium	Metamucil	Laxative	8
Diphenhydramine	Benadryl	Antihistamine	7	Docusate	Colace	Laxative	8
Chlorpheniramine	Chlor-Trimeton	Antihistamine	7	Magnesium Citrate	Evac-Q-Kwik	Laxative	8
Triprolidine/ Pseudoephedrine	Actifed Cold and Allergy	Antihistamine	7	Sodium Phosphate	Fleet Ready-to-use Enema	Laxative	8
Loratadine	Claritin	Antihistamine	7	Glycerin	Fleet Babylax	Laxative	8
Fexofenadine	Allegra	Antihistamine	7	Bisacodyl	Dulcolax	Laxative	8
Cetirizine	Zyrtec	Antihistamine	7	Senna	Ex-Lax	Laxative	8
Oxymetazoline	Afrin	Decongestant	7	Simethicone	Gas-X	Antiflatulent	8
Phenylephrine	Neo-Synephrine	Decongestant	7	Alpha-Galactoside	Beano	Antiflatulent	8
Guaifenesin	Robitussin	Expectorant	7	Loperamide	Imodium	Antidiarrheal	8
Benzonatate	Tessalon	Antitussive	7	Metronidazole	Flagyl	Antibiotic	8
Dextromethorphan	Vicks Formula 44	Antitussive	7	Penicillin V Potassium	Veetids	Antibiotic	8
Pseudoephedrine	Sudafed	Decongestant	7	Ampicillin	Omnipen	Antibiotic	9
Bismuth	Pepto-Bismol	Antidiarrheal	7	Amoxicillin	Amoxil	Antibiotic	9
Cimetidine	Tagamet	Antiulcerative	8	Amoxicillin plus clavulanate	Augmentin	Antibiotic	9
Famotidine	Pepcid	Antiulcerative	8	Cephalexin	Keflex	Antibiotic	9
Ranitidine	Zantac	Antiulcerative	8	Cefadroxil	Duricef	Antibiotic	9
Nizatidine	Axid	Antiulcerative	8	Cefprozil	Cefzil	Antibiotic	9
Omeprazole	Prilosec	Antiulcerative	8	Cefaclor	Ceclor	Antibiotic	9
Lansoprazole	Prevacid	Antiulcerative	8	Loracarbef	Lorabid	Antibiotic	9
Rabeprazole	Aciphex	Antiulcerative	8	Cefixime	Suprax	Antibiotic	9
Pantoprazole	Protonix	Antiulcerative	8	Cefpodoxime	Vantin	Antibiotic	9
Esomeprazole	Nexium	Antiulcerative	8	Cefepime	Maxipime	Antibiotic	9
Sucralfate	Carafate	Antiulcerative	8	Tobramycin	Nebcin	Antibiotic	9
Metoclopramide	Reglan	GI stimulant	8	Amikacin	Amikin	Antibiotic	9
Sodium Bicarbonate	Alka-Seltzer	Antacid	8	Neomycin	Neo-Fradin	Antibiotic	9
Aluminum Hydroxide	Amphojel	Antacid	8	Clindamycin	Cleocin	Antibiotic	9
Aluminum Hydroxide/ Magnesium Carbonate	Gavison	Antacid	8	Norfloxacin	Noroxin	Antibiotic	9
				Ciprofloxacin	Cipro	Antibiotic	9
Aluminum Hydroxide/ Magnesium Hydroxide	Maalox	Antacid	8	Levofloxacin	Levaquin	Antibiotic	9
				Gatifloxacin	Tequin	Antibiotic	9
				Moxifloxacin	Avelox	Antibiotic	9

Generic	Brand	Class	Chapter
Minocycline	Minocin	Antibiotic	9
Doxycycline	Vibramycin	Antibiotic	9
Tetracycline	Sumycin	Antibiotic	9
Erythromycin	E-Mycin	Antibiotic	9
Azithromycin	Zithromax	Antibiotic	9
Clarithromycin	Biaxin	Antibiotic	9
Sulfamethoxazole/ Trimethoprim	Bactrim	Antibiotic	9
Quinupristin- Dalfopristin	Synercid	Antibiotic	9
Acyclovir	Zovirax	Antibiotic	9
Docosanol	Abreva	Antiviral	9
Famciclovir	Famvir	Antiviral	9
Valacyclovir	Valtrex	Antiviral	9
Amantadine	Symmetrel	Antiviral	9
Oseltamivir	Tamiflu	Antiviral	9
Zanamivir	Relenza	Antiviral	9
Rimantadine	Flumadine	Antiviral	9
Tolnaftate	Tinactin	Antifungal	9
Econazole	Spectazole	Antifungal	9
Terbinafine	Lamisil	Antifungal	9
Miconazole	Micatin	Antifungal	9
Clotrimazole	Lotrimin AF	Antifungal	9
Ketoconazole	Nizoral	Antifungal	9
Naftifine	Naftin	Antifungal	9
Itraconazole	Sporanox	Antifungal	9

Generic	Brand	Class	Chapter
Capsaicin	Zostrix	Topical Analgesic	9
Codeine	Codeine	Narcotic Analgesic	10
Morphine	MS IR	Narcotic Analgesic	10
Oxycodone	OxyContin	Narcotic Analgesic	10
Fentanyl	Duragesic	Narcotic Analgesic	10
Meperidine	Demerol	Narcotic Analgesic	10
Methadone	Dolophine	Narcotic Analgesic	10
Hydrocodone	Hycodan	Narcotic Analgesic	10
Pentazocine	Talwin	Narcotic Analgesic	10
Propoxyphene	Darvon	Analgesic	10
Procaine	Novocaine	Local Anesthetic	10
Lidocaine	Xylocaine	Local Anesthetic	10
Bupivacaine	Marcaine	Local Anesthetic	10
Hydrocortisone	Cortizone	Anti-inflammatory	10
Triamcinolone	Kenalog-10	Anti-inflammatory	
Dexamethasone	Decadron	Anti-inflammatory	
Fluoxymesterone	Halotestin	Steroid	
Methandrostenolone	Dianabol	Steroid	11
Oxandrolone	Anavar	Steroid	11
Oxymetholone	Anadrol-50	Steroid	11
Stanozolol	Winstrol	Steroid	11
Ethylestrenol	Maxibolin	Steroid	11
Nandrolone Decanoate	Deca-Durabolin	Steroid	11
Testosterone	Depo- Testosterone	Steroid	11

Adenomatous—pertaining to a benign tumor composed of epithelial cells

Adulteration—the addition or substitution of an impure, weaker, cheaper, or possibly toxic substance in a formulation or product

Affinity—a force causing agents to combine

Agonist—a drug that binds to the receptor and stimulates the receptor's function

Alimentary—pertaining to the digestive tract

Alopecia—the absence or loss of hair

Anabolic—the building of tissues

Anaerobe—a microorganism that can live and grow in the absence of oxygen

Androgenic—causing masculinization

Antigenic—the ability to produce antibodies

Antiperistaltic—the loss of the wave of contractions in the gastrointestinal tract moving toward the end point

Antagonists—a drug that has affinity for a cell receptor and, by binding to it, prevents the cell from responding to an agonist

Arthropathy—general term for joint disease

Ataxia—defective muscular coordination

Atrial fibrillation—quivering or spontaneous contraction of individual cardiac muscle fibers

Attenuated—to make less virulent

Autoimmune—a condition in which antibodies are produced against the body's own tissues

Bactericidal—capable of killing bacteria

Bacteriostatic—inhibiting or retarding bacterial growth

Basal—baseline or resting

Bioavailability—the rate and extent to which an active drug or metabolite enters the general circulation, permitting access to the site of action

Bioequivalence—pertaining to a drug that has the same effect on the body as another drug, usually one nearly identical in its chemical formulation

Bolus—dose of medication administered rapidly or all at once to decrease the response time

Buccal—relating to the cheek or mouth

Capsid—the protein covering around the central core of a virus

Capsule—a special container made of gelatin, sized for a single dose of a drug

Centrally acting— pertaining to a drug or medication that works through the central nervous system

Cardiomyopathy—any disease that affects the heart muscle, diminishing cardiac performance

Chemotactic—the movement of additional white blood cells to an area of inflammation in response to the release of chemical mediators by neutrophils, monocytes, and injured tissue

Device—an instrument, apparatus, implement, machine, implant, in vitro reagent, or other similar or related article, including any component, part, or accessory, which is intended for the use in the diagnosis of disease or other conditions, or in the cure, mitigation, treatment, or prevention of disease in man or other animals

Direct acting—pertaining to a drug or medication that works directly on a specific site or tissue

Dissolution—the process by which a solid enters into solution

Dyslipidemia—abnormal amount of lipids in the blood

Efficacy—the ability to produce a desired effect

Elixir—a clear liquid containing water, alcohol, sweeteners, or flavors; used in the compounding of oral medicines

Endogenous—produced or originating from within a cell or organism

Enkephalin—a peptide produced in the brain, which acts as an opioid to produce analgesia

Enteral—within or by way of the intestine

Ergogenic—having the ability to increase work, especially to increase the potential for work output

Exogenous—originating outside an organ or part

Formulary—a continually revised compilation of pharmaceuticals

Gluconeogenesis—the formation of glucose from excess amino acids, fats, or other noncarbohydrate sources

Glucocorticoid—a general classification of adrenal cortical hormones that are primarily active in protecting against stress and in affecting protein and carbohydrate metabolism

Glycogenolysis—a biochemical process occurring chiefly in the liver and the muscles by which glycogen is broken down into glucose

Gram-negative—pertaining to inability of bacteria to retain the color of the staining procedure

Gram-positive—pertaining to ability of bacteria to retain the color of the violet staining procedure

Guild—an association of people with similar interests or pursuits

Gynecomastia—enlargement of breast tissue in a male

Hematocrit—the volume of erythrocytes packed by centrifugation in a given volume of blood. It is expressed as the percentage of total blood volume that consists of erythrocytes

Hepatotoxic—toxic to the liver

Hirsutism—condition characterized by excessive growth of hair or the presence of hair in unusual places

Hyperglycemia—increase in blood glucose

Hyperinsulinism—a relative or absolute excess of insulin in the blood

Hyperplasia—increase in the number of cells

Hypertension— abnormally high blood pressure

Hypertrophic cardiomyopathy—impaired filling of the left ventricular chamber of the heart caused by a disorganized growth of the myofibrils and a thickening of the ventricular wall, leading to arrhythmic activity.

Hypertrophy—an increase in the size of an organ or structure

Hypoglycemia—decrease of blood glucose

Jaundice—a condition marked by yellow staining of body tissues and fluids as a result of excessive levels of bilirubin in the bloodstream

Ketoacidosis—acidosis produced by the presence of excessive amounts of ketones in the body

Ketone—a substance containing the carbonyl group attached to hydrocarbon groups

Latency—the period of inactivity between the time a stimulus is presented and the moment a response occurs

Lipogenic—producing fat

Macrotrauma—tissue damage from a single, high-force traumatic event

Microtrauma—tissue damage as a result of chronic, repetitive stresses to local tissues (most often tendons)

Nephrotoxicity—toxicity to the kidneys

Neutrophil—the most common type of white blood cell, responsible for the majority of the body's protection from infection

Non-productive cough—a dry, hacking cough that keeps one up at night and does not produce any mucus or excessive lung drainage

Nonproprietary—the name of a drug other than its trademarked name

Ointment—a viscous, semisolid vehicle used to apply medicines to the skin

Opioids—any drug containing or derived from opium.

Parenteral—denoting any medication route other than the alimentary canal

Pharmacodynamics—the study of drugs and their actions on living organisms

Pharmacokinetics—the study of metabolism and action of drugs with particular emphasis on the time required for absorption, duration of action, distribution in the body, and method of excretion

Pharmacopeia—a book containing formulas and information that provides a standard for preparation and dispensation of drugs

Phocomelia—a congenital malformation in which the proximal portions of the extremities are poorly developed or absent

Photosensitivity—increased sensitivity to light

Postprandial—following a meal

Potency—the relative pharmacologic activity of a dose of a compound compared with the dose of a different agent producing the same effects

Potentiation—the synergistic action of two substances, such as hormones or drugs, in which the total effects are greater than the sum of the independent effects of the two substances

Precipitation—the process of a substance being separated from a solution

Prohormone—a precursor of a hormone

Proprietary—pertaining to the trade name of a drug

Purity—state of being free of contamination

Rebound effect—a reflex response in which there is a sudden increase in activity when a stimulus is withdrawn

Recombinant—pertains to the genetic material combined from different sources

Reconstitution—the return of a substance previously altered from preservation and storage to its original state

Rescue inhaler—a bronchodilating metered dose inhaler used during an asthma exacerbation

Rhabdomyolysis—an acute, sometimes fatal disease in which the byproducts of skeletal muscle destruction accumulate in the renal tubules and produce acute renal failure

Sinus arrhythmia—cardiac irregularity marked by a variation in the interval between the sinus beats, evidenced by alternately long and short intervals between the P waves on the electrocardiogram

Solubility—the capability of being dissolved

Solution—a liquid containing a dissolved substance

Somnolence—prolonged drowsiness or sleepiness

Suppository—a semisolid substance for introduction into the rectum, vagina, or urethra, where it dissolves

Tablet—a small disk-like mass of medicinal powder

Threshold—point at which a physiological effect begins to be produced

Tinea—any fungal skin disease

Tolerance—decreased sensitivity to subsequent doses of the same drug

Vehicle—an inert agent that carries the active ingredient in a medicine

Answers to Chapter Questions

Chapter 1
1. B
2. A
3. A
4. A
5. B
6. D
7. D
8. B
9. A
10. D

Chapter 2
1. D
2. B
3. D
4. C
5. B
6. E
7. B
8. A
9. D
10. A

Chapter 3
1. Chemical mediators
2. Leukotrienes
3. True
4. Reye's
5. Antipyretic and analgesic
6. Improve efficacy and limit toxicity
7. Willow bark
8. Gastric toxicity
9. C
10. B

Chapter 4
1. A
2. A
3. A
4. A
5. A

Chapter 5
1. B
2. B
3. D
4. A
5. D
6. C
7. D
8. A
9. C
10. A
11. D
12. D

Chapter 6
1. True
2. D
3. C
4. A
5. D
6. False
7. B
8. A
9. C
10. B

Chapter 7

1. Respiration = exchange of gases; ventilation = movement of air
2. Cholinergic = increased salivation and gastric activity; andrenergic = exciting and relaxing various tissues
3. Asthma = bronchoconstriction and inflammation; EIA = bronchoconstriction and inflammation resulting from exercise; EIB = bronchoconstriction only
4. Increase in mucus production and contraction of smooth muscles of the airways
5. Athlete returns to normal shortly after exacerbation
6. Antihistamines = prevent histamine production; decongestants = vasoconstrictor to reduce nasal mucus production; antitussives = cough reduction; expectorants = facilitate mucus movement out of system
7. Increase in the need for medication dosage
8. Cold is viral based and allergies result from exogenous stimulants
9. Drowsiness, excessive mucosal drying, tachycardia, nausea
10. Antihistamines = drowsiness, cardiac stimulation; decongestants = excessive mucosal drying, nausea

Chapter 8

1. A
2. C
3. A
4. C
5. A
6. B
7. C
8. D
9. B
10. A

Chapter 9

1. D
2. B
3. D
4. B
5. A
6. A
7. B
8. B
9. C
10. D
11. A
12. C

Chapter 10

1. A
2. A
3. C
4. C
5. D
6. B
7. True
8. True
9. D
10. False

Chapter 11

1. C
2. D
3. False
4. A
5. C
6. B
7. A
8. D
9. C
10. A
11. D
12. B

Chapter 12

1. True
2. False
3. False
4. False
5. B
6. True
7. D
8. C
9. B
10. A

Chapter 13

1. D
2. C
3. A
4. A
5. False
6. C
7. B
8. A
9. B
10. False
11. D

Chapter 14

1. B
2. D
3. B
4. D
5. B
6. B
7. D
8. D
9. B
10. A
11. A

Chapter 15

1. False
2. True
3. A
4. A
5. False
6. False

Index

Note: Page numbers followed by the letter b refer to boxed material. Those followed by the letter f refer to figures; those followed by t refer to tables.